G000109883

BIOCHEMICAL SOCIETY SYMPOSIA

No. 67

NEURONAL SIGNAL TRANSDUCTION AND ALZHEIMER'S DISEASE

BIOCHEMICAL SOCIETY SYMPOSIUM No. 67
held at University College Cork, September 1999

Neuronal Signal Transduction and Alzheimer's Disease

ORGANIZED AND EDITED BY

C. O'NEILL AND B. ANDERTON

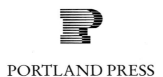

PORTLAND PRESS

Published by Portland Press,
59 Portland Place, London W1B 1QW, U.K.
on behalf of The Biochemical Society
Tel: (+44) 20 7580 5530; e-mail: editorial@portlandpress.com
http://www.portlandpress.com

ISBN 1 85578 133 6   ISSN 0067-8694

British Library Cataloguing in Publication Data
A catalogue record for this book is available from the British Library

Typeset by Portland Press Ltd
Printed in Great Britain by Information Press Ltd, Eynsham, UK

Contents

Preface

Alzheimer's disease research has undergone a major revolution over the last 10 years, and a combination of molecular genetics and biochemical pathology has identified key proteins involved in the pathological sequence of events that cause the disease. These proteins are: the amyloid precursor protein (APP) and its proteolytic fragments, particularly the β-amyloid peptide; the microtubular-associated protein tau; the presenilin proteins; and apolipoprotein E (ApoE). We are now at an exciting point, at which we are close to defining and integrating the neuronal signal-transduction events that impinge on, or emanate from, these proteins to cause the brain degeneration in Alzheimer's disease. Progress in this area has identified, and will hopefully continue to identify, specific therapeutic targets for treatment of Alzheimer's disease, while also providing a model for elucidating other neurodegenerative disorders. In September 1999 the Biochemical Society devoted its Annual Symposium at University College Cork, Ireland, to the topic of Neuronal Signal Transduction and Alzheimer's Disease. The Symposium, sponsored by Elan Corporation, Novartis and Pfizer, was attended by many of the key researchers in this area. This book aims to present and integrate the latest research on this topic from some of the major researchers in this field.

Genetic studies have been invaluable in uncovering the fundamental molecular defects that can cause Alzheimer's disease. Chapter 5 discusses the role of genetics in deciphering the molecular causes of Alzheimer's disease and other primary neurodegenerative disorders. Chapter 6 looks at how knowledge of *tau* gene mutations enables us to understand the signals that lead to brain degeneration and dementia. Chapters 18 and 19 examine the application of molecular genetics to the creation of transgenic mouse models of Alzheimer's disease.

Specific chapters consider various aspects of APP, tau, presenilin and ApoE signal-transduction biology.

Understanding the mechanisms controlling APP proteolysis and function is a crucial area of Alzheimer's disease research, as the excessive production and deposition of β-amyloid in neuritic plaques is considered by many to be the central driving force for the disease. Chapter 1 discusses progress towards identification of inhibitors of β-amyloid production and fibrillization. Chapters 2 and 4 examine the signalling role of β-amyloid and the C-100 terminus of APP, respectively. Chapter 14 explores the role of β-amyloid-induced oxidative and inflammatory pathways in Alzheimer's disease, while Chapters 18 and 19 look at the potential of overexpressing mutant APP to create transgenic animal models of Alzheimer's disease. Chapter 3 considers the importance of post-translational modifications in APP processing and function, and Chapters 15–17 discuss the role of endoplasmic reticular function, receptor–G-protein signalling and intracellular calcium homeostasis in APP processing, and β-amyloid deposition in the Alzheimer's disease brain.

The microtubular-associated protein tau is the main component of the neurofibrillary tangle lesions that are a defining neuropathological characteristic of Alzheimer's disease. The recent discovery that mutations in the *tau* gene can cause fronto-temporal dementia with Parkinsonism (FTDP-17) has drawn even more attention to identifying the cellular mechanisms by which this protein contributes to brain degeneration in Alzheimer's disease and other dementia disorders. Chapter 7 reviews the role of *tau* gene mutations in neurodegeneration and Alzheimer's disease. Chapters 8 and 9 discuss the latest research on the signalling mechanisms underlying tau phosphorylation and the role this may play in tau function and neurodegeneration. Chapter 11 considers evidence for interactions between ApoE and the neuronal cytoskeleton, with particular reference to tau. Chapters 16 and 17 discuss data suggesting that dysfunctional receptor–G-protein function and altered intracellular calcium homeostasis are related to tau hyperphosphorylation and neurofibrillary tangle formation in the Alzheimer's disease brain. Chapter 19 reflects on work attempting to make transgenic models that recapitulate Alzheimer's disease pathology by overexpressing tau.

Mis-sense mutations in presenilin genes are the most common cause of early onset, familial Alzheimer's disease. The presenilin proteins have been discovered to impact on a number of diverse signal-transduction pathways involved in development, apoptosis and calcium ion homoeostasis. The discovery that presenilin mutations cause an overproduction of β-amyloid-42, is of central importance when considering the role of these proteins in the pathogenesis of Alzheimer's disease. Chapter 9 reviews the signal-transduction function of presenilin proteins and their involvement in the development of Alzheimer's disease. Chapters 18 and 19 contemplate the transgenic Alzheimer's disease mouse models which overexpress mutant presenilin.

The finding that polymorphic variation in *APOE* (the gene encoding ApoE) was associated with an altered risk of developing Alzheimer's disease was a significant advance in Alzheimer's disease research. This immediately prompted a search for the mechanisms by which different *APOE* alleles can cause an increased propensity to develop Alzheimer's disease. The complex signal-transduction mechanisms by which ApoE functions are described in Chapter 10. Chapter 11 reviews evidence for and against the interaction of ApoE with the cytoskeleton, with particular focus on the tau protein. Chapter 12 considers the mechanisms by which ApoE might influence neuronal and glial signalling, as well as the possible interaction of ApoE with β-amyloid. Chapter 19 describes phenotypic effects of ApoE4 overexpression in transgenic mice.

Other chapters in the book discuss central signal-transduction events which are aberrant in the Alzheimer's disease post-mortem brain, and which may underly both plaque and tau pathology, and the progresive neurodegeneration associated with the disease. These events are receptor–G-protein function

(Chapter 16) and intracellular calcium homeostasis (Chapter 17). The role of calcium in Alzheimer's disease is also reviewed in Chapter 15, which presents data suggesting that the endoplasmic reticulum may be a focal point for the neurodegenerative cascade that is Alzheimer's disease.

Therapies that ameliorate the pathogenesis of Alzheimer's disease are a primary goal of research into the sequence of molecular events that cause the disease. Many chapters discuss possible treatment strategies emanating from research findings. Current therapies attempt to upregulate acetylcholine cholinergic signal transduction using cholinomimetic drugs. Chapter 13 presents data exploring the key genes that are regulated by activation of muscarinic acetylcholine receptors, pointing to possible novel therapeutic targets. Chapter 14 describes the key role of oxidative stress and inflammatory pathways in Alzheimer's disease, and provides some ideas about possible therapeutic targets. In an invited lecture, Professor I. Lieberburg (Elan Corporation) presented exciting findings which suggest that administering β-amyloid may block the excessive build-up of β-amyloid in Alzheimer's disease.

Unravelling and identifying the primary and central signal transduction events that lead to Alzheimer's disease provides many future challenges for scientific research. This book aims to summarize the current status of research in this area and will hopefully stimulate further investigation in this vital research field.

Cora O'Neill
Brian Anderton

Abbreviations

ABAD	β-amyloid peptide binding alcohol dehydrogenase
AC	adenylate cyclase
ACh	acetylcholine
AChE	acetylcholinesterase
AD	Alzheimer's disease
AGE	advanced glycation endproducts
ApoE	apolipoprotein E
APP	β-amyloid precursor protein
Aβ	β-amyloid
Aβ40	40-amino-acid form of β-amyloid
$[Ca^{2+}]i$	intracellular calcium
CaM kinase II	calcium/calmodulin-dependent kinase II
CBD	corticobasal degeneration
CDK	cyclin-dependent kinase
CLIP	chymotrypsin-like activity of the proteasome
CNS	central nervous system
COX	cyclo-oxygenase
CSF	cerebrospinal fluid
DLB	dementia with Lewy bodies
EGF	epidermal growth factor
ER	endoplasmic reticulum
ERK	extracellular signal-related kinase
FAD	familial Alzheimer's disease
FTDP-17	frontotemporal dementia with Parkinsonism linked to chromosome 17
GFP	green fluorescent protein
GSK-3	glycogen synthase kinase-3
HDL	high-density lipoprotein
IL-1	interleukin-1
iNOS	inducible nitric oxide synthase
JNK	c-Jun N-terminal kinase
KPI	Kunitz protease inhibitor
LDL	low-density lipoprotein
LPS	lipopolysaccharide
LRP	low-density lipoprotein receptor-related protein
LTP	long-term potentiation
mAChR	muscarinic acetylcholine receptor
MAP	mitogen-activated protein

M-CSF	macrophage-colony stimulating factor
NCAM	neural cell adhesion molecule
NFT	neurofibrillary tangle
NF-κB	nuclear factor κB
NGF	nerve growth factor
NMDA	N-methyl-D-aspartate
NO	nitric oxide
NPRAP	neuron-specific plakophilin-related armadillo protein
NSAID	non-steroidal anti-inflammatory drug
Par-4	prostate apoptosis response-4
PHF	paired helical filament
PI-3K	phosphoinositide 3-kinase
PKA	cAMP-dependent protein kinase
PKC	protein kinase C
PLA_2	phospholipase A_2
PS	presenilin
PSA	polysialic acid
PSP	progressive supranuclear palsy
RAGE	receptor for advanced glycation endproducts
RAP	receptor-associated protein
RyR	ryanodine receptor
sAPPα	secreted form of β-amyloid precursor protein
SERCA	sarcoplasmic/endoplasmic reticulum Ca^{2+}-ATPase
SOD	superoxide dismutase
TM	transmembrane
TNF-α	tumour necrosis factor-α
VLDL	very-low-density lipoprotein

Biochem. Soc. Symp. **67**, 1–14
(Printed in Great Britain)

Modulation of β-amyloid production and fibrillization

David Allsop*[1], Lance J. Twyman†, Yvonne Davies*, Susan Moore*, Amber York*, Linda Swanson† and Ian Soutar†

*Department of Biological Sciences and †School of Physics and Chemistry, Lancaster University, Lancaster LA1 4YQ, U.K.

Abstract

Alzheimer's disease (AD) is the most common cause of dementia in old age and presently affects an estimated 4 million people in the U.S.A. and 0.75 million people in the U.K. It is a relentless, degenerative brain disease, characterized by progressive cognitive impairment. In the final stages of the disease, patients are often bedridden, doubly incontinent and unable to speak or to recognize close relatives. Pathological changes of Alzheimer's disease include extensive neuronal loss and the presence of numerous neurofibrillary tangles and senile plaques in the brain. The senile plaques contain amyloid fibrils derived from a 39–43-amino-acid peptide referred to as β-amyloid or Aβ. The basic theory of the so-called 'amyloid hypothesis' is that the deposition of aggregated forms of Aβ in the brain parenchyma triggers a pathological cascade of events that leads to neurofibrillary tangle formation, neuronal loss and the associated dementia [1]. Here we discuss progress towards the identification of inhibitors of Aβ production and fibrillization.

Alzheimer's disease and the amyloid hypothesis

The most convincing evidence in support of the amyloid hypothesis has come from molecular genetic studies of the mutations responsible for familial Alzheimer's disease (AD), and associated biochemical studies into the effects of these mutations on the properties of β-amyloid (Aβ) or its production from the β-amyloid precursor protein (APP). Familial AD mutations in the genes encoding APP, presenilin 1 (PS1) and presenilin 2 (PS2) have all been shown to result in either, enhanced fibrillogenic properties of Aβ [2–4], increased total

[1]To whom correspondence should be addressed.

Aβ production [5,6], or increased production of the longer 42-amino-acid form of Aβ (Aβ42) relative to the shorter 40-amino-acid form (Aβ40) [7]. The latter effect has been demonstrated *in vitro* in cell culture systems and *in vivo* in patients and in transgenic mice [7–11]. Synthetic Aβ42 aggregates much more rapidly than Aβ40 *in vitro* [12], suggesting that one crucial effect of the familial AD mutations is to influence Aβ aggregation and amyloid deposition by diverting the proteolytic processing of APP towards production of longer, more amyloidogenic forms of Aβ. Since all of the APP, PS1 and PS2 mutations influence either the production or properties of Aβ, and since some of them give rise to familial AD with large numbers of neurofibrillary tangles (NFTs), this suggests that Aβ deposition precedes and precipitates the formation of NFTs in these patients. One puzzle remains concerning the effects of the Ala^{21}→Gly mutation found in a Dutch family with a history of both cerebro-vascular amyloidosis and AD. *In vitro* we have found that synthetic peptides incorporating this mutation have consistently refused to aggregate [4], and this has also been reported by others [13]. However, cells transfected with this mutant form of APP do produce more Aβ than cells transfected with wild-type APP [14]. Nevertheless, the effects of this particular mutation seem worthy of further investigation.

The following observations, among others, provide further support for the amyloid hypothesis:

- Down's syndrome sufferers (with three copies of chromosome 21 and hence of the *APP* gene) develop Aβ deposits in the brain before any other recognizable pathology, such as NFTs [15].
- Aggregated or fibrillar forms of synthetic Aβ are toxic to cultured neurons and neuronal-like cells [16], and inhibiting Aβ aggregation blocks this toxicity; Aβ in an aggregated form also shows neurotoxic properties *in vivo* when injected into the brains of aged primates [17].
- Exposure of primary neuronal cultures to fibrillar Aβ leads to tau phosphorylation [18,19], as does the injection of fibrillar Aβ into aged rhesus monkey cerebral cortex [17].
- Knockout of the *APOE* gene in the V717F PDAPP transgenic mouse model results in a dramatic reduction in brain Aβ deposition and senile plaque formation, so providing compelling evidence of a link between apolipoprotein (ApoE) and the deposition of β-amyloid [20].
- Mutations in the *tau* gene do not give rise to AD but instead give rise to frontotemporal dementia, which is characterized by the presence of tau-derived inclusions without significant β-amyloid deposits [21–23].
- Fibrillar protein aggregates are increasingly thought to play an important role in other neurodegenerative diseases, for example α-synuclein in Parkinson's disease, prion protein in the transmissible spongiform encephalopathies and Huntingtin protein in Huntington's disease [24].

The idea that aggregated forms of Aβ are responsible for neurodegeneration in AD is a basic principle of the amyloid hypothesis. The molecular mechanisms underlying the observed toxicity of Aβ to cultured neurons are not fully understood, but current evidence suggests that exposure of cells to Aβ induces the production of reactive oxygen species and free radical damage [16], either via non-receptor-mediated intercalation of Aβ into membranes [25], or via specific binding of Aβ to a receptor such as the RAGE receptor (receptor for advanced glycation endproducts) [26]. The peptide has also been shown to disrupt calcium homoeostasis [27,28] and to induce apoptosis [29]. In an important series of experiments, Geula and colleagues [17] have found that the injection of fibrillar Aβ into the cerebral cortex of aged monkeys results in neuronal loss, microglial proliferation and tau phosphorylation. These effects were not seen to the same extent in younger monkeys, or in rodents, suggesting that the aged primate brain is particularly vulnerable to Aβ-mediated neuronal damage. This might explain the fact that transgenic mouse models of AD with substantial deposits of Aβ can show little evidence of neuronal loss, which is frequently cited as an argument against the amyloid hypothesis.

It is important to realize that the β-amyloid fibrils themselves do not necessarily initiate the cascade of events that leads to neurodegeneration and dementia. The precise nature of the cytotoxic species of Aβ is unclear with small oligomers, protofibrils and higher-molecular-mass species being implicated [30–32]. Aβ that has been 'aged' for several days eventually loses its neurotoxicity, so the real culprit in AD could be an intermediate aggregate *en route* to mature fibril formation, such as the recently described protofibrils [13]. Indeed, the culpable form of Aβ need not be extracellular. Given data on the intracellular formation of Aβ42 [33] and the detection of intracellular aggregates of Aβ [34], it is possible that aggregation of Aβ within cells initiates NFT formation and neurodegeneration. Whether intracellular aggregates of Aβ can be regarded as 'amyloid' is a matter of semantics. Figure 1 shows an updated version of the amyloid hypothesis.

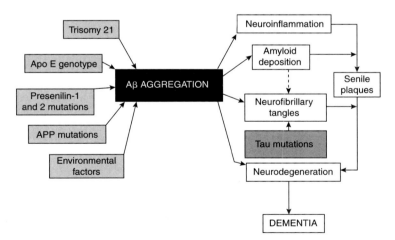

Figure 1 The amyloid hypothesis. Version of the 'amyloid hypothesis' stressing the central role of Aβ aggregation in the pathogenesis of AD, rather than the mature amyloid fibrils. Note that neurotoxic Aβ can precipitate the formation of NFTs, but in frontotemporal dementia linked to chromosome 17, intracellular aggregates of tau can also be induced directly by mutations in the tau gene.

New approaches to drug therapy

Marketed drugs for AD (acetylcholinesterase inhibitors, muscarinic agonists) are designed to increase cholinergic input to the brain, so as to enhance
aspects of memory and cognition. Although it is possible that these drugs
might influence the progression of AD via effects on APP processing and Aβ
formation, this effect has only been demonstrated in cell culture and in brain
slices and has not been reported in animal models or patients. These drugs also
suffer from undesirable side effects. A prediction of the amyloid hypothesis is
that drugs designed to inhibit the formation of Aβ, or its aggregation into cytotoxic forms, will be effective in halting or slowing the progression of AD. The
remainder of this chapter briefly reviews progress in these two areas.

Inhibitors of Aβ formation

One of the most straightforward ways to prevent the formation of Aβ
would be to inhibit the proteinases (β- and γ-secretase) involved in its release
from APP. However, despite more than 10 years of intensive research in this
area, these enzymes have still not been conclusively identified. In the case of α-
secretase, which cleaves in the middle of the Aβ sequence and so precludes Aβ
formation, it is becoming increasingly likely that this enzyme is a member of
the ADAMs (a disintegrin and metalloproteinase-like) family of membrane-
associated zinc metalloproteinases that are similar to, but distinct from, the
matrix metalloproteinases [35,36]. The suggestion that α-secretase is the matrix
metalloproteinase gelatinase A [37] has not been substantiated [38,39].

There are numerous reports claiming the identification of β-secretase
and/or γ-secretase. The metallopeptidase 'thimet' and the aspartyl protease
cathepsin D, which were once considered as reasonable candidates for β-secretase, now appear unlikely [40,41]. In the case of γ-secretase, the situation is
complicated by the fact that there may be different enzymes responsible for the
generation of Aβ40 and Aβ42 [42,43], and this has been highlighted by the
finding that Aβ40 and Aβ42 are formed in different subcellular compartments
[33]. Again, the question of whether one or more γ-secretases exist has not
been clearly resolved. Two interesting possibilities that have arisen recently are
that the metalloproteinase S2P or the presenilin PS1 may in fact be γ-secretase.
The former candidate was identified through similarities between the proteolytic cleavage of APP and cleavage of the sterol regulatory element binding
protein [44–46]. However, the fact that production of Aβ40 and Aβ42 is the
same in CHO cell variant M19 cells that lack S2P as it is in wild-type cells, indicates that S2P cannot be γ-secretase [44,45]. Mutagenesis of two transmembrane aspartate residues in PS1 has been found to abolish APP cleavage at the
γ-secretase site, suggesting that PS1 may be γ-secretase [47]. However, these
data are not conclusive as a role for PS1 upstream of the actual cleavage event
(e.g. in presenting γ-secretase to its APP substrate) cannot be ruled out. One
possibility is that PS1 interacts with γ-secretase and that the aspartate residues
mentioned above are important in modulating this interaction. In this context,
it is interesting to note that recent independent studies, which have been the
subject of commercial patent applications, have identified two different serine

proteases that have been picked out as interacting partners with PS1 in the yeast two-hybrid system [48,49]. The relationship of these proteases to γ-secretase is unknown.

In the absence of clear data on the identity of the secretases, an alternative approach to the identification of secretase inhibitors has been to test the effects of various known protease inhibitors on Aβ production from whole cells in culture. In this way, several independent groups have found that certain peptide aldehydes, in particular Cbz-Phe-Leu-H (MDL-28170), Cbz-Leu-Leu-Leu-H (calpain inhibitor 1), Cbz-Leu-Leu-Nle-H, and Cbz-Leu-Nle-H (calpeptin), can inhibit Aβ formation [42,43,50–52]. These compounds have been proposed as inhibitors of γ-secretase, based on the fact that they block p3 (residues 17–40/42 of Aβ) as well as Aβ formation, with little effect on the release of sAPPα or sAPPβ (secreted forms of APP), and also inhibit the formation of Aβ from cells transfected with the C-terminal 100 amino acids of APP. However, since these inhibitors were identified in whole-cell systems, their effects on APP processing could be indirect. Therefore, their precise molecular target has not been established. Peptide aldehydes of this type are known to be potent inhibitors of both cysteine proteases (such as the calpains) and serine proteases.

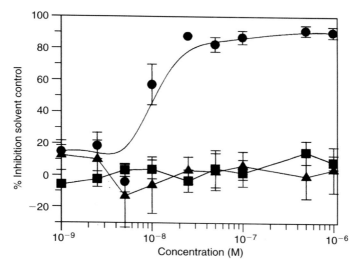

Figure 2 Effect of Bz-Phe-boroLeu on total Aβ secretion. Data show % inhibition of the accumulation of Aβ (●) and sAPPα (▲) in conditioned medium, and also effects on MTT turnover (■). Values are means ± S.D. of triplicate determinations. Reproduced from Christie, G., Markwell, R.E., Gray, C.W., Smith, L., Godfrey, F., Mansfield, F., Wadsworth, H., King, R., McLaughlin, M., Cooper, D.G., et al. Alzheimer's disease: correlation of the suppression of beta-amyloid peptide secretion from cultured cells with inhibition of the chymotrypsin-like activity of the proteosome. J. Neurochem. **73**(1), 195–204 with permission. © (1999) Lippincott, Williams & Wilkins.

It has recently been shown that peptide boronic acids, which are inhibitors of serine proteases only, are considerably more potent inhibitors of Aβ formation than their parent aldehydes [53] (Figure 2). The boronates showed very similar properties to the aldehydes, suggesting that they both inhibit Aβ formation by the same mechanism. At active concentrations of these inhibitors, there was little or no effect on MTT turnover (a marker of mitochondrial dehydrogenase activity), or on the production of sAPPα, indicating that these compounds do not inhibit Aβ by an overtly toxic effect (Figure 2). However, it was noted with all of the effective inhibitors that there was a change in cell morphology and adhesion (rounding up and detachment from plates) at the higher concentrations of inhibitor and over prolonged exposure times (>18 hours). This suggests that these compounds might be inhibiting Aβ formation via a more subtle, indirect mechanism. The activity of these compounds as inhibitors of Aβ production was shown to correlate remarkably well with their potency as inhibitors of the chymotrypsin-like activity of the proteasome (CLIP), suggesting that they exert their effects on Aβ through inhibition of CLIP [53]. Proteasomes are involved in the destruction of aberrant proteins, progression through the cell cycle, tumorigenesis and inflammation, and they also play an important role in antigen presentation. The 26S proteasome/ubiquitin system has been shown to be capable of degrading not only cytoplasmic proteins, but also certain membrane-spanning proteins, including mutant proteins found in the endoplasmic reticulum (ER) such as the cystic fibrosis transmembrane regulatory protein [54]. The precise molecular mechanism of the latter process is unclear, but presumably it involves proteasomes attached to the cytoplasmic side of the ER membrane. Thus, the possibility that the proteasome is involved directly in the proteolytic processing of APP cannot be entirely ruled out. Regardless of the precise mechanism of action of these aldehyde and boronate inhibitors, it is clear that this type of compound is unlikely to be a viable therapeutic agent for AD since inhibition of the proteasome is likely to have unacceptable side effects/toxicity.

Wolfe and colleagues have recently described a series of difluoroketones that also appear to be inhibitors of γ-secretase [55,56]. This was demonstrated not only in a cell-based assay system but also in a cell-free membrane system, which makes these compounds more convincing as direct-acting γ-secretase inhibitors. Some of the effective compounds proved to be potent inhibitors of the aspartyl protease cathepsin D, but poor inhibitors of the cysteine protease calpain 1. This rules out the possibility that γ-secretase is a calpain-like enzyme. However, from the published data [56] it is clear that there was a very poor correlation between the potency of these compounds as cathepsin D inhibitors and their activity as inhibitors of Aβ production. This supports the previous conclusion from cathepsin D knockout mice that this enzyme cannot be γ-secretase [41]. However, it is possible that γ-secretase is another aspartyl protease. This is certainly intriguing given the link between the two aspartyl residues in PS-1 and the activity of γ-secretase [47]. We are currently investigating the effects of these difluoroketone inhibitors on CLIP.

Inhibitors of Aβ aggregation

Known details of the Aβ fibrillogenesis process are drawn almost entirely from work with synthetic peptides [57,58]. Peptide fragments of Aβ from 9–43 amino acid residues in length will aggregate to form fibrils, with the longer peptides tending to produce fibrils that are most similar in appearance to amyloid in the brain itself. The mature β-amyloid fibril appears to be constructed from a small number of 'protofibrils' arranged in lateral association, with the Aβ molecules within the protofibrils taking up the cross-β configuration that is typical of all amyloids [57]. Data on the mechanism and kinetics of Aβ fibrillization are consistent with a nucleation-dependent model of fibril formation [12,59] where soluble peptide monomers (or dimers) combine to form 'nuclei' which themselves combine to form an early fibrillar intermediate or protofibril, with mature amyloid fibrils probably being formed by the lateral association of protofibrils [57–61] (Figure 3). The slow formation of nuclei is the rate-limiting step in this process, but this step can be bypassed or greatly accelerated by the presence of amyloid 'seed' in the form of preaggregated Aβ. Hence, control of nucleation-dependent oligomer formation may be an important determinant of disease development in AD.

A number of compounds have now been described which can inhibit Aβ fibrillization. These include β-cyclodextrin, rifamycins, laminin, a series of charged sulphonates, nicotine, melatonin, the anthracycline 4′-deoxy-4′-iododoxorubicin (IDOX) and short synthetic peptide fragments based on the central hydrophobic region of Aβ [62,63]. There have been no reports of the effects of any of these compounds on Aβ deposition in the available transgenic mouse models of AD, but Soto and colleagues [64] have claimed that a synthetic 'β-sheet breaker peptide' can prevent Aβ deposition when co-injected with Aβ directly into rat brain. However, it is not clear from this study whether Aβ aggregation was actually inhibited *in vivo* or prior to/during the course of the injection. More recently, it has been reported that immunization of V717F PDAPP transgenic mice with aggregated forms of Aβ42 can block

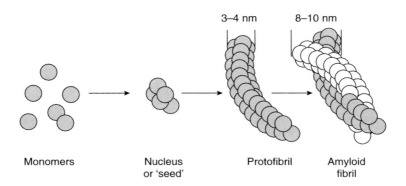

Figure 3 Likely pathway of Aβ fibril formation.

and even reverse the formation of β-amyloid fibrils and senile plaques [65]. It is impossible to determine in this model whether blocking the formation of Aβ fibrils prevents neurodegeneration because significant neuronal loss has not been detected in these mice. As noted above, this is most likely due to rodent brains being inherently less sensitive than primate brains to the toxic effects of Aβ aggregates. The mechanism by which β-amyloid deposition is blocked and reversed in the immunized mice is unknown, but it has been shown that the formation of synthetic Aβ fibrils can be inhibited and even reversed by anti-Aβ antibodies [66–69] suggesting that antibodies induced by the injections might have the same effect. This possibility will only serve to accelerate the search for brain-penetrant, low-molecular-mass inhibitors of Aβ aggregation.

We have recently been involved in the study of a number of benzofuran derivatives (Figure 4) that have been identified as inhibitors of Aβ aggregation [70–72]. These compounds have been shown to inhibit Aβ fibril formation by means of a standard Congo Red binding assay, and also as assessed by a novel sandwich immunoassay that detects only aggregated forms of Aβ [32,72]. The latter assay is based on the capture of synthetic Aβ peptide with a monoclonal antibody (mAb) directed at residues 1–16 (e.g. the commercially available 6E10), followed by detection with a biotinylated form of the same mAb. This immunoassay has been shown to give a strong signal only when the Aβ peptide has been incubated under conditions in which some aggregation occurs [32,72]. This is presumably because multiple copies of the same mAb epitope are available for capture and detection only when the Aβ is in an aggregated state (Figure 5). Interestingly, we have demonstrated, by dot blotting, that antibodies to the N-terminus of Aβ react weakly with Aβ40 monomers or dimers, but immunoreactivity is greatly enhanced following peptide incubation and aggregation [73]. This might also explain the fact that a sandwich immunoassay configured with two antibodies directed at the N-terminus of Aβ detects only aggregated forms of Aβ. The biotinylated secondary antibody is detected with streptavidin-europium, with quantification by the DELFIA system (delayed enhanced lanthanide fluorescence immunoassay). The precise point of intervention of the benzofuran inhibitors along the Aβ aggregation pathway is

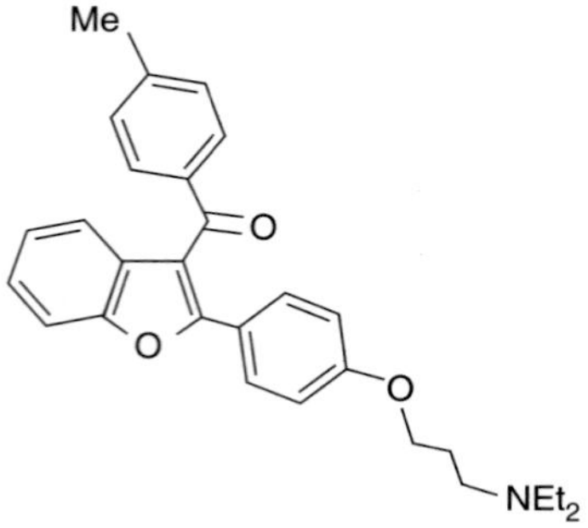

Figure 4 3-p-Toluoyl-2-[4'-(3-diethylaminopropoxy)-phenyl]-benzofuran, an inhibitor of Aβ aggregation [70–72].

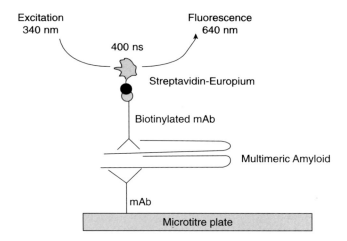

Excitation
340 nm

Fluorescence
640 nm

400 ns

Streptavidin-Europium

Biotinylated mAb

Multimeric Amyloid

mAb

Microtitre plate

Figure 5 Immunoassay for the detection of aggregated forms of Aβ.

unknown, but these compounds have been shown to block the cytotoxicity of Aβ [72] and so appear to act at a point prior to formation of the cytotoxic amyloid species. Unlike many of the other reported anti-aggregation inhibitors, these benzofurans are responsive to chemical modification using a high-speed parallel synthetic approach. Interestingly, they are similar in structure to amiodarone, an iodinated benzofuran derivative that is a potent, orally bioavailable drug for heart arrhythmia and angina [74]. Amiodarone is also known to be a brain penetrant but we have found that amiodarone itself is a poor inhibitor of Aβ aggregation (D. Allsop and Y. Davies, unpublished work). However, if the more active benzofuran derivatives have a similar bioavailability profile to amiodarone, then they may be suitable as test compounds to determine if it is feasible to inhibit Aβ aggregation with a small molecule inhibitor in a transgenic mouse model. With this in mind, we have developed a novel synthetic route to the target benzofuran inhibitor 3-*p*-Toluoyl-2-[4′-(3-diethylamino-propoxy)-phenyl]-benzofuran [74a] (Figure 4). In an effort to obtain more potent inhibitors, we are developing a combinatorial approach towards the synthesis of other related benzofurans, which will be tested against a variety of amyloid-forming proteins and peptides.

Fluorescence anisotropy as a method of monitoring Aβ aggregation

We have also been interested in developing more sensitive methods than those available at present for monitoring Aβ aggregation and for determining the point of intervention of inhibitors in the Aβ aggregation and fibril assembly pathway (Figure 3). One technique that we have begun to look at is fluorescence anisotropy, which can be used to determine the rate at which a fluorescent species tumbles in solution. Since the rate of reorientation of a particle is a function of its size, fluorescence anisotropy measurements, particularly time-resolved experiments, offer a very sensitive and informative means of interrogating interactions between molecules [75–77]. We have carried out some preliminary experiments with the fluorescein-labelled form of β-amyloid (so-called fluo-β-amyloid) recently marketed by New England Nuclear. In a time-resolved anisotropy experiment, a pulse of polarized light is used to excite (a proportion of) those fluorescent molecules which are orientated within the plane of polarization at the instant of excitation. Fluorescence emitted shortly after absorption will be highly polarized. However, since the molecules reorientate to regain a random distribution within the system, the fluorescence observed as time progresses becomes less and less polarized. Once randomization is complete, light emitted from the molecular assembly is unpolarized. The degree of polarization of the fluorescence, expressed as the anisotropy, r, will decay from a characteristic initial value to zero, at a rate determined by the rate at which molecular reorientation occurs. The rate of anisotropy decay and, thence, of molecular motion, can be expressed as a 'correlation time', τ_c. The more slowly the particle tumbles, the longer the value of τ_c. Figure 6(a) shows that the anisotropy of the fluorescence from a dilute solution (1 μM) of fluorescently labelled β-peptide on its own decays rapidly to zero (τ_c~1 ns). Upon addition of unlabelled peptide, at a concentration which will induce aggregation (in this case 125 μM), a much more slowly decaying component appears and the anisotropy, r, no longer attains zero within the time range over which fluorescence can be observed. The relative magnitude of this longer-lived, i.e. greater τ_c value, component of the anisotropy increases with incubation time and this component is clearly associated with the presence of aggregated forms of Aβ and amyloid fibrils in the system (Figure 6b). These results demonstrate that fluorescently labelled Aβ is incorporated into synthetic β-amyloid fibrils and that this process can be monitored very effectively and at early time points by measuring changes in fluorescence polarization. There are reports in the literature involving the use of energy transfer measurements or fluorescence correlation spectroscopy to study Aβ peptide aggregation [78–81] but there are no reported studies using fluorescence anisotropy for this purpose. We now intend to develop the method further and to investigate the effects of aggregation inhibitors in this system.

Conclusion

Recent developments in understanding of the genetics of the 'tauopathies' and the emergence of protein aggregation as a common theme in various neurodegenerative disorders such as AD, Parkinson's disease, prion disease and Huntington's disease, have only acted to strengthen the amyloid hypothesis. The same applies to the finding of a clear link between the presence of ApoE and the deposition of Aβ in the brains of transgenic mice, and the demonstration that the aged primate brain is particularly vulnerable to the toxic effects of Aβ. However, emphasis has now shifted away from mature amyloid fibrils and towards intermediates in the fibril assembly pathway, since it is becoming

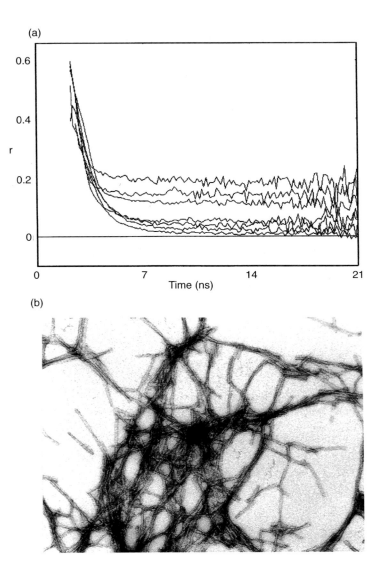

Figure 6 Fluorescence anisotropy experiments. (a) Anisotropy decay of Aβ40 following incubation in 50 mM Tris buffer, pH 7.4, for various times at 37°C. The traces, in order of increased 'r' values after anisotropy decay, are due to: 1 μM fluo-peptide only (r decays rapidly to zero); then 1 μM fluo-peptide plus 125 μM normal peptide after incubation for 0, 1, 24, 72, 96, 120 hours. (b) Appearance of amyloid fibrils at the end of the experiment, as demonstrated by negative-stain (uranyl acetate) electron microscopy. Magnification × 100,000.

increasingly likely that the latter are responsible for the neurotoxic properties of Aβ. It has been argued that these intermediates cannot be regarded as 'amyloid' if their effects are due to accumulation within cells, but in our opinion this is purely a matter of semantics and is, therefore, a sterile argument. The dramatic demonstration that immunization of transgenic mice with Aβ can block and even reverse the formation of senile plaques suggests that the time is fast approaching when the amyloid hypothesis will be tested in human patients.

We are grateful to The Wellcome Trust for continued support of our research.

References

1. Hardy, J. and Allsop, D. (1991) *Trends Pharmacol. Sci.* **12**, 383–388
2. Wisniewski, T., Ghiso, J. and Frangione, B. (1991) *Biochem. Biophys. Res. Commun.* **179**, 1247–1254
3. Clements, A., Walsh, D.M., Williams, C.H. and Allsop, D. (1993) *Neurosci. Lett.* **161**, 17–20
4. Clements, A., Allsop, D., Walsh, D.M. and Williams, C.H. (1996) *J. Neurochem.* **66**, 740–747
5. Citron, M., Oltersdorf, T., Haass, C., McConlogue, L., Hung, A.Y., Seubert, P., Vigo-Pelfrey, C., Lieberburg, I. and Selkoe, D.J. (1992) *Nature (London)* **360**, 672–674
6. Cai, X.D., Golde, T.E. and Younkin, S.G. (1993) *Science* **25**, 514–516
7. Younkin, S.G. (1995) *Ann. Neurol.* **37**, 287–288
8. Scheuner, D., Eckman, C., Jensen, M., Song, X., Citron, M., Suzuki, N., Bird, T.D., Hardy, J., Hutton, M., Kukull, W., et al. (1996) *Nat. Med. (N.Y.)* **2**, 864–870
9. Duff, K., Eckman, C., Zehr, C., Yu, X., Prada, C.M., Perez-tur, J., Hutton, M., Buee, L., Harigaya, Y., Yager, D., et al. (1996) *Nature (London)* **383**, 710–713
10. Borchelt, D.R., Thinakaran, G., Eckman, C.B., Lee, M.K., Davenport, F., Ratovitsky, T., Prada, C.M., Kim, G., Seekins, S., Yager, D., et al. (1996) *Neuron* **17**, 1005–1013
11. Citron, M., Westaway, D., Xia, W., Carlson, G., Diehl, T., Levesque, G., Johnson-Wood, K., Lee, M., Seubert, P., Davis, A., et al. (1997) *Nat. Med. (N.Y.)* **3**, 67–72
12. Jarrett, J.T., Berger, E.P. and Lansbury, P.T. (1993) *Biochemistry* **32**, 4693–4697
13. Walsh, D.M., Lomakin, A., Benedek, G.B., Condron, M.M. and Teplow, D.B. (1997) *J. Biol. Chem.* **272**, 22364–22372
14. Haass, C., Hung, A.Y., Selkoe, D.J. and Teplow, D.B. (1994) *J. Biol. Chem.* **269**, 17741–17748
15. Iwatsubo, T., Mann, D.M., Odaka, A., Suzuki, N. and Ihara, Y. (1995) *Ann. Neurol.* **37**, 294–299
16. Iversen, L.L., Mortishiresmith, R.J., Pollack, S.J. and Shearman, M.S. (1995) *Biochem. J.* **311**, 1–16
17. Geula, C., Wu, C.K., Saroff, D., Lorenzo, A., Yuan, M.L. and Yankner, B.A. (1998) *Nat. Med. (N.Y.)* **4**, 827–831
18. Busciglio, J., Lorenzo, A., Yeh, J. and Yankner, B.A. (1995) *Neuron* **14**, 879–888
19. Takashima, A., Noguchi, K., Michel, G., Mercken, M., Hoshi, M., Ishiguro, K. and Imahori, K. (1996) *Neurosci. Lett.* **203**, 33–36
20. Bales, K.R., Verina, T., Dodel, R.C., Du, Y., Altstiel, L., Bender, M., Hyslop, P., Johnstone, E.M., Little, S.P., Cummins, D.J., et al. (1997) *Nat. Genet.* **17**, 263–264
21. Hutton, M., Lendon, C.L., Rizzu, P., Baker, M., Froelich, S., Houlden, H., Pickering-Brown, S., Chakraverty, S., Isaacs, A., Grover, A., et al. (1998) *Nature (London)* **393**, 702–705
22. Poorkaj, P., Bird, T.D., Wijsman, E., Nemens, E., Garruto, R.M., Anderson, L., Andreadis, A., Wiederholt, W.C., Raskind, M. and Schellenberg, G.D. (1998) *Ann. Neurol.* **43**, 815–825
23. Spillantini, M.G., Bird, T.D. and Ghetti, B. (1998) *Brain Pathol.* **8**, 387–402

24. Kakizuka, A. (1998) *Trends Genet.* **14**, 396–402
25. McLaurin, J. and Chakrabartty, A. (1996) *J. Biol. Chem.* **271**, 26482–26489
26. Yan, S.D., Chen, X., Fu, J., Chen, M., Zhu, H., Roher, A., Slattery, T., Zhao, L., Nagashima, M., Morser, J., et al. (1996) *Nature (London)* **382**, 685–691
27. Mattson, M.P., Cheng, B., Davis, D., Bryant, K., Lieberberg, I. and Rydel, R.E. (1992) *J. Neurosci.* **12**, 376–389
28. Arispe, N., Rojas, E. and Pollard, H.B. (1993) *Proc. Natl. Acad. Sci. U.S.A.* **90**, 567–571
29. Loo, D.T., Copani, A., Pike, C.J., Whittemore, E.R., Walencewicz, A.J. and Cotman, C.W. (1993) *Proc. Natl. Acad. Sci. U.S.A.* **90**, 7951–7955
30. Roher, A.E., Chaney, M.O., Kuo, Y.M., Webster, S.D., Stine, W.B., Haverkamp, L.J., Woods, A.S., Cotter, R.J., Tuohy, J.M., Krafft, G.A., et al. (1996) *J. Biol. Chem.* **271**, 20631–20635
31. Lambert, M.P., Barlow, A.K., Chromy, B.A., Edwards, C., Freed, R., Liosatos, M., Morgan, T.E., Rozovsky, I., Trommer, B., Viola, K.L., et al. (1998) *Proc. Natl. Acad. Sci. U.S.A.* **95**, 6448–6453
32. Howlett, D.R., Ward, R.V., Bresciani, L., Jennings, K.H., Christie, G., Allsop, D., Gray, C.W. and Karran, E.H. (1999) *Alzheimer Rep.* **2**, 171–177
33. Hartmann, T., Bieger, S.C., Bruhl, B., Tienari, P.J., Ida, N., Allsop, D., Roberts, G.W., Masters, C.L., Dotti, C.G., Unsicker, K. and Beyreuther, K. (1997) *Nat. Med. (N.Y.)* **3**, 1016–1020
34. Podlisny, M.B., Ostaszewski, B.L., Squazzo, S.L., Koo, E.H., Rydell, R.E., Teplow, D.B. and Selkoe, D.J. (1995) *J. Biol. Chem.* **270**, 9564–9570
35. Parvathy, S., Hussain, I., Karran, E.H., Turner, A.J. and Hooper, N.M. (1998) *Biochemistry* **37**, 1680–1685
36. Parvathy, S., Karran, E.H., Turner, A.J. and Hooper, N.M. (1998) *FEBS Lett.* **431**, 63–65
37. Miyazaki, K., Hasegawa, M., Funahashi, K. and Umeda, M. (1993) *Nature (London)* **362**, 839–841
38. Walsh, D.M., Williams, C.H., Kennedy, H.E., Allsop, D. and Murphy, G. (1994) *Nature (London)* **367**, 27–28
39. Lepage, R.N., Fosang, A.J., Fuller, S.J., Murphy, G., Evin, G., Beyreuther, K., Masters C.L. and Small, D.H. (1995) *FEBS Lett.* **377**, 267–270
40. Chevallier, N., Jiracek, J., Vincent, B., Baur, C.P., Spillantini, M.G., Goedert, M., Dive, V. and Checler, F. (1997) *Br. J. Pharmacol.* **121**, 556–562
41. Saftig, P., Peters, C., von Figura, K., Craessaerts, K., Van Leuven, F. and De Strooper, B. (1996) *J. Biol. Chem.* **271**, 27241–27244
42. Citron, M., Diehl, T.S., Gordon, G., Biere, A.L., Seubert, P. and Selkoe, D.J. (1996) *Proc. Natl. Acad. Sci. U.S.A.* **93**, 13170–13175
43. Klafki, H., Abramowski, D., Swoboda, R., Paganetti, P.A. and Staufenbiel, M. (1996) *J. Biol. Chem.* **271**, 28655–28659
44. Ross, S.L., Martin, F., Simonet, L., Jacobsen, F., Deshpande, R., Vassar, R., Bennett, B., Luo, Y., Wooden, S., Hu, S., et al. (1998) *J. Biol. Chem.* **273**, 15309–15312
45. Tomita, T., Chang, T.Y., Kodama, T. and Iwatsubo, T. (1998) *NeuroReport* **9**, 911–913
46. Manni, M.E., Cescato, R., and Paganetti, P.A. (1998) *FEBS Lett.* **427**, 367–370
47. Wolfe, M.S., Xia, W., Ostaszewski, B.L., Diehl, T.S., Kimberly, W.T. and Selkoe, D.J. (1999) *Nature (London)* **398**, 513–517
48. Karran, E.H., Clinkenbeard, H.E., Browne, M.J., Southan, C.D., Creasy, C. L. and Livi, G.P. (1998) European Patent EP 828003
49. St. George-Hyslop, P.H., Fraser, P. and Rommens, J.M. (1998) International Patent WÖ 98/01549
50. Higaki, J., Quon, D., Zhong, Z.Y. and Cordell, B. (1995) *Neuron* **14**, 651–659
51. Klafki, H., Paganetti, P.A., Sommer, B. and Staufenbiel, M. (1995) *Neurosci. Lett.* **201**, 29–32

52. Allsop, D., Christie, G., Gray, C., Holmes, S., Markwell, R., Owen, D., Smith, L., Wadsworth, H., Ward, R.V., Hartmann, T., et al. (1997) in *Alzheimer's Disease: Biology, Diagnostics and Therapeutics* (Iqbal, K., Winblad, B., Nishimura,T., Takeda, M. and Wisniewski, H.M., eds.), pp. 717–727, John Wiley, Chichester

53. Christie, G., Markwell, R.E., Gray, C.W., Smith, L., Godfrey, F., Mansfield, F., Wadsworth, H., King, R., McLaughlin, M., Cooper, D.G., et al. (1999) *J. Neurochem.* **73**, 195–204

54. Jensen, T.J., Loo, M.A., Pind, S., Williams, D.B., Goldberg, A.L. and Riordan, J.R. (1995) *Cell* **83**, 129–135

55. Wolfe, M.S., Citron, M., Diehl, T.S., Xia, W., Donkor, I.O., and Selkoe, D.J. (1998) *J. Med. Chem.* **41**, 6–9

56. Wolfe, M.S., Xia, W., Moore, C.L., Leatherwood, D.D., Ostaszewski, B., Rahmati, T., Donkor, I.O. and Selkoe, D.J. (1999) *Biochemistry* **38**, 4720–4727

57. Teplow, D.B. (1998) *Int. J. Exp. Clin. Invest.* **5**, 121–142

58. Forloni, G., Tagliavini, F., Bugiani, O. and Salmona, M. (1996) Prog. Neurobiol. **49**, 287–315

59. Harper, J.D., Liber, C.M. and Lansbury, P.T. (1997) *Chem. Biol.* **4**, 951–959

60. Harper, J.D., Wong, S.S., Lieber, C.M. and Lansbury, P.T. (1997) *Chem. Biol.* **4**, 119–125

61. Walsh, D.M., Lomakin, A., Benedek, G.B., Condron, M.M. and Teplow, D.B. (1997) *J. Biol. Chem.* **272**, 22364–22372

62. Bandiera, T., Lansen, J., Post, C. and Varasi, M. (1997) *Current Med. Chem.* **4**, 159–170

63. Soto, C. (1999) *Mol. Med. Today* **5**, 343–350

64. Soto, C., Sigurdsson, E.M., Morelli, L., Kumar, R.A., Castano, E.M. and Frangione, B. (1998) *Nat. Med. (N.Y.)* **4**, 822–826

65. Schenk, D., Barbour, R., Dunn, W., Gordon, G., Grajeda, H., Guido, T., Hu, K., Huang, J., Johnson-Wood, K., Khan, K., et al. (1999) *Nature (London)* **400**, 173–177

66. Solomon, B., Koppel, R., Hanan, E. and Katzav, T. (1996) *Proc. Natl. Acad. Sci. U.S.A.* **93**, 452–455

67. Solomon, B., Koppel, R., Frankel, D. and Hanan-Aharon, E. (1997) *Proc. Natl. Acad. Sci. U.S.A.* **94**, 4109–4112

68. Frenkel, D., Balass, M. and Solomon, B. (1998) *J. Neuroimmunol.* **88**, 85–90

69. Frenkel, D., Balass, M., Katchalski-Katzir, E. and Solomon, B. (1999) *J. Neuroimmunol.* **95**, 136–142

70. Allsop, D., Howlett, D., Christie, G. and Karran, E. (1998) *Biochem. Soc. Trans.* **26**, 459–462

71. Howlett, D.R., Allsop, D. and Karran, E.H. (2000) in *Neurobiology of Alzheimer's Disease* (Dawbarn, D. and Allen, S.J., eds.) Oxford University Press, Oxford. In press.

72. Howlett, D.R., Perry, A.E., Godfrey, F., Swatton, J.E., Jennings, K.H., Spitzfaden, C., Wadsworth, H., Wood, S.J. and Markwell, R.E. (1999) *Biochem. J.* **340**, 283–289

73. Kametani, F., Tanaka, K., Tokuda, T. and Allsop, D. (1995) *Brain Res.* **703**, 237–241

74. Podrid, P.J. (1995) *Ann. Intern. Med.* **122**, 689–700

74a Twyman, L.J. and Allsop, D. (1999) *Tetrahedron Lett.* **40**, 9383–9384

75. Soutar, I., Swanson, L., Wallace, S.J.L., Ghiggino, K.P., Haines, D.J. and Smith, T.A. (1995) *ACS Symp. Ser.* **598**, 363–378

76. Soutar, I. and Swanson, L. (1990) *Macromolecules* **23**, 5170–5172

77. Soutar, I., Swanson, L., Thorpe, F.G. and Zhou, C. (1996) *Macromolecules* **29**, 918–924

78. Jackson Huang, T.H., Fraser, P.E. and Chakrabartty, A. (1997) *J. Mol. Biol.* **269**, 214–224

79. Garzon-Rodriguez, W., Sepulveda-Becerra, M., Milton, S. and Glabe, C.G. (1997) *J. Biol. Chem* **272**, 21037–21044

80. Pitschke, M., Prior, R., Haupt, M. and Riesner, D. (1998) *Nat. Med. (N.Y.)* **4**, 832–834

81. Tjernberg, L.O., Pramanik, A., Björling, S., Thyberg, P., Thyberg, J., Nordstedt, C., Berndt, K.D., Terenius, L. and Rigler, R. (1999) *Chem. Biol.* **6**, 53–62

Biochem. Soc. Symp. **67**, 15–22
(Printed in Great Britain)

2

Alzheimer's disease:
inside, outside, upside down

Shi Du Yan*[1], Ann M. Schmidt† and David Stern‡

Departments of *Pathology, †Physiology and Cellular Biophysics and ‡Surgery,
College of Physicians and Surgeons, Columbia University, 630 West 168th Street,
New York, NY 10032, U.S.A.

Abstract

Neurotoxicity of β-amyloid peptide (Aβ) in Alzheimer's disease (AD) is usually thought to arise from the nonspecific effects of high concentrations of Aβ on vunerable neurons, resulting in membrane destabilization and increasing intracellular calcium concentration. This review advances the hypothesis that at early stages of AD, when Aβ is present in lower amounts, its ability to perturb the function of cellular targets is mediated by specific cofactors present on the cell surface and intracellularly. Receptor for advanced glycation endproducts (RAGE) is a cell-surface receptor which binds Aβ and amplifies its effects on cells in the nanomolar range. The intracellular enzyme Aβ-binding alcohol dehydrogenase (ABAD) is likely to engage nascent Aβ formed in the endoplasmic reticulum, and to mediate cell stress from this site. The analysis of Aβ interaction with RAGE and ABAD, as well as other cofactors, provides insight into new mechanisms and, potentially, identifies therapeutic targets relevent to neuronal dysfunction in AD.

Introduction

Extracellular accumulations of amyloid in neuritic plaques, composed predominately of β-amyloid (Aβ) peptide and intracellular neurofibrillary tangles, composed in large part of hyperphosphorylated paired helical filament tau, are pathognomonic features of Alzheimer's disease (AD) [1–5]. With time, these lesions increase in number and volume, concomitant with neuronal toxicity and death [1–6]. While amyloidogenic peptides are condensed into copious fibrillar deposits in the middle to late stages of AD, the relationship of such lesions to mechanisms of early cellular dysfunction is undefined. It is possible that the densely packed deposits of Aβ found at the centre of neuritic plaques

---

[1]To whom correspondence should be addressed.

may have a protective function by sequestering toxic amyloid from cellular elements.

Aβ interaction with cell surface receptors

In AD it is widely accepted that later in the course of the disease, when Aβ fibrils are abundant, non-specific interactions of such fibrils with the cell surface may be frequent and disruptive for cellular functions [7-12] (Figure 1, left). Aβ fibrils can destroy plasma membranes, causing changes in ionic homoeostasis, and could trigger cell death by several mechanisms. However, earlier in the course of the disease when Aβ fibrils are present at lower levels, and Aβ is presumably present principally in oligomeric soluble forms, higher affinity interactions with cellular surface molecules are more likely to be relevant (Figure 1, right). One such molecule is the immunoglobulin superfamily receptor RAGE (receptor for advanced glycation endproducts). In the AD brain, this receptor is expressed at higher levels in neurons and microglia proximate to neuritic plaques and in cells of Aβ-loaded blood vessels, than in those areas free of pathology or in control brains [13]. RAGE binds Aβ in its soluble monomeric/oligomeric and insoluble fibrillar forms with nanomolar affinity, targeting the amyloidogenic peptide to the cell surface. In culture, cells expressing RAGE are more susceptible to Aβ-induced cellular dysfunction than those with lower levels of RAGE, or those in which the receptor is blocked.

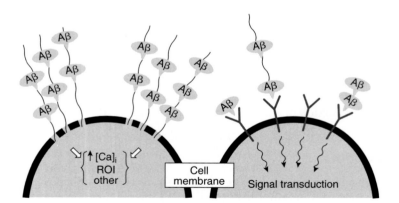

Figure 1 Schematic depiction of non-specific (left) and specific (right) interactions of Aβ with cellular elements. Aβ monomer/oligomers/fibrils and cell binding proteins for Aβ (Y) are shown in relation to the cell membrane. Resulting increases in cytosolic free calcium [Ca]$_i$ and reactive oxygen intermediates (ROI) are also noted. Reprinted from Biochim. Biophys. Acta, **1502**, Yan, S.D., Roher, A., Chaney, M., Zlokovic, B., Schmidt, A.M. and Stern, D., Cellular cofactors potentiating induction of stress and cytotoxicity by amyloid beta-peptide, 145–157. © (2000) with permission from Elsevier Science.

Consistent with a role for Aβ-receptor interactions in the early disruption of neuronal functions, are the findings that Aβ binding to neuronal RAGE results in activation of nuclear factor κB (NF-κB), induction of haem oxygenase type 1 and expression of macrophage-colony stimulating factor (M-CSF), each of which can be demonstrated in AD brain [13,14]. In contrast, cells expressing low levels of RAGE require greater concentrations of Aβ to bring about changes in cellular properties. Cellular disruption resulting from low levels of Aβ binding to RAGE reflects active redirection of cellular biosynthetic mechanisms, not non-specific and rapid induction of cell death, which is observed at high levels of Aβ (the latter is independent of RAGE). Therefore, Aβ–RAGE interaction could contribute to the well-recognized chronic inflammatory component underlying AD. Aβ stimulation of RAGE causes nuclear translocation of NF-κB, thereby increasing the expression of M-CSF by neurons (which also spills over into cerebrospinal fluid) and resulting in the recruitment and activation of microglia to early sites of cellular disruption [14] (Figure 2).

In view of the multiple conformational structures into which Aβ assembles, it is to be expected that the amyloidogenic peptide will interact with several cell-surface recognition sites, potentially opportunistic receptors whose activation could engender varied alterations in cellular phenotype. Consistent with this theory, the macrophage scavenger receptor, expressed selectively in the brain on microglia, has been shown to bind and internalize Aβ fibrils [15,16]. Such endocytosis of Aβ could enhance a protective function, by sequestering and disposing of toxic peptides, or alternatively could contribute to pathogenicity by promoting chronic cellular dysfunction. In this context, increased expression of megalin/gp330, a lipoprotein receptor that serves as an acceptor site for apolipoprotein E (ApoE) [17], in neurons that display intracellular ApoE and Aβ as well as evidence of DNA fragmentation suggests that

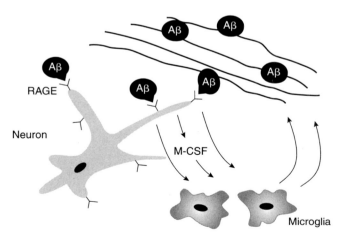

Figure 2 Schematic depiction of M-CSF and AD [14]. Reprinted from Biochim. Biophys. Acta, **1502**, Yan, S.D., Roher, A., Chaney, M., Zlokovic, B., Schmidt, A.M. and Stern, D., Cellular cofactors potentiating induction of stress and cytotoxicity by amyloid beta-peptide, 145–157. © (2000) with permission from Elsevier Science.

uptake of the ApoE/Aβ complex via this receptor system may load cells with intracellular Aβ in a relatively stable complex that promotes toxicity, and eventually apoptosis [17]. Although cell-surface RAGE [18], and presumably other Aβ cellular binding sites, are not necessary or even sufficient mediators of Aβ-induced cytotoxicity (which can occur in the absence of RAGE given a sufficiently high concentration of Aβ), the presence of such receptors may serve to focus and amplify the toxic effects of Aβ, especially at relatively low amounts of peptide and when Aβ is in filamentous form. If only by sustained approximation of Aβ to the cell surface, RAGE can effectively increase toxicity but, in addition, binding of Aβ to RAGE may trigger intracellular signals deleterious to cell function and viability. Finally, RAGE can also serve to assist clearance of very small amounts of Aβ (or filaments) through interaction of the Aβ–RAGE complex. The ability of RAGE to bind Aβ and advanced glycation endproducts (AGEs) [19] is in all likelihood an accident of evolution due to molecular mimicry with other RAGE ligands such as amphoterin [20], which promotes neurite outgrowth in the developing brain. A result of the proposed involvement of Aβ receptors in the pathogenesis of AD is that early in the course of this disorder, before irreversible cellular events occur, inhibition of Aβ–cell-surface interactions could be neuroprotective, and potentially therapeutic. However, this hypothesis must await development of appropriate transgenic animal models that imitate the pathophysiology of AD to be proved completely. In this context, mice overexpressing RAGE and/or the scavenger receptor, along with other susceptibility factors such as presenilins or β-amyloid precursor protein (APP) mutants, may represent excellent candidates for such models.

Aβ interaction with the intracellular enzyme ABAD (Aβ-binding alcohol dehydrogenase)

Evidence linking increased production of Aβ, in culture and in the brains of transgenic mice that are overexpressing presenilins or which have mutations in APP, with early-onset familial AD have highlighted a role for Aβ in the pathogenesis of neurodegeneration [1-3,21–24]. Processing of APP may occur by several pathways [1], including generation of the amyloidogenic peptide within the endoplasmic reticulum [25–28], also a site for localization of presenilin [29]. Immunoprecipitation of APP–presenilin complexes formed within the cell indicates that these two molecules may interact *in vivo*, potentially affecting the processing of APP [30]. Using the yeast two-hybrid system, we have identified a polypeptide, ABAD, which specifically binds Aβ. ABAD was found in the endoplasmic reticulum and in mitochondria and was originally named ERAB (endoplasmic reticulum-associated Aβ binding protein), after its first site of intracellular localization within the endoplasmic reticulum. However, it is now refered to as ABAD in view of its functional properties and presence in multiple subcellular compartments [31]. ABAD binds with nanomolar affinity to the Aβ monomer/oligomer, as well as to Aβ assembled into fibrils, and it potentiates Aβ-induced cellular toxicity, assessed by induction of apoptosis. The blockage of ABAD–Aβ interaction, through the introduction of anti-ABAD F(ab')^2 into cells, using liposomes, suppressed Aβ-induced apoptosis at lower concentrations of amyloidogenic peptide (up to 1 μM). However, at higher concentrations of Aβ (<10 μM), the effects of ABAD were not discernible, presumably due to an excess of non-specific Aβ–cellular interactions. Immunohistochemical analysis of the AD brain shows ABAD at low levels in normal cortical neurons, but with substantially increased expression in AD neurons in the brains of patients with AD. ABAD is an intriguing cellular target of Aβ as it is the human counterpart of type II 3-hydroxyacyl-CoA dehydrogenase, an enzyme which participates in the third reaction of the β-oxidation spiral [32], and is therefore integral to cellular energy and fatty acid metabolism. Based on protein sequence homologies, ABAD could also be a short chain-alcohol dehydrogenase, which suggests its potential to generate toxic aldehydes within disrupted cells. Of course, the discovery of ABAD raises many questions with respect to how such an intracellular polypeptide gains access to Aβ, whether ABAD enzymic activity is related to its potential role in cellular toxicity, and, if this is not the case, whether its activity is modulated by Aβ. These considerations indicate the extent to which further studies will be required to determine a possible role for ABAD in Aβ-mediated neurotoxicity. In this context, it is possible that intracellular Aβ, concentrated in cellular compartments such as the endoplasmic reticulum and Golgi or in the endosomal–lysosomal pathway, damages cell membranes and gains access to otherwise remote subcellular targets [33]. Other neurotoxic species also interact with enzymes fundamental in cellular metabolism, as illustrated by the binding of huntingtin and other proteins containing polyglutamine domains to glyceraldehyde-3-phosphate dehydrogenase [34–36]. The potential of Aβ, an enzyme that can participate in cellular homoeostasis, to modulate properties of an intracellular target (Figure 3) opens a new view to

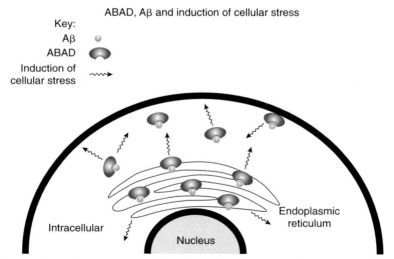

Figure 3 Schematic depiction of Aβ interaction with intracellular targets.

possible early cellular events signalling trouble within neurons at a time when intervention might reverse early functional perturbations.

Conclusion

There is still much unknown about the pathogenesis and even pathological manifestations of sporadic AD. This is exemplified by the recent recognition of distinct hitherto unsuspected extracellular proteinaceous deposits of ~100 kDa polypeptide in AD with monoclonal antibodies to plaque-derived substances [37]. The identification and characterization of specific cellular targets of Aβ, such as RAGE, scavenger receptor, megalin/gp330 and ABAD provides a context for considering early cellular perturbations due to Aβ, in relation to both cell-surface binding sites/receptors and intracellular targets, and may provide new insights into molecular mechanisms and future therapeutic approaches.

Dr Gabriel Godman and Dr Giuseppe Andres (Department of Pathology) provided invaluable suggestions during planning and preparation of this manuscript.

References

1. Haass, C. and Selkoe, D. (1994) Cellular processing of β-amyloid precursor protein and the genesis of amyloid β-peptide. *Cell* 75, 1039–1042
2. Kosik, K. (1994) Alzheimer's disease sphinx: a riddle with plaques and tangles. *J. Cell Biol.* 127, 1501–1504
3. Yankner, B. (1996) Mechanisms of neuronal degeneration in Alzheimer's disease. *Neuron* 16, 921–932
4. Goedert, M. (1993) Tau protein and the neurofibrillary pathology of Alzheimer's disease. *Trends Neurosci.* 16, 460–465
5. Trojanowski, J. and Lee, V. (1994) Paired helical filament tau in Alzheimer's disease, the kinase connection. *Am. J. Pathol.* 144, 449–453
6. Cummings, B. and Cotman, C. (1995) Image analysis of β-amyloid load in Alzheimer's dissease and relation to dementia severity. *Lancet* 346, 1524–1528
7. Yankner, B., Duffy, L. and Kirschner, D. (1990) Neurotrophic and neurotoxic effects of amyloid β protein: reversal by tachykinin neuropeptides. *Science* 250, 279–282
8. Cotman, C. and Anderson, A. (1995) A potential role for apoptosis in neurodegeneration and Alzheimer's disease. *Mol. Neurobiol.* 10, 19–45
9. Mattson, M. (1995) Free radicals and disruption of neuronal ion homeostasis in AD: a role for Aβ? *Neurobiol. Aging* 16, 679–682
10. Hensley, K., Carney, J.M., Mattson, M.P., Aksenova, M., Harris, M., Wu, J.F., Floyd, R.A. and Butterfield, D.A. (1994) A model for β-amyloid aggregation and neurotoxicity based on free radical generation by the peptide; relevance to Alzheimer disease. *Proc. Natl. Acad. Sci. U.S.A.* 91, 3270–3274
11. Behl, C., Davis, J., Lesley, R. and Schubert, D. (1994) Hydrogen peroxide mediates amyloid Aβ protein toxicity. *Cell* 77, 817–827
12. Younkin, S. (1995) Evidence that Aβ is the real culprit in Alzheimer's disease. *Ann. Neurol.* 37, 287–288
13. Yan, S.D., Chen, X., Fu, J., Chen, M., Zhu, H., Roher, A., Slattery, T., Zhao, L., Nagashima, M., Morser, J., et al. (1996) RAGE and amyloid-Aβ peptide neurotoxicity in Alzheimer's disease. *Nature (London)* 382, 685–691

14. Yan, S.-D., Zhu, H., Fu, J., Yan, S.D., Roher, A., Tourtellotte, W.W., Rajavashisth, T., Chen, X., Godman, G.C., Stern, D. and Schmidt, A. (1997) Amyloid-β peptide-RAGE interaction elicits neuronal expression of M-CSF: a proinflammatory pathway in Alzheimer disease. *Proc. Natl. Acad. Sci. U.S.A.* **94**, 5296–5301

15. Paresce, D., Ghosh, R. and Maxfield, F. (1996) Microglial cells internalize aggregates of the Alzheimer's disease Aβ via a scavenger receptor. *Neuron* **17**, 553–565

16. El Khoury, J., Hickman, S.E., Thomas, C.A., Cao, L., Silverstein, S.C. and Loike, J.D. (1996) Scavenger receptor-mediated adhesion of mciroglia to Aβ fibrils. *Nature (London)* **382**, 716–719

17. La Ferla, F., Troncoso, J., Strickland, D., Kawas, C. and Jay, G. (1997) Neuronal cell death in Alzheimer's disease correlates with apoE uptake and intracellular Aβ stabilization. *J. Clin. Invest.* **100**, 310–320

18. Liu, Y., Cargusch, R. and Schubert, D. (1997) Aβ toxicity does not require RAGE protein. *Biochem. Biophys. Res. Commun.* **237**, 37–40

19. Schmidt, A.M., Vianna, M., Gerlach, M., Brett, J., Ryan, J., Kao, J., Esposito, C., Hegarty, H., Hurley, W., Clauss, M., et al. (1992) Isolation and characterization of binding proteins for advanced glycosylation endproducts from lung tissue which are present on the endothelial cell surface. *J. Biol. Chem.* **267**, 14987–14997

20. Hori, O., Brett, J., Slattery, T., Cao, R., Zhang, J., Chen, J.X., Nagashima, M., Lundh, E.R., Vigay, S., Nitecki, D., et al. (1995) RAGE is a cellular binding site for amphoterin: mediation of neurite outgrowth and coexpression of RAGE and amphoterin in the developing nervous system. *J. Biol. Chem.* **270**, 25752–25761

21. Haass, C. (1996) Presenile because of presenilin: the presenilin genes and early onset Alzheimer's disease. *Curr. Opin. Neurol.* **9**, 254–259

22. Dewji, N. and Singer, S. (1996) Genetic clues to Alzheimer's disease. *Science* **271**, 159–160

23. Tanzi, R., Kovacs, D., Kim, T., Moir, R., Guenette, S. and Wasco, W. (1996) The gene defects responsible for familial Alzheimer's disease. *Neurobiol. Dis.* **3**, 159–168

24. Hardy, J. (1997) Amyloid, the presenilins and Alzheimer's disease. *Trends Neurosci.* **20**, 154–159

25. Wild-Bode, C., Yamnzaki, T., Capeil, A., Leimer, U., Stainer, H., Ihara, Y. and Haass, C. (1997) Intracellular generation and accumulation of Aβ terminating at amino acid 42. *J. Biol. Chem.* **272**, 16085–16088

26. Tienari, P., Ida, N., Ikonen, E., Simons, M., Wepdemann, A., Multhaup, G., Masters, C.L., Dotti, C.G. and Beyreuther, K. (1997) Intracellular and secreted Alzheimer Aβ species are generated by distinct mechanisms in cultured hippocampal neurons. *Proc. Natl. Acad. Sci. U.S.A.* **94**, 4125–4130

27. Hartmann, T., Bieger, S.C., Bruhi, B., Tienari, P.J., Ida, N., Allsop, D., Roberts, G.W., Masters, C.L., Dotti, C.G., Unsicker, K. and Beyreuther, K. (1997) Distinct sites of intracellular production for Alzheimer's disease Aβ40/42 amyloid peptides. *Nat. Med. (N.Y.)* **3**, 1016–1020

28. Cook, D., Forman, M.S., Sung, J.C., Leight, S., Kolson, D.L., Inatsubo, T., Lee, V.M.Y. and Doms, R.W. (1997) Alzheimer's Aβ(1-42) is generated in the endoplasmic reticulum/intermediate compartment of NT2N cells. *Nat. Med. (N.Y.)* **3**, 1021–1023

29. Kovacs, D., Fausett, H.J., Page, K.J., Kim, T.W., Mopr, R.D., Merriam, D.E., Hollister, R.D., Hallmark, O.G., Mancini, R., Felsenstein, K.M., et al. (1996) Alzheimer-associated presenilins 1 and 2: neuronal expression in brain and localization to intracellular membranes in mammalian cells. *Nat. Med. (N.Y.)* **2**, 224–229

30. Weidemann, A., Paliga, K., Durrwang, U., Czech, C., Evin, G., Master, C.L. and Beyreuther, K. (1997) Formation of stable complexes between two Alzheimer's disease gene products: presenilin-2 and β-amyloid precursor protein. *Nat. Med. (N.Y.)* **3**, 328–332

31. Yan, S.-D., Fu, J., Soto, C., Chen, X. and Zhu, H. (1997) ERAB: an intracellular protein that binds Aβ and mediates neurotoxicity in Alzheimer's disease. *Nature (London)* **389**, 689–695

32.   Furuta, S., Kobayashi, A., Miyazawa, S. and Hashimoto, T. (1997) Cloning and expression
       of cDNA for a newly identified isozyme of bovine liver 3-hydroxyacyl-CoA dehydro-
       geanse and its import into mitochondria. *Biochim. Biophys. Acta* **1350**, 317–324

33.   Yang, A., Chandswangbhuvana, D., Shu, T., Margol, L. and Glabe, C.G. (1997) Lysosomal
       membrane damage is one of earliest pathological events in β-amyloid-mediated neurotoxic-
       ity, in *Molecular Mechanisms in Alzheimer's Disease*, pp. 29, Keystone Symposia
       Proceedings, C1

34.   MacDonald, M.E., Ambrose, C.M., Duyao, M.P., Myers, R.H., Lin, C., Srinidhi, L., Barnes,
       G., Taylor, S.A., James, M., Groot, N., et al. (1993) Huntington's disease collaborative
       research group. A novel gene containing a trinucleotide repeat that is expanded and unstable
       in Huntington's disease chromosomes. *Cell* **72**, 971–983

35.   Li, X.-J., Li, S.H., Sharp, A.H., Nucifora, F.C., Schilling, J.G., Lanahan, A., Wowey, P.,
       Snyder, S.H. and Ross, C.A. (1995) A huntingtin-associated protein enriched in brain with
       implications for pathology. *Nature (London)* **378**, 398–402

36.   Burke, J., Enghild, J.J., Martin, M.E., Jou, Y.S., Myers, R.M., Ross, A.D., Vance, J.M. and
       Strittmatter, W.J. (1996) Huntingtin and DRPLA proteins selectively interact with the
       enzyme GAPDH. *Nat. Med. (N.Y.)* **2**, 347–350

37.   Schmidt, M.-L., Lee, V.M.Y., Forman, M., Chiu, T.S. and Trojanouski, J.Q. (1997)
       Monoclonal antiboides to a 100 kDa protein reveal abundant amyloid-beta peptide-negative
       plaques throughout gray matter of Alzheimer's disease brains. *Am. J. Pathol.* **151**, 69–80

Biochem. Soc. Symp. **67**, 23–36
(Printed in Great Britain)

3

The role of post-translational modification in β-amyloid precursor protein processing

Niki Georgopoulou, Mark McLaughlin, Ian McFarlane and Kieran C. Breen[1]

Department of Pharmacology and Neuroscience, University of Dundee,
Ninewells Hospital Medical School, Dundee DD1 9SY, U.K.

Abstract

The β-amyloid precursor protein (APP) plays a pivotal role in the early stages of neurodegeneration associated with Alzheimer's disease. An alteration in the processing pattern of the protein results in an increase in the generation of the 40–42-amino-acid β-amyloid (Aβ) peptide, which coalesces to form insoluble, extracellular amyloid deposits. A greater understanding of the factors that influence APP processing may assist in the design of effective therapeutic agents to halt progression of Alzheimer's disease. APP is a sialoglycoprotein with two potential N-linked glycosylation sites, one of which may contain a complex oligosaccharide chain. An alteration in the glycosylation state of APP by the generation of oligomannosyl oligosaccharides results in a decrease in the secretion of the neuroprotective, soluble form of the protein and a parallel increase in the deposition of the cellular protein within the perinuclear region of the cell. Conversely, the attachment of additional terminal sialic acid residues on to the oligosaccharide chain results in an increase in secretion of soluble APP (sAPPα). One factor that has been widely reported to alter APP processing is the activation of protein kinase C (PKC). This process has been characterized using synaptosomal preparations, which suggests that the PKC action is occurring at the level of the plasma membrane. Furthermore, when cells are transfected with the sialyltransferase enzyme, there is a direct relationship between the sialylation potential of APP and the fold stimulation of sAPPα, after PKC activation. These results suggest that the post-translational modification of APP by glycosylation is a key event in determining the processing of the protein.

[1]To whom correspondence should be addressed.

Protein glycosylation

The post-translational modification of cell-surface and secreted glycoproteins is a key event in protein processing. These modifications, which include glycosylation, myristoylation, palmitoylation, sulphation and phosphorylation, result in the covalent linkage of additional chemical structures to the amino acid backbone, which in turn may directly influence the structure and associated function of the protein backbone. Post-translational processing may also act indirectly to modify the protein structure, function and processing [1].

Glycosylation is one of the most common post-translational covalent modifications undertaken by newly synthesized proteins passing through the endoplasmic reticulum (ER) and the Golgi network. Glycoproteins are defined as conjugated proteins containing one or more heterosaccharides covalently bound to the polypeptide chain as a prosthetic group [1]. They are either integral-membrane or secreted proteins and may contain up to 85% carbohydrate by weight. Glycoproteins make up several important classes of macromolecule with a variety of functions, including enzymes, hormones, immunoglobulins, transport proteins, cell-adhesion molecules, neurotransmitter receptors and structural proteins [1]. In contrast, very few of the proteins found in the nucleus and cytosol are glycosylated, and those that are carry a different sugar modification [2]. These proteins, which contain a single O-linked N-acetyl-glucosamine (O-GlcNAc) residue, include elements of the cytoskeleton such as the microtubule-associated protein tau [3]. Since the O-GlcNAc residues may be attached to sites that additionally serve as phosphorylation sites, there may be a competition between the two modifications, with both groups competing for the same sites [4,5].

Glycosylation is one of the most diverse post-translational modifications owing to the variety of amino acids that can be modified and the myriad oligosaccharide structures and components. Glycosylation is species, tissue and cell specific, and differential glycosylation may lead to functional diversity, due to the existence of multiple glycoforms of an individual glycoprotein. It plays a major role in the processing of the protein backbone, and the trafficking of cell-surface proteins in polarized cells is also influenced by the glycosylation state of the protein [6,7]. The generation of multiple glycoforms of a protein depends on the cellular environment in which the protein is glycosylated and may, therefore, vary with the type, as well as with the physiological state, of the organism, tissue or cell in which the glycoprotein is synthesized [8,9].

The oligosaccharide side-chains of glycoproteins can be classified into two groups according to the amino acid to which they are attached: N-linked oligosaccharides are attached to asparagine (Asn) residues, whereas O-linked sugars can be linked to serine (Ser) or threonine (Thr) residues. The structural variation of oligosaccharide chains is influenced by the levels of activity and the specificity of the individual glycosyltransferase enzymes in the Golgi. Indeed, many proteins can have both N-linked and O-linked glycans on the same polypeptide chain [1].

The N-linked glycans act predominantly to provide recognition signals at the level of the cell surface to regulate biological functions such as cell adhesion. All N-linked carbohydrates share a common pentasaccharide core structure called the trimannosyl core, which consists of two GlcNAc residues (one of which is attached to Asn of the polypeptide chain) and three mannose (Man) residues in the format Manα1,3-(Manα1,6)-Manα1,4-GlcNAcβ1,4-GlcNAc-Asn. N-linked sugar chains can be subdivided subsequently into three main categories according to the variation and linkage point of the peripheral sugar residues: high-mannose, complex and hybrid N-linked oligosaccharides (Figure 1).

The high-mannose-type glycans contain only α-mannosyl residues outside the pentasaccharide core (Figure 1a), whereas complex oligosaccharides contain either lactosamine units (Galα1,4-GlcNAc or Galα1,3-GlcNAc) or sialolactosamine units (NeuNAc linked via an α2,3 to lactosamine) attached to the mannose residues of the trimannosyl core (Figure 1b). Complex-type oligosaccharides can be highly branched, depending on the substitution pattern of the GlcNAc residues to the mannose residues in the core. The complex sugar chains may also be sulphated, fucosylated or phosphorylated, and usually con-

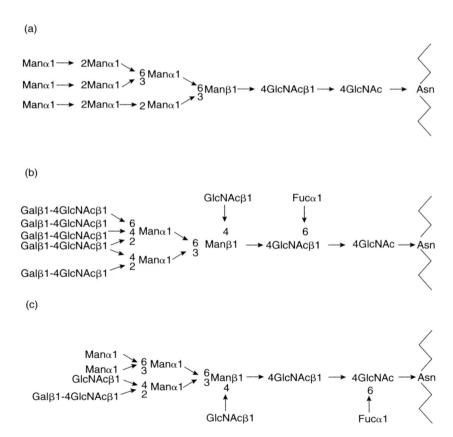

Figure 1 Diagrammatic structure of (a) high-mannose, (b) complex and (c) hybrid N-linked oligosaccharides. Abbreviations used: gal, galactose; fuc, fucose.

tain a negatively charged terminal sialic acid (NeuNAc) residue. The hybrid-type glycans combine certain structural features of both the high-mannose and the complex types. For example, one arm of the trimannosyl core may be of high-mannose-type glycan, whereas the other arm may be of a complex-type glycan (Figure 1c).

Because of their negative charge, the terminal NeuNAc residues play a particular role in influencing the structure and function of the protein back-bone. The role of NeuNAc residues is illustrated well in the structure and function of the neural cell adhesion molecule (NCAM). NCAM plays a pivotal role in the mediation of cell–cell interaction. During embryogenesis, and again coincident with plastic events in the mature central nervous system (CNS), NCAM contains polysialic acid (PSA) chains in which up to 50 NeuNAc residues are attached by $\alpha 2,8$ linkages in an N-linked oligosaccharide chain. PSA acts to prevent the homophilic binding of the NCAM backbone and this serves to prevent the premature formation of synapses during development. It also allows for synaptic rearrangement in the adult. PSA has been shown to play a role in memory formation [10], as well as in long-term potentiation (LTP), which is an electrophysiological paradigm of synaptic plasticity [11]. In fact, recent studies have proposed that PSA plays a role in the maintenance of LTP (which is associated with synaptic rearrangement) rather than in its induction (which is receptor mediated) [12].

Glycosylation of β-amyloid precursor protein (APP)

APP is a transcribed sialoglycoprotein that exists as three primary iso-forms: APP_{695}, APP_{751} and APP_{770} (the numbers referring to the number of amino acids in the protein). Both APP_{751} and APP_{770} contain the 56-amino-acid Kunitz protease inhibitor (KPI) domain and, in addition, APP_{770} contains a 19-amino-acid insert that codes for an Ox-2 (the MRC Ox-2 antigen) domain [13–15].

There are two mutually exclusive pathways which serve to process APP: cleavage at Lys^{16}, within the β-amyloid (Aβ) region of the protein, by the α-secretase results in the generation of soluble APP (sAPPα); alternatively, it can be cleaved by the β- and γ-secretases to generate the 40–42-amino-acid Aβ peptide [16,17]. Furthermore, the processing mechanisms may be cell, tissue or species specific.

APP trafficking in non-polarized cells indicates that the protein is delivered to the cell surface via a constitutive biosynthetic pathway, where it can be cleaved by α-secretase and secreted as sAPPα. Alternatively, it can be internalized by endocytosis and eventually degraded by an endosomal/lysosomal pathway, with the generation of the Aβ peptide [18–20]. However, there is an increasing body of evidence to suggest that Aβ may also be generated at the level of the ER and Golgi [21–23].

The APP holoprotein is multifunctional, with the membrane-bound form playing a role in cell–cell adhesion and in cellular interaction with the extracellular matrix [24,25]. The soluble (secreted) form of the protein exhibits both neuroprotective and neurotropic effects [26]. These functions of the protein may be responsible, at least in part, for its role in memory/learning [27,28] and in the induction of LTP [29,30]. Transgenic mice overexpressing the mutated human APP$_{695}$ (APP$_{695}$SWE), which exhibit some of the pathological hallmarks of AD, also demonstrate an impairment in synaptic plasticity [31].

APP contains two potential N-linked oligosaccharide attachment sites (Asn[467] and Asn[496]), although the available evidence suggests that only the former may be occupied under normal conditions [32]. APP may also contain O-linked oligosaccharide chains [33,34]. Previous studies have proposed that the N-linked oligosaccharide chain on sAPPα is of the complex type, with a fuco-sylated core [35] and a terminal NeuNAc residue [36]. These results have been confirmed by lectin blot analysis of sAPPα labelled with the *Lens culinaris* (LcH), *Phaseolus vulgaris* (PHA-L) and *Maackia amurensis* (MAA) lectins (Figure 2). Each of the lectins recognizes a specific sugar residue or short oligosaccharide sequence, and the use of multiple lectins allows for the genera-tion of a composite profile of the oligosaccharide structure. The cellular holo-protein, however, exhibits a different oligosaccharide profile and, in particular, is labelled by the *Datura stramonium* lectin, which detects high-mannose-type oligosaccharides. This labelling, however, may reflect the diverse sugar profiles of the protein as it undergoes different stages of glycosylation on its pathway through the cell. The fact that the cellular form of APP contains a high-man-nose-type (immature) oligosaccharide side-chain suggests that the majority of the particulate form of the protein is likely to be retained within the perinuclear region of the cell. In order for APP to be released from the ER/Golgi, for trans-portation to the plasma membrane and ultimately secretion, the predominant oligosaccharide side-chain is of the complex type. Since the protein has a very high turnover rate at the level of the plasma membrane, it is likely that only very low levels of the protein are actually expressed at the level of the cell sur-face at any one time. This is in good agreement with previous studies that have reported a relatively short half-life for the protein within the cell [37–39]. The rapid turnover of the protein at the level of the plasma membrane may explain

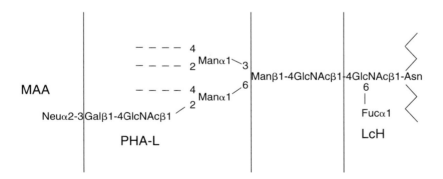

Figure 2 Proposed structure of the N-linked oligosaccharide attached to the secreted form of APP based on lectin blot analysis. APP was labelled with the LcH, PHA-L and MAA lectins, each of which detect specific sugar residues.

the differences between the glycosylation patterns of the particulate APP (which is largely retained within the ER/Golgi and is of the high-mannose type) and the secreted form of the protein.

APP processing

It has been proposed that the oligosaccharide side-chains of APP play a pivotal role in the processing of the protein and a number of different model systems have been employed to determine the effect of altered glycosylation on APP processing. The Lec8 strain of mutant CHO cell lines have a defect in the CMP-NeuNAc transport system resulting in the expression of asialo-oligosaccharides [40]. Soluble inhibitors of the early stages of glycosylation, including tunicamycin and brefeldin A, have also been used to study the role of glycosylation in APP processing. APP secretion was diminished when core N-glycosylation or N-glycan processing (and particularly sialylation) was blocked [41]. It was proposed, however, that in addition to APP glycosylation itself, the glycosylation of other proteins may also be involved in APP processing. Alterations in protein glycosylation, either by tunicamycin or through the inhibition of mannosidase, also upset the axonal sorting of the protein both *in vitro* and *in vivo* [42]. A similar result was observed when the asparagine residues, to which the complex sugars are attached, were deleted [43]. Studies in this lab have used the mannosidase I and II inhibitors 2-deoxymannojirimycin (dMan) and swainsonine to investigate the differential effects of high mannose and complex sugars on APP processing [44]. Treatment of AtT-20 mouse pituitary cells *in vitro* with dMan or swainsonine, which prevents maturation of N-linked sugars, resulted in a significant decrease in the translocation of APP from the perinuclear region of the cell to the cell membrane and therefore in ultimate secretion (Figure 3). In addition, parallel *in vivo* studies were carried out using the hamster retinotectal projection as a model system. The dMan was injected intraocularly and the axonal transport of APP along the retinal ganglion cells was determined following dissection of the superior colliculus [45]. The prevention of oligosaccharide maturation by the inhibition of mannosidase action, significantly decreased the axonal transport of APP [46]. Taken together, these results confirm the earlier lectin studies that suggest the preferential transfer of APP, containing mature complex N-linked oligosaccharide chains, from the perinuclear region of the cell to the plasma membrane, with the high-mannose-containing forms of the protein being retained in the ER/Golgi complex. Although the presence of complex oligosaccharides may not be an absolute requirement for protein transport to the cell surface [47], it certainly plays a significant role in APP processing and trafficking within the cell.

The retention of APP in the perinuclear region of the cell may also have implications for the final processing of the protein and in particular on the generation of the Aβ peptide. There is increasing evidence to suggest that Aβ may be generated, at least in part, at the level of the Golgi or ER [21–23]. Thus any factors, such as the impairment of oligosaccharide maturation, which retain the protein in the perinuclear region, preventing translocation to the plasma mem-

(a)

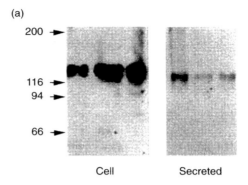

(b)

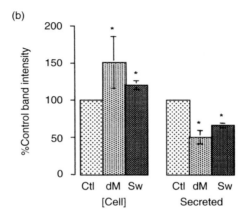

Figure 3 The effect of altered glycosylation on APP processing.
(a) Immunoblot analysis for 18 hours in serum-free medium with the 22C11 antibody of cellular and secreted APP from control (Ctl) 6A1 mouse pituitary cells and cells treated with dMan (dM; 1mM) or swainsonine (Sw; 10μM). Lanes were loaded with equivalent amounts of protein. The numbers represent the migration of molecular weight standards. (b) Densitometric quantification of APP following the different treatments. Values are means ± S.E.M. (n=4). * indicates P<0.05 vs. control (ANOVA followed by Tukey test). Reproduced from Neuroscience, **90**, McFarlane, I., Georgopoulou, N., Coughlan, C.M., Gillian, A.M. and Breen, K.C., The role of protein glycosylation state in the control of cellular transport of the amyloid-β precursor protein, 15–25, © (1999) with permission from Elsevier Science.

brane, may lead to an increase in cellular Aβ concentration due to the build up of the holoprotein in the intermediate cellular compartment [16,48].

The pivotal role of the terminal sialic acid residue in APP processing has been confirmed using cells that overexpress the α2,6(N) sialyltransferase (ST6N) enzyme. Stably-transfected B104 rat neuroblastoma cells that overexpress the ST6N enzyme have been generated. These cells have specific enzyme activities reaching up to 20 times that of control (mock-transfected) cells and

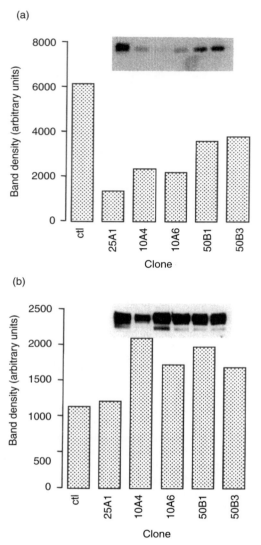

Figure 4 Expression of (a) particulate and (b) secreted APP in control B104 rat neuroblastoma cells and cells transfected with the ST6N enzyme. ST6N enzyme activity increases from left to right [49]. APP was detected using the 790 antibody (directed against the Aβ region of the protein) and quantified by densitometric analysis [61].

show a parallel increase in protein-bound α2,6 linked sialic acid [49,50]. There was a marked decrease in the levels of particulate (cellular) APP in the transfected cells, which was accompanied by an increase in the secreted form of the protein (Figure 4). Furthermore, there was a subtle change in the banding pattern of the secreted form of the protein. APP existed as a doublet (with a predominant upper band) in the control cells. In the cells with the high ST activity, there was a tendency towards a decrease in the intensity of the lower band. Previous studies have proposed that the existence of multiple APP immunoreactive bands may reflect the expression of different glycoforms of the protein [36,41]. Therefore, it is likely that the upper band is more highly glycosylated and the increase in its intensity reflects an increase in the sialic acid content of the protein.

Second messenger systems

The processing of APP can also be modulated by the action of extracellular stimuli such as metabotropic glutamate [51,52] and cholinergic [53,54] agonists, and also by various growth factors including epidermal growth factor [55] and nerve growth factor [56]. The activation of these receptors induces a potentiation of sAPPα secretion. The detailed mechanisms of the signalling pathways that are coupled to receptor-mediated sAPPα secretion remain to be clearly defined, although evidence implicates the hydrolysis of inositol phospholipid by phospholipase C in response to G-protein-coupled receptor activation [51]. The mitogen-activated protein kinase kinase (MEK) inhibitor PD 98059 [17,56] blocks growth-factor-stimulation of sAPPα secretion, thus providing strong evidence that the action of growth factors operates via a tyrosine-kinase cascade. However, stimulation of sAPPα secretion by phorbol esters, which directly activate protein kinase C (PKC) by mimicking its physiological activator diacylglycerol, can also be blocked by the actions of PD 98059 [17,56].

From these studies, it is likely that PKC (or specific isoforms thereof) may serve as a convergent point for the pathways that stimulate sAPPα secretion. The mechanisms by which PKC activation potentiate sAPPα secretion, however, remain unknown. Although the C-terminus of sAPPα can be phosphorylated [57–59], the degree of phosphorylation does not correlate with the PKC-mediated enhanced secretion [60,61] and, in fact, deletion of the C-terminus of APP increased the basal rate of secretion [62]. This observation is of particular interest since one group has proposed that the basal secretion of sAPPα is independent of the PKC-induced stimulatory pathway [63]; this theory is based on evidence generated using inhibitors of a proteasome complex which may contain the α-secretase. Recently, Racchi and colleagues [64] reported that both the constitutive and stimulatory pathways converge on a proteolytic complex which may represent the α-secretase. Perhaps, therefore, there is a cross-regulation between the two pools of APP that feed into PKC-dependent and independent pathways.

Since the activation of PKC has also been shown to cause an accompanying reduction in the production of Aβ peptide [65,66], identifying the loci of its action could have significant therapeutic benefits. It has been shown that phorbol esters can act by stimulating vesicle budding from the Golgi apparatus [67] but, since phorbol esters can also enhance sAPPα secretion from isolated nerve terminals (synaptosomes) (Figure 5) [61], this would suggest that an additional PKC target may be at, or in close proximity to, the plasma membrane. However, *in vivo*, it is possible that events occurring at the level of the Golgi

N. Georgopoulou et al.

(a)

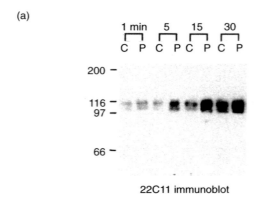

22C11 immunoblot

(b)

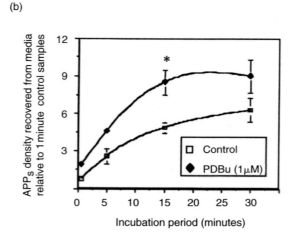

Figure 5 Effect of PKC activation on the time course of sAPPα secretion from synaptosomal membranes. (a) A representative immunoblot, using antibody 22C11, of the APP content of the secretion media of synaptosomes incubated in the presence (P) and absence (C) of phorbol ester (PDBu; 1 μM). (b) The optical density of the immunoblots. Symbols represent means ± S.E.M., n=4; * indicates P< 0.05, ANOVA with Bonferroni t-test. Reproduced from [61] with permission. © (1999) Lippincott, Williams & Wilkins.

apparatus, such as glycosylation, can influence the subsequent transportation of APP to the nerve terminal [68].

Recently it has been reported that PKC activation can influence cellular ST activity [69–71]. Therefore, as transfection of cells with ST6N results in increased trafficking of APP to the cell membrane (with a parallel up-regulation of sAPPα secretion) (Figure 4), and PKC activation modulates the protein secretion at the level of the cell membrane, the transfected cells were used to

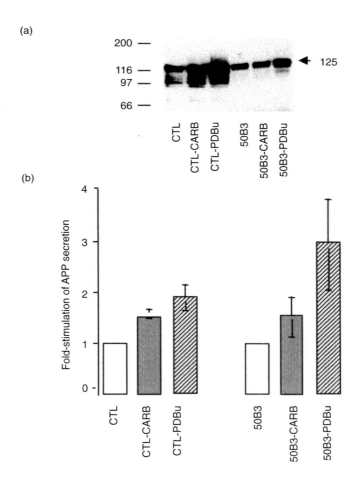

Figure 6 Effect of carbachol (CARB; 1mM) and phorbol ester (PDBu; 1μM) on the secretion of APP from control B104 mouse neuroblastoma cells (CTL) and cells transfected with the ST6N enzyme (50B3). Values are means ± S.E.M.
The graphs represent the densitometric analyses of the Western blots.

investigate whether there may be an additive effect of the two controlling factors. In the control cells, treatment with carbachol (to activate muscarinic receptors) or phorbol esters resulted in increased APP secretion (Figure 6a). The carbachol stimulation of sAPPα secretion from cells with high ST6N activity was similar to that observed in control cells. The phorbol-stimulated protein secretion, however, was markedly increased over the control cells (Figure 6b). This suggests that glycosylation (and specifically sialylation) not only stimulates the intracellular transport of APP, but also influences its subsequent processing at the level of the cell membrane.

Conclusion

Because of the neuroprotective role of soluble APP and the role of the membrane-bound form in cell adhesion, both of which may modulate the role of the protein in synaptic plasticity, any changes in the glycosylation state of the cell that result in an increase in the intracellular protein levels, and a parallel decrease in the rate of secretion, may have a significant effect on neuronal function. Indeed, there is some evidence for an association between altered protein glycosylation and Alzheimer's disease pathology, although it is not clear whether this is an early or late event in the disease [72,73]. Further studies will need to be carried out in order to gain a clearer understanding of the role of glycosylation in APP processing and Aβ generation and to determine whether altered protein glycosylation may be a key early event in the onset of Alzheimer's disease.

These studies were supported by the Scottish Hospital Endowments Research Trust, the Association for International Cancer Research, The Caledonian Research Foundation and a local trust through a Tenovus initiative.

References

1.   Breen, K.C., Coughlan, C.M. and Hayes, F.D. (1998) *Mol. Neurobiol.* **16**, 163–220
2.   Hart, G.W. (1997) *Annu. Rev. Biochem.* **66**, 315–335
3.   Arnold, C.S., Johnson, G.V.W., Cole, R.N., Dong, D.L.Y., Lee, M. and Hart, G.W. (1996) *J. Biol. Chem.* **271**, 28741–28744
4.   Hart, G.W., Kreppal, L.K., Comer, F.I., Arnold, C.S., Snow, D.M., Ye, Z., Cheng, X., DellaManna, D., Caine, D.S., Earles, B.J., et al. (1996) *Glycobiology* **6**, 711–716
5.   Cole, R.N. and Hart, G.W. (1999) *J. Neurochem.* **73**, 418–428
6.   Hwang, J.B. and Frost, S.C. (1999) *J. Biol. Chem.* **274**, 22813–22820
7.   Ramanathan, Z.K. and Hall, Z.W. (1999) *J. Biol. Chem.* **274**, 20513–20520
8.   Lis, H. and Sharon, N. (1993) *Eur. J. Biochem.* **218**, 1–27
9.   Coughlan, C.M. and Breen, K.C. (1998) *J. Neurosci. Res.* **51**, 619–626
10.   Fox, G.B., O'Connell, A.W., Murphy, K.J. and Regan, C.M. (1995) *J. Neurochem.* **65**, 2796–2799
11.   Becker, C.G., Artola, A., GerardySchahn, R., Becker, T., Welzl, H. and Schachner, M. (1996) *J. Neurosci. Res.* **45**, 143–152
12.   Matthies, H., Kretlow, J., Matthies, H., Smalla, K.–H., Staak, S. and Krug, M. (1999) *Neuroscience* **91**, 175–183
13.   Ponte, P., Gonzalez-DeWhitt, P., Schilling, J., Miller, J., Hsu, D., Greenberg, B., Davis, K., Wallace, W., Lieberburg, I., Fuller, F. and Cordell, B. (1988) *Nature (London)* **331**, 525–527
14.   Tanzi, R.E., McClatchey, A.I., Lamperti, E.D., Gusella, J.F. and Neve, R.L. (1988) *Nature (London)* **331**, 528–530
15.   Kitaguchi, N., Takahashi, Y., Tokushima, Y., Shiojiri, S. and Ito, H. (1988) *Nature (London)* **331**, 530–532
16.   Busciglio, J., Gabuzda, D.H., Matsudaira, P. and Yankner, B.A. (1993) *Proc. Natl. Acad. Sci. U.S.A.* **90**, 2092–2096
17.   Mills, J. and Reiner, P.B. (1999) *J. Neurochem.* **72**, 443–460
18.   Haass, C., Koo, E.H., Mellon, A., Hung, A.Y. and Selkoe, D.J. (1992) *Nature (London)* **357**, 500–503

19. Nordstedt, C., Caporoso, G.L., Thyberg, J., Gandy, S.E. and Greengard, P. (1993) *J. Biol. Chem.* **268**, 608–612

20. Koo, E.H. and Squazzo, S.L. (1994) *J. Biol. Chem.* **269**, 17386–17389

21. Chyung, A.S.C., Greenberg, B.D., Cook, D.G., Doms, R.W. and Lee, V.M.Y. (1997) *J. Cell Biol.* **138**, 671–680

22. Cook, D.G., Forman, M.S., Sung, J.C., Leight, S., Kolson, D.L., Iwatsubo, T., Lee, V.M.Y. and Doms, R.W. (1997) *Nat. Med. (N.Y.)* **3**, 1021–1023

23. Xu, H., Sweeney, D., Wang, R., Thinakaran, G., Lo, A.C.Y., Sisodia, S.S., Greengard, P. and Gandy, S. (1997) *Proc. Natl. Acad. Sci. U.S.A.* **94**, 3748–3752

24. Breen, K.C., Bruce, M.T. and Anderton, B.H. (1991) *J. Neurosci. Res.* **28**, 90–100

25. Gillian, A.M., McFarlane, I., Lucy, F.M., Overly, C.C., McConlogue, L. and Breen, K.C. (1997) *J. Neurosci. Res.* **49**, 154–160

26. Mattson, M.P. (1997) *Physiol. Rev.* **77**, 1081–1132

27. Doyle, E., Bruce, M.T., Breen, K.C., Smith, D.C., Anderton, B.H. and Regan, C. M. (1990) *Neurosci. Lett.* **115**, 97–102

28. Meziane, H., Dodart, J.-C., Mathias, C., Little, S., Clemens, J., Paul, S.M. and Ungerer, A. (1998) *Proc. Natl. Acad. Sci. U.S.A.* **95**, 12683–12688

29. Fazeli, M.S., Breen, K.C., Errington, M.L. and Bliss, T.V.P. (1994) *Neurosci. Lett.* **169**, 77–80

30. Ishida, A., Furukawa, K., Keller, J.N. and Mattson, M.P. (1997) *NeuroReport* **8**, 2133–2137

31. Chapman, P.F., White, G.I., Jones, M.W., Cooper-Blacketer, D., Marshall, V.J., Irizarry, M., Younkin, L., Good, M.A., Bliss, T.V.P., Hyman, B.T., et al. (1999) *Nat. Neurosci.* **2**, 271–276

32. Pahlsson, P., Shakin-Eschleman, S.H. and Spitalnik, S.L. (1992) *Biochem. Biophys. Res. Commun.* **189**, 1667–1673

33. Griffith, L.S., Mathes, M. and Schmitz, B. (1995) *J. Neurosci. Res.* **41**, 270–278

34. Tomita, S., Kirino, Y. and Suzuki, T. (1998) *J. Biol. Chem.* **273**, 6277–6284

35. Saito, F., Tani, A., Miyatake, T. and Yanagisawa, K. (1995) *Biochem. Biophys. Res. Commun.* **210**, 703–710

36. Dichgans, M., Monning, U., Konig, G., Sandbrink, R., Masters, C.L. and Beyreuther, K. (1993) *Dementia* **4**, 301–307

37. Leblanc, A.C., Xue, R. and Gambetti, P. (1996) *J. Neurochem.* **66**, 2300–2310

38. Siaodia, S.S., Koo, E.H., Beyreuther, K., Unterbeck, A. and Price, D.L. (1990) *Science* **248**, 492–495

39. Lyckman, A.W., Confaloni, A., Thinaharan, G., Sisodia, S.S. and Moya, K.L. (1998) *J. Biol. Chem.* **273**, 11100–11106

40. Stanley, P. (1989) *Mol. Cell Biol.* **9**, 377–383

41. Pahlsson, P. and Spitalnik, S.L. (1996) *Arch. Biochem. Biophys.* **331**, 177–186

42. Tienari, P.J., De Strooper, B., Ikonen, E., Simons, M., Weidemann, A., Czech, C., Hartmann, T., Ida, N., Multhaup, G., Masters, C.L., et al. (1996) *EMBO J.* **15**, 5218–5229

43. Yazaki, M., Tagawa, K., Maruyama, K., Sorimachi, H., Tsuchiya, T., Ishiura, S. and Suzuki, K. (1996) *Neurosci. Lett.* **221**, 57–60

44. McFarlane, I., Georgopoulou, N., Coughlan, C.M., Gillin, A.M. and Breen, K.C. (1999) *Neuroscience* **90**, 15–25

45. Moya, K.L., Confaloni, A. and Allinquant, B. (1994) *J. Neurochem.* **63**, 1971–1974

46. McFarlane, I., Breen, K.C., DiGiamberardino, L. and Moya, K.L. (1997) *Soc. Neurosci Abstr.* **23**, 640

47. Bagriacik, E.U., Kirkpatrick, A. and Miller, K.S. (1996) *Glycobiology* **6**, 413–421

48. Haass, C., Hung, A.V., Schlossmacher, M.G., Teplow, D.B. and Selkoe, D.J. (1993) *J. Biol. Chem.* **268**, 3021–3024

49. Georgopoulou, N. and Breen, K.C. (1999) *J. Neurosci. Res.*, **58**, 641–651

50. Breen, K.C., Potratz, A., Georgopoulou, N. and Sandhoff, K. (1998) *Glyco. J.* **15**, 199–202

51. Jolly-Tornetta, C., Gao, Z.Y., Lee, V.M.Y. and Wolf, B.A. (1998) *J. Biol. Chem.* **273**, 14015–14021

52. Nitsch, R.M., Deng, A., Wurtman, R.J. and Growdon, J.H. (1997) *J. Neurochem.* **69**, 704–712

53. Buxbaum, J.D., Oishi, M., Chen, H.I., Pinkaskramarski, R., Jaffe, E.A., Gandy, S. E. and Greengard, P. (1992) *Proc. Natl. Acad. Sci. U.S.A.* **89**, 10075–10078

54. Kim, S.H., Kim, Y.K., Jeong, S.J., Haass, C., Kim, Y.H. and Suh, Y.H. (1997) *Mol. Pharmacol.* **52**, 430–436

55. Slack, B.E., Breu, J., Muchnicki, L. and Wurtman, R.J. (1997) *Biochem. J.* **327**, 245–249

56. DesdouitsMagnen, J., Desdouits, F., Takeda, S., Syu, L.J., Saltiel, A.R., Buxbaum, J.D., Czernik, A.J., Nairn, A.C. and Greengard, P. (1998) *J. Neurochem.* **70**, 524–530

57. Aplin, A.E., Gibb, G.M., Jacobsen, J.S., Gallo, J.M. and Anderton, B.H. (1996) *J. Neurochem.* **67**, 699–707

58. Ando, K., Oishi, M., Takeda, S., Iijima, K., Isohara, T., Nairn, A.C., Kirino, Y., Greengard, P. and Suzuki, T. (1999) *J. Neurosci.* **19**, 4421–4427

59. Isohara, T., Horiuchi, A., Watanabe, T., Ando, K., Czernik, A.J., Uno, I., Greengard, P., Nairn, A.C. and Suzuki, T. (1999) *Biochem. Biophys. Res. Commun.* **258**, 300–305

60. Hung, A.Y. and Selkoe, D.J. (1994) *EMBO J.* **13**, 534–542

61. McLaughlin, M. and Breen, K.C. (1999) *J. Neurochem.* **72**, 273–281

62. Koo, E.H., Squazzo, S.L., Selkoe, D.J. and Koo, C.H. (1996) *J. Cell Sci.* **109**, 991–998

63. Marambaud, P., LopezPerez, E., Wilk, S. and Checler, F. (1997) *J. Neurochem.* **69**, 2500–2505

64. Racchi, M., Solano, D.C., Sironi, M. and Govoni, S. (1999) *J. Neurochem.* **72**, 2464–2470

65. Hung, A.Y., Haass, C., Nitsch, R.M., Qiu, W.Q., Citron, M., Wurtman, R.J., Growdon, J.H. and Selkoe, D.J. (1993) *J. Biol. Chem.* **268**, 22959–22962

66. Savage, M.J., Trusko, S.P., Howland, D.S., Pinsker, L.R., Mistretta, S., Reaume, A.G., Greenberg, B.D., Siman, R. and Scott, R.W. (1998) *J. Neurosci.* **18**, 1743–1752

67. Xu, H., Greengard, P. and Gandy, S. (1995) *J. Biol. Chem.* **270**, 23243–23245

68. Koo, E.H., Sisodia, S.S., Archer, D.R., Martin, L.J., Weidemann, A., Beyreuther, K., Fischer, P., Masters, C.L. and Price, D.L. (1990) *Proc. Natl. Acad. Sci. U.S.A.* **87**, 1561–1565

69. Gu, X., Preub, U., Gu, T. and Yu, R.K. (1995) *J. Neurochem.* **64**, 2295–2302

70. Bieberich, E., Freischutz, B., Liour, S.S. and Yu, R.K. (1998) *J. Neurochem.* **71**, 972–979

71. Ma, J.Y., Simonovic, M., Qian, R. and Colley, K.J. (1999) *J. Biol. Chem.* **274**, 8046–8052

72. Gillian, A.M. and Breen, K.C. (1995) in *Research Advances in Alzheimer's Disease and Related Disorders* (Iqbal, K., Mortimer, J., Winblad, B. and Wisniewski, H., eds.), pp. 429–436, Wiley, New York

73. Maguire, T.M. and Breen, K.C. (1995) *Dementia* **6**, 185–190

Biochem. Soc. Symp. **67**, 37–50
(Printed in Great Britain)

4

Alzheimer's disease: dysfunction of a signalling pathway mediated by the amyloid precursor protein?

Rachael L. Neve[1], Donna L. McPhie and Yuzhi Chen

Department of Psychiatry, Harvard Medical School, McLean Hospital, Belmont, MA 02478, U.S.A.

Abstract

All individuals with Alzheimer's disease (AD) experience a progressive loss of cognitive function, resulting from a neurodegenerative process characterized by the deposition of β-amyloid (Aβ) in plaques and in the cerebrovasculature, and by the formation of neurofibrillary tangles in neurons. The cause of the neuronal death is unknown but it is thought to be linked in some way to the β-amyloid precursor protein (APP), which is the source of the Aβ that accumulates in the AD brain. There are two pieces of supporting data for this: first, APP is overexpressed in Down's syndrome, which leads to AD-like neuropathology by the age of 40 in virtually all affected individuals; secondly, specific point mutations in APP cause some forms of familial AD. Our laboratory has focused on a specific aspect of APP and its connection with the neuronal destruction seen in AD. We have hypothesized that AD results from a progressive dysfunction of APP. In addition, on the basis of recent data generated by our laboratory and others, we propose that in the normal brain a percentage of APP is present as an integral protein of the plasma membrane that mediates the transduction of extracellular signals into the cell via its Aβ-containing C-terminal tail. In AD, accumulation of abnormal levels of the C-terminus in the neuron disturbs this signal-transduction function of APP, causing disorders in the cell-cycle machinery and consequent apoptosis. Here, we discuss the key findings that support this hypothesis, and discuss its therapeutic implications for AD.

[1]Address for correspondence: MRC 223, McLean Hospital, 115 Mill St., Belmont, MA 02478, U.S.A.

β-amyloid precursor protein, β-amyloid and Alzheimer's disease

Alzheimer's disease (AD) is characterized by a progressive loss of cognitive function, resulting from a neurodegenerative process characterized classically by the deposition of β-amyloid (Aβ) in plaques and in the cerebrovasculature, and the formation of neurofibrillary tangles in neurons. Additional pathological hallmarks of AD include granulovacular degeneration, loss of synapses and decreases in cell density in distinct regions of the brain. AD does not have a simple aetiology. It can occur as a 'sporadic' event, it can result from the possession of an extra copy of chromosome 21 (Down's syndrome), or it can be caused by mutations in the β-amyloid precursor protein (APP) gene on chromosome 21 or in the presenilin genes on chromosomes 1 and 14. Additional genetic complexity is conferred on it by the fact that the ε4 allele of the *APOE* gene is a major risk factor for the development of AD. Thus it is unlikely that AD is caused by a single molecular event.

Numerous mechanisms for the neuronal cell death in AD have been proposed. One of these is the amyloid hypothesis, which suggests that deposition of Aβ is a primary event in the pathological cascade for AD. This argument is based on studies *in vitro* showing that Aβ is toxic to neurons and on the measurement of the increase in release of Aβ by cells carrying familial AD (FAD) mutant genes.

There are two major C-terminal variants of Aβ: Aβ40 is the major species secreted from cultured cells and is found in cerebrospinal fluid, whereas Aβ42 is the major component of amyloid deposits [1]. Cells expressing FAD mutants of APP and the presenilins are reported to secrete increased amounts of Aβ42, suggesting a link of this variant of Aβ to AD pathogenesis. Consequently, a leading hypothesis for the aetiology of AD is that increased Aβ42 is a shared molecular correlate of FAD mutations, and that it represents a gain of deleterious function that can cause FAD [2] and may be an essential-early event in AD [1]. Although this 'amyloid hypothesis' is attractive, molecular mechanisms other than those mediated by extracellular Aβ could also lead to AD neurodegeneration.

These mechanisms are likely to be linked in some way to APP, the source of Aβ. One of the most compelling pieces of evidence that links AD neurodegeneration to APP and/or its Aβ-containing derivatives is the early finding that the APP gene is on chromosome 21: virtually all individuals trisomic for this chromosome show AD-like neuropathology by 40 years of age. Additionally, it has been discovered that specific mutations in APP cause some forms of familial FAD. These data have raised the possibility that AD may result from an alteration in the normal function of APP [3,4], and have refocused attention on the delineation of the function that APP subserves in the brain. It has been shown [5,6] that in the brain a percentage of APP is present on the cell surface, and it is proposed [4,6] that this cell-surface APP mediates the transduction of extracellular signals into the cell via its C-terminal tail.

Nishimoto and colleagues [7] showed that APP binds to the brain-specific, signal-transducing G-protein, G_o; independent confirmation of this finding has subsequently been published [8,9]. It was then discovered [10] that Val[642] ('London') FAD mutants of APP induce neuronal DNA fragmentation, a feature of apoptosis, in a neuronal cell line. This fragmentation is independent of Aβ42 production [10] and is mediated by the $G\beta_2\gamma_2$ complex of G_o [11]. These data support the notion that APP has an intrinsic signalling function in the neuron, which becomes ligand independent when APP is mutated at Val[642].

To examine the mechanism by which FAD APP might cause apoptosis in neurons, we expressed five different Alzheimer mutations of APP in primary neurons via recombinant herpes simplex virus (HSV) vectors, and quantified the levels of APP metabolites [12]. The predominant intracellular accumulation product was a C-terminal fragment of APP that co-migrated with the protein product of an HSV recombinant expressing the C-terminal 100 amino acids (C-100) of APP. Interestingly, we had proposed previously that C-100 is involved in the aetiology of AD [13]. It is neurotoxic *in vitro* [14–18] and is amyloidogenic [19–25]. In addition, expression of C-100 *in vivo* can cause neuropathology that is similar in some ways to that in AD, including neurodegeneration and cognitive dysfunction [26–33], as well as increases in acetylcholinesterase [34] and abnormalities in synaptic transmission [35]. There has been some question of whether C-100 exerts its neurotoxic effects from inside or outside the cell [36,37]. Our data of the past 6 years suggest strongly that C-100 kills from inside the cell; this is supported by the observation that C-100 is not secreted, even when it carries a signal peptide [12,22,38]. Although at least one group has reported neurotoxicity resulting from the addition of C-100 to the culture medium [39], we believe that this type of neurotoxicity is mechanistically different from the neurodegeneration caused by the expression of C-100 within neurons.

The fact that APP interacts with the signalling molecule G_o, that FAD mutants of APP can cause G_o-mediated apoptosis in neuronal cells and that the same FAD mutants of APP cause the intracellular accumulation of C-100 suggested to us the following working hypothesis: in the brain a portion of APP is present as an integral plasma membrane protein that mediates the transduction of extracellular signals into the cell via its C-terminal tail; abnormal accumulation of its Aβ-containing C-terminus in the neuron causes progressive dysfunction of APP signalling in AD, resulting in apoptosis. This hypothesis was further supported by the finding that the intracellular C-terminal tail of APP also interacts with the protein APP-BP1 [40], and with members of the Fe65 family of adaptor proteins [41].

Processing of APP

Most of what is known about APP processing has come from work with cultured cells. APP matures through the constitutive secretory pathway. Some of the APP is endoproteolytically cleaved at the cell surface within the Aβ sequence by the α-secretase, which generates the neuroprotective, secreted APP and non-amyloidogenic, 3 kDa Aβ-secreted products [42–44]. Secreted APP is readily detected in human plasma and cerebrospinal fluid.

Endocytosis of cell-surface APP generates C-terminal fragments of 8–12 kDa that are degraded in the lysosomes [45,46]; some of these, generated by β-secretase cleavage at the N-terminus of the Aβ sequence, are analogous to C-100 and are amyloidogenic. Activity of a second protease, γ-secretase, cleaves these C-terminal fragments of APP to release the full-length Aβ protein. Thus both Aβ and C-100-like fragments of APP are produced normally at low levels by the cell. Most of the Aβ that is generated is secreted, although small amounts can be detected intracellularly. C-100-like amyloidogenic fragments have only been detected intracellularly.

It is important to note that APP processing is cell-type specific. LeBlanc and colleagues have reported that human neurons secrete more 4 kDa Aβ than 3 kDa Aβ, and metabolize approximately 40% of newly synthesized APP through the α-secretase pathway [47,48]. Moreover, human neurons produce five C-terminal fragments of APP, in a pattern seen uniquely in the human brain [47,49]. The two largest C-terminal derivatives have the entire Aβ sequence at or near their N-terminus [49], and probably represent endogenous C-100 fragments. Thus C-100 is a physiologically relevant fragment of APP in the human brain. In contrast with human neurons, most APP-transfected human or non-human cell lines produce more 3 kDa Aβ than 4 kDa Aβ, and show a relatively non-amyloidogenic pattern of C-terminal fragments [45,46,50,51].

Analyses of Aβ in genetically engineered cell lines expressing FAD mutations in both APP and the presenilins have shown that all of the mutations cause either increased overall secretion of Aβ or increased secretion of the long (42–43-amino-acid) form of Aβ (Aβ42) relative to the shorter 40-amino-acid form [2]. Increases in Aβ42 have also been detected in transgenic mice expressing FAD mutations of both APP and presenilin (PS) [2]. Aβ42 is the major component of brain amyloid deposits in AD. Consequently, a leading hypothesis for the aetiology of AD is that increased Aβ42 is a shared molecular correlate of FAD mutations which may also be operative in 'sporadic' AD. Increases in Aβ42 have not been shown directly in human AD brain homogenates, although it is clear that amyloid plaques contain a disproportionate amount of Aβ42. Furthermore, analyses of levels of this peptide in the plasma and cerebrospinal fluid of AD patients have revealed no differences between AD patients and controls in the plasma [52], and a reduction of Aβ42 in the cerebrospinal fluid of AD patients relative to controls [52,53]. However, increased release of Aβ42 from fibroblasts of AD patients with mutations in the presenilins, as well as increased levels of Aβ42 in their plasma, has been demonstrated [54].

The β-secretase cleavage product of APP, C-100, is increased in cell lines expressing the Swedish FAD mutation of APP [55,56], but not in cell lines expressing the London Val[642] mutation of APP [57]. Since neurons process APP differently from cell lines, we expressed all known FAD mutants of APP in primary neurons in culture, and analysed APP processing in the infected neurons. We showed that all the mutants caused increases in the intracellular levels of C-100 [12]. We have not yet determined whether FAD mutations in the presenilins cause the same alterations in C-100 levels. Although increases of

C-100 in FAD APP transgenic animal models have not been published, at least one such model, expressing the Val^{642}→Phe (V642F) mutation of APP (numbered according to the APP$_{695}$ of APP) [58], shows a significant increase in C-100 in brain homogenates. We have hypothesized that abnormal accumulation of C-100 in the neuron occurs in AD; however, it has not yet been shown whether the level of C-100 protein is increased in human AD versus control brains *post mortem*.

Even if C-100 levels are increased in AD brains, this does not prove that C-100 causes the neuropathology of AD. One issue is whether the neurodegeneration is caused by intact C-100 or by the Aβ that is generated from C-100. To answer this question, it will be necessary to create mutants of C-100 and of FAD APPs that inhibit γ-secretase cleavage and production of Aβ [59], and determine whether these mutants cause neurodegeneration *in vitro* or AD-like pathology *in vivo*. This leads us to the question of whether the apoptosis caused by FAD mutants of APP in neuronal cells [10] is due to the increased intracellular C-100 that results from expression of these mutants. To answer this, it will be necessary to mutate the β-secretase cleavage site in the London FAD mutant of APP, show that it inhibits the production of C-100, and assay this mutant relative to the non-mutated London FAD mutant for its ability to cause apoptosis in neurons. If inhibition of γ-secretase cleavage of C-100 increases the accumulation of C-100 in the neurons, and does not inhibit apoptosis caused by C-100 or by the FAD APP mutants, the safety of therapeutic agents that inhibit γ-secretase is called into question.

APP as a signalling molecule

The possibility that APP may act as a signalling receptor was first proposed on the basis of its predicted amino acid sequence, which suggested that APP was a type-1 intrinsic membrane protein consistent with the structure of a cell-surface receptor [60]. However, subsequent studies of the function of APP concentrated largely on the secreted ectodomain, because of a lack of direct evidence that mature APP exists on the cell surface with intact intracellular, transmembrane and extracellular domains. APP was inferred to exist on the surface of a variety of cultured cells [46,61,62], but some laboratories could not detect it [63]. Nevertheless, some reports demonstrating involvement of APP in neuronal development, synaptogenesis and synaptic plasticity [64–69] did not restrict the observed function to secreted APP, raising the possibility that some aspects of synaptic plasticity are mediated by cell-associated APP. Indeed, it has now been demonstrated directly that some APP is found on the cell surface in neurons [5,6,70]. Cell-surface APP possesses a neurite-promoting activity that is distinct from that of the secreted APP [69], co-localizes with adhesion plaque components [70,71] and participates in synaptic vesicle recycling [72], suggesting that a percentage of APP may function as a cell-surface receptor, transducing signals from the extracellular matrix to the interior of the cell (Figure 1).

The growth cone G-protein, G$_o$ [7], the presumptive adaptor proteins Fe65 and X11 [41], and APP-BP1 [40] have been reported to interact with the

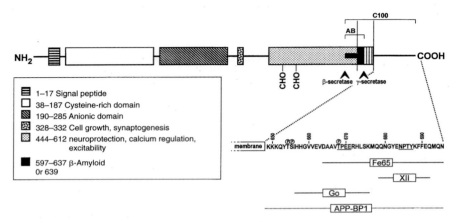

Figure 1　Structural and functional domains of APP₆₉₅.

C-terminus of APP, presumably to initiate intracellular signalling (Figure 1). Although the functions of Fe65 and X11 are not known, Fe65 has the characteristics of adaptor proteins, which are thought to link signal-transduction events emanating from plasma membrane receptors to intracellular molecules by forming complexes of these proteins. Therefore, one could envisage APP as being part of a G_o-protein-centred complex that transduces extracellular signals to the cytoplasm and the nucleus, with Fe65 linking APP to molecules downstream in the pathway. APP-BP1 could be one of the downstream molecules.

The molecule whose interaction with APP has been defined in greatest detail is G_o. Nishimoto and colleagues have demonstrated that the His^{657}–Lys^{676} domain of the APP_{695} isoform activates the heterotrimeric G_o in a $GTP_\gamma S$-inhibitable manner [7,73]. Their demonstration that an antibody to the extracellular domain of APP that acts as a ligand mimetic [74] causes activation of G_o, provides an argument for APP being a G-protein-coupled receptor. As noted earlier, the London mutation of APP, V642I, causes DNA fragmentation when expressed in a neuronal cell line [10]. Notably, expression in the cells of V642I APP deleted for residues His^{657}–Lys^{676} did not cause DNA fragmentation. Pertussis toxin, an inhibitor of G_o and G_i, blocked the DNA fragmentation caused by V642I, as did co-transfection of V642I APP and a cDNA encoding a dominant-negative mutant of $G\alpha_o$, but not with a cDNA encoding a dominant-negative mutant of $G\alpha_i$. Inhibition of Aβ42 production from the V642I APP by mutating the γ-secretase cleavage site did not have any effect on the DNA fragmentation caused by V642I.

These data suggest that G_o mediates the DNA fragmentation caused by the V642I mutants of APP; indeed, a subsequent study by Nishimoto's group revealed that the DNA fragmentation was mediated by the βγ complex of G_o [11]. Aβ does not appear to play a causative role in inducing DNA fragmentation in this experimental paradigm. The data support the notion that these mutants act by causing unregulated activation of G_o and, by inference, of a cellular signalling pathway downstream of G_o.

Apoptosis and the cell cycle in AD

The notion that a form of cell suicide called apoptosis participates in the neuropathology of AD was raised by Su et al. [75], when they reported evidence for DNA fragmentation in neurons in the AD brain. Although other groups have also detected this feature of apoptosis in the AD brain, many in the field have been sceptical of the idea that the neurons that die in AD undergo apoptosis, partly because DNA fragmentation can also be caused by oxidative damage [76] or by autolysis *post mortem* [77]. However, a recent report from the laboratory of Mark Mattson [78] has revived interest in the possibility that apoptosis is operative in AD. These investigators found that levels of a marker of apoptosis, prostate apoptosis response-4 protein (Par-4), are increased 15–20-fold in vulnerable neurons in AD brain compared with controls. They also showed that Par-4 expression is increased in cultured neurons undergoing apoptosis, and that inhibition of Par-4 expression in these neurons blocks apoptosis.

These findings provide the strongest evidence to date that neuronal death in AD may be due to apoptosis, and they are consistent with the increasing awareness in the field that at least one of the normal functions of APP is to regulate apoptosis in the neuron. As noted earlier, Nishimoto's group showed that the V642I mutation of APP causes DNA fragmentation when expressed in a neuronal cell line [10]. Zhao and co-workers [79] showed that the same mutation, as well as two additional FAD APP mutations, induced apoptosis in differentiated PC12 cells. Barnes and colleagues [80] reported that levels of APP are increased in motor neurons dying of apoptosis, and that APP is cleaved by caspase-3, a caspase activated in apoptotic motor neurons. Interestingly, we [81] and others [82] have shown that overexpression of wild-type APP causes apoptotic death of neurons, although to a lesser degree than does expression of FAD mutants of APP.

Approximately 50% of inherited AD cases are caused by mutations in the presenilin genes *PS1* and *PS2*. It has been reported that overexpression of these genes in transfected cell lines can cause apoptosis [83] or result in an increased susceptibility to apoptosis [78,84–86]. On the other hand, we have found [81] that expression of PS1 in primary neurons does not cause or enhance apoptosis; rather, it protects neurons against experimentally induced apoptosis. Thus the ability of PS1 to induce apoptosis appears to be cell-type specific; and this may have important implications for the pathogenesis in AD, in which neurons are differentially affected. PS1 is reported to be expressed primarily in central nervous system neurons in the brain, suggesting that this protein may perform a neuron-specific function [87]. In fact, in AD, neurons that express PS1 antigen are less vulnerable to the disease than neurons that do not express it [88], and inhibition of PS1 expression results in apoptosis [89], suggesting a protective role for this protein. Although the precise role of presenilins in regulation of apoptosis in the neuron is still unclear, the evidence that they do play a role in this pathway is strong. These data implicate both APP and presenilins in the control of apoptotic death in the brain, and it is not unreasonable to suppose that FAD mutations in these genes may cause dysfunction in this pathway.

The implication of apoptosis in AD aetiology is consistent with the numerous findings of cell-cycle abnormalities in AD. Apoptosis and the cell cycle are closely coupled, and the re-expression of cell-cycle markers has been linked with the occurrence of certain types of neuronal cell death [90–92]. The interpretation of these findings [92] is that a neuron is committed to the permanent cessation of cell division, so if, for any reason, it is forced to re-enter the cell cycle after this commitment, it dies. Notably, ectopic expression of cell-cycle proteins and their associated kinases in the AD brain has been reported [94–97]. Most recently, Busser and co-workers [98] found abnormal appearance of cell-cycle markers in regions of the AD brain where cell death is extensive; in addition, Chow and colleagues [99] found increases in the expression of genes encoding cell-cycle proteins in single neurons in late-stage relative to early-stage AD brain. The phosphoepitope Ser^{214} of the microtubule-associated protein tau, which appears in the neurofibrillary tangles in AD, is a prominent phosphorylation site in metaphase, but not in interphase, of dividing cells expressing tau [100]. This supports the view that reactivation of the cell-cycle machinery may be involved in hyperphosphorylation of tau in AD brain. The possibility that phosphorylation-dependent events occurring during the cell cycle affect the normal function of APP is suggested by the finding that regulation of the phosphorylation and metabolism of this protein occurs in a cell-cycle-dependent manner [101,102].

We hypothesize that dysfunction of pathways mediated by APP may be one cause of the reactivation of cell-cycle proteins in the AD brain. It is important to increase our understanding of the normal function of APP in the brain, identify which fragment(s) of APP causes apoptotic neuronal death and clarify some of the molecular events that lead to this apoptosis. Given the recent evidence that apoptosis and cell-cycle abnormalities occur in the AD brain, the data that are obtained may suggest a mechanism by which neurons die in AD.

References

1. Younkin, S.G. (1995) Evidence that Aβ 42 is the real culprit in Alzheimer's disease. *Ann. Neurol.* **37**, 287–288
2. Hardy, J. (1997) The Alzheimer family of diseases: many etiologies, one pathogenesis? *Proc. Natl. Acad. Sci. U.S.A.* **18**, 2095–2097
3. Neve, R.L. and Robakis, N.K. (1998) Alzheimer disease: A re-examination of the amyloid hypothesis. *Trends Neurosci.* **21**, 15–19
4. Nishimoto, I. (1998) A new paradigm for neurotoxicity by FAD mutants of βAPP: a signaling abnormality. *Neurobiol. Aging* **19**, S33–S38
5. Jung, S.S., Nalbantoglu, J. and Cashman, N.R. (1996) Alzheimer's β-amyloid precursor protein is expressed on the surface of immediately *ex vivo* brain cells: a flow cytometric study. *J. Neurosci. Res.* **46**, 336–348
6. Perez, R.G., Zheng, H., Van der Ploeg, L.H.T. and Koo, E.H. (1997) The β-amyloid precursor protein of Alzheimer's disease enhances neuron viability and modulates neuronal polarity. *J. Neurosci.* **17**, 9407–9414

7.   Nishimoto, I., Okamoto, T., Matsuura, Y., Okamoto, T., Murayama, Y. and Ogata, E. (1993) Alzheimer amyloid protein precursor complexes with brain GTP-binding protein G(o). *Nature (London)* **362**, 75–79

8.   Borowicz, S.L. and Dokas, L.A. (1995) Association of the amyloid precursor protein, B-50 (GAP-43), and G_o in neuronal membranes. *Soc. Neurosci. Abstr.* **21**, 207

9.   Brouillet, E., Trembleau, A., Galanaud, D., Volovitch, M., Bouillot, C., Valenza, C., Prochiantz, A. and Allinquant, B. (1999) The amyloid precursor protein interacts with G_o heterotrimeric protein within a cell compartment specialized in signal transduction. *J. Neurosci.* **19**, 1717–1727

10. Yamatsuji, T., Okamoto, T., Takeda, S., Fukumoto, H., Iwatsubo, T., Suzuki, N., Asami-Odaka, A., Ireland, S., Kinane, T.B. and Nishimoto, I. (1996) G protein-mediated neuronal DNA fragmentation induced by familial Alzheimer's disease-associated mutants of APP. *Science* **272**, 1349–1352

11. Giambarella, U., Yamatsuji, T., Okamoto, T., Matsui, T., Ikezu, T., Murayama, Y., Levine, M.A., Katz, A., Gautam, N. and Nishimoto, I. (1997) G protein βγ complex-mediated apoptosis by familial Alzheimer's disease mutant of APP. *EMBO J.* **16**, 4897–4907

12. McPhie, D.L., Lee, R.K.K., Eckman, C.B., Olstein, D.H., Durham, S.P., Yager, D., Younkin, S.G., Wurtman, R.J. and Neve, R.L. (1997) Neuronal expression of β-amyloid precursor protein Alzheimer mutations causes intracellular accumulation of a C-terminal fragment containing both the amyloid β and cytoplasmic domains. *J. Biol. Chem.* **272**, 24743–24746

13. Neve, R.L. and Kozlowski, M.R. (1995) The carboxyl-terminal 100 amino acids of the β-amyloid protein precursor: Role in Alzheimer disease neurodegeneration. *Dev. Brain Dysfunction* **8**, 13–24

14. Yankner, B.A., Dawes, L.R., Fisher, S., Villa-Komaroff, L., Oster-Granite, M.L. and Neve, R.L. (1989) Neurotoxocity of a fragment of the amyloid precursor associated with Alzheimer's disease. *Science* **245**, 417–420

15. Fukuchi, K., Sopher, B., Furlong, C.E., Smith, A.C., Dang, N.T. and Martin, G.M. (1993) Selective neurotoxicity of COOH-terminal fragments of the β-amyloid precursor protein. *Neurosci. Lett.* **154**, 145–148

16. Sopher, B.L., Fukuchi, K., Smith, A.C., Leppig, K.A., Furlong, C.E. and Martin, G.M. (1994) Cytotoxicity mediated by conditional expression of a carboxyl-terminal derivative of the β-amyloid precursor protein. *Mol. Brain Res.* **26**, 207–217

17. Suh, Y.-H. (1997) An etiological role of amyloidogenic carboxyl-terminal fragments of the β-amyloid precursor protein in Alzheimer's disease. *J. Neurochem.* **68**, 1781–1791

18. Li, Q.-X., Maynard, C., Cappai, R., McLean, C.A., Cherny, R.A., Lynch, T., Culvenor, J.G., Trevaskis, J., Tanner, J.E., Bailey, K.A., et al. (1999) Intracellular accumulation of detergent-soluble amyloidogenic Aβ fragment of Alzheimer's disease precursor protein in the hippocampus of aged transgenic mice. *J. Neurochem.* **72**, 2479–2487

19. Dyrks, T., Weidemann, A., Multhaup, G., Salbaum, J.M., Lemaire, H.G., Kang, J., Muller-Hill, B., Masters, C.L. and Beyreuther, K. (1988) Identification, transmembrane orientation and biogenesis of the amyloid A4 precursor of Alzheimer's disease. *EMBO J.* **7**, 949–957

20. Dyrks, T., Dyrks, E., Hartmann, T., Masters, C. and Beyreuther, K. (1992) Amyloidogenicity of βA4 and βA4-bearing amyloid protein precursor fragments by metal-catalyzed oxidation. *J. Biol. Chem.* **267**, 18210–18217

21. Dyrks, T., Dyrks, E., Monning, U., Urmoneit, B., Turner, J. and Beyreuther, K. (1993) Generation of βA4 from the amyloid protein precursor and fragments thereof. *FEBS Lett.* **335**, 89–93

22. Maruyama, K., Terakado, K., Usami, M. and Yoshikawa, K. (1990) Formation of amyloid-like fibrils in COS cells overexpressing part of the Alzheimer amyloid protein precursor. *Nature (London)* **347**, 566–569

23.   Wolf, D., Quon, D., Wang, Y. and Cordell, B. (1990) Identification and characterization of
      C-terminal fragments of the β-amyloid precursor produced in cell culture. *EMBO J.* **9**,
      2079–2084

24.   Gardella, J.E., Gorgone, G.A., Candela, L., Ghiso, J., Castano, E.M., Frangione, B. and
      Gorevic, P.D. (1993) High-level expression and in vitro mutagenesis of a fibrillogenic 109-
      amino-acid C-terminal fragment of Alzheimer's disease amyloid precursor protein.
      Biochem. J. **294**, 667–674

25.   Tjernberg, L.O., Naslund, J., Thyberg, J., Gandy, S.E., Terenius, L. and Nordstedt, C.
      (1997) Generation of Alzheimer amyloid β peptide through nonspecific proteolysis. *J. Biol.*
      Chem. **272**, 1870–1875

26.   Neve, R.L., Kammesheidt, A. and Hohmann, C.F. (1992) Brain transplants of cells express-
      ing the carboxyterminal fragment of the Alzheimer amyloid protein precursor cause specific
      neuropathology *in vivo. Proc. Natl. Acad. Sci. U.S.A.* **89**, 3448–3452

27.   Kammesheidt, A., Boyce, F.M., Spanoyannis, A.F., Cummings, B.J., Ortegon, M., Cotman,
      C.W., Vaught, J.L. and Neve, R.L. (1992) Amyloid deposition and neuronal pathology in
      transgenic mice expressing the carboxyterminal fragment of the Alzheimer amyloid precur-
      sor in the brain. *Proc. Natl. Acad. Sci. U.S.A.* **89**, 10857–10861

28.   Tate, B., Aboody-Guterman, K.S., Morris, A.M., Walcott, E.C., Majocha, R.E. and
      Marotta, C.A. (1992) Disruption of circadian regulation by brain grafts that overexpress
      Alzheimer β/A4 amyloid. *Proc. Natl. Acad. Sci. U.S.A.* **89**, 7090–7094

29.   Fukuchi, K., Kunkel, D.D., Schwartzkroin, P.A., Kamino, K., Ogburn, C.E., Furlong, C.E.
      and Martin, G.M. (1994) Overexpression of a C-terminal portion of the β-amyloid precur-
      sor protein in mouse brains by transplantation of transformed neuronal cells. *Exp. Neurol.*
      127, 253–264

30.   Oster-Granite, M.L., McPhie, D.L., Greenan, J. and Neve, R.L. (1996) Age-dependent neu-
      ronal and synaptic degeneration in mice transgenic for the carboxyl-terminus of the
      amyloid precursor protein. *J. Neurosci.* **16**, 6732–6741

31.   Nalbantoglu, J., Tirado-Santiago, G., Lahsaini, A., Poirier, J., Goncalves, O., Verge, G.,
      Momoli, F., Weiner, S.A., Massicotte, G., Julien, J.-P. and Shapiro, M.L. (1997) Impaired
      learning and LTP in mice expressing the carboxy terminus of the Alzheimer amyloid pre-
      cursor protein. *Nature (London)* **387**, 500–505

32.   Sato, M., Kawarabashi, T., Shoji, M., Kobayashi, T., Tada, N., Matsubara, E. and Hirai, S.
      (1997) Neurodegeneration and gliosis in transgenic mice overexpressing a carboxy-terminal
      fragment of Alzheimer amyloid-beta protein precursor. *Dementia Geriatr. Cognit. Disord.*
      8, 296–307

33.   Berger-Sweeney, J., McPhie, D.L., Arters, J.A., Greenan, J., Oster-Granite, M.L. and Neve,
      R.L. (1999) Impairment in spatial learning accompanied by neurodegeneration in mice
      transgenic for the carboxyl-terminus of the amyloid precursor protein. *Mol. Brain Res.* **66**,
      150–162

34.   Sberna, G., Saez-Valero, J., Li, Q.X., Czech, C., Beyreuther, K., Masters, C.L., McLean,
      C.A. and Small, D.H. (1998) Acetylcholinesterase is increased in the brains of transgenic
      mice expressing the C-terminal fragment (CT100) of the β-amyloid protein precursor of
      Alzheimer's disease. *J. Neurochem.* **71**, 723–731

35.   Ghiribi, O., Lapierre, L., Girard, M., Ohayon, M., Nalbantoglu, J. and Massicotte, G.
      (1999) Hypoxia-induced loss of synaptic transmission is exacerbated in hippocampal slices
      of transgenic mice expressing C-terminal fragments of Alzheimer amyloid precursor pro-
      tein. *Hippocampus* **9**, 201–205

36.   Fukuchi, K., Sopher, B. and Martin, G.M. (1993) Neurotoxicity of β-amyloid. *Nature*
      (London) **361**, 122

37.   Yoshikawa, K. (1993) Neurotoxicity of β-amyloid (reply). *Nature (London)* **361**, 122–123

38. Citron, M., Diehl, T.S., Capell, A., Haass, C., Teplow, D.B. and Selkoe, D.J. (1996) Inhibition of amyloid β-protein production in neural cells by the serine protease inhibitor AEBSF. *Neuron* **17**, 1–9

39. Kim, S.-H. and Suh, Y.-H. (1996) Neurotoxicity of a carboxy-terminal fragment of the Alzheimer's amyloid precursor protein. *J. Neurochem.* **67**, 1172–1182

40. Chow, N., Korenberg, J.R., Chen, X.-N. and Neve, R.L. (1996) APP-BP1, a novel protein that binds to the carboxyl-terminal region of the amyloid precursor protein. *J. Biol. Chem.* **271**, 11339–11346

41. Russo, T., Faraonio, R., Minopoli, G., De Candia, P., De Renzis, S. and Zambrano, N. (1998) Fe65 and the protein network centered around the cytosolic domain of the Alzheimer's β-amyloid precursor protein. *FEBS Lett.* **434**, 1–7

42. Palmert, M., Siedlak, S., Podlisny, M., Greenberg, B., Shelton, E., Chan, H., Usiak, M., Selkoe, D., Perry, G. and Younkin, S. (1989) Soluble derivatives of the β-amyloid protein precursor of Alzheimer's disease are labeled by antisera to the β-amyloid protein. *Biochem. Biophys. Res. Commun.* **165**, 7533–7539

43. Haass, C., Hung, A., Schlossmacher, M., Teplow, D. and Selkoe, D. (1993) β-amyloid peptide and a 3 kDa fragment are derived by distinct cellular mechanisms. *J. Biol. Chem.* **268**, 3021–3024

44. Mattson, M., Cheng, B., Culwell, A., Esch, F., Lieberburg, I. and Rydel, R. (1993) Evidence for excitoprotective and intraneuronal calcium-regulating roles for secreted forms of the β-amyloid precursor protein. *Neuron* **10**, 243–254

45. Golde, T., Estus, S. and Younkin, S.G. (1992) Processing of the amyloid protein precursor to potentially amyloidogenic derivatives. *Science* **255**, 728–730

46. Haass, C., Koo, E., Mellon, A., Jung, A. and Selkoe, D. (1992) Targeting of cell-surface β-amyloid precursor protein to lysosomes: alternative processing into amyloid-bearing fragments. *Nature (London)* **357**, 500–503

47. LeBlanc, A.C. (1995) Increased production of 4 kDa amyloid β peptide in serum deprived human primary neuron cultures: possible involvement of apoptosis. *J. Neurosci.* **15**, 7837–7846

48. LeBlanc, A.C., Papadopoulos, M., Belair, C., Chu, W., Crosato, M., Powell, J. and Goodyer, C. (1997) Amyloid precursor protein metabolism in human neurons, astrocytes and microglia. *J. Neurochem.* **68**, 1183–1190

49. Estus, S., Golde, T., Kunishita, T., Blades, D., Lowery, D., Eisen, M., Usiak, M., Qu, X., Tabira, T., Greenberg, B. and Younkin, S. (1992) Potentially amyloidogenic, carboxy-terminal derivatives of the amyloid protein precursor. *Science* **255**, 726–728

50. Haass, C., Hung, A., Schlossmacher, M., Teplow, D. and Selkoe, D. (1993) β-amyloid peptide and a 3 kDa fragment are derived by distinct cellular mechanisms. *J. Biol. Chem.* **268**, 3021–3024

51. LeBlanc, A.C., Xue, R. and Gambetti, P. (1996) APP metabolism in primary cell cultures of neurons, astrocytes and microglia. *J. Neurochem.* **66**, 2300–2310

52. Ida, N., Hartmann, T., Pantel, J., Schroder, J., Zerfass, R., Forstl, H., Sandbrink, R., Masters, C.L. and Beyreuther, K. (1996) Analysis of heterogeneous βA4 peptides in human cerebrospinal fluid and blood by a newly developed sensitive western blot assay. *J. Biol. Chem.* **271**, 22908–22914

53. Motter, R., Vigo-Pelfrey, C., Kholodenko, D., Barbour, R., Johnson-Wood, K., Galasko, D., Chang, L., Miller, B., Clark, C., Green, R., et al. (1995) Reduction of β-amyloid peptide$_{42}$ in the cerebrospinal fluid of patients with Alzheimer's disease. *Ann. Neurol.* **38**, 643–648

54. Scheuner, D., Eckman, C., Jensen, M., Song, X., Citron, M., Suzuki, N., Bird, T.D., Hardy, J., Hutton, M., Kukull, W., et al. (1996) Secreted amyloid β-protein similar to that in the senile plaques of Alzheimer's disease is increased in vivo by the presenilin 1 and 2 and APP mutations linked to familial Alzheimer's disease. *Nat. Med. (N.Y.)* **2**, 864–870

55.   Citron, M., Oltersdorf, T., Haas, C., McConlogue, L., Hung, A.Y., Seubert, P., Vigo-
       Pelfrey, C., Lieberburg, I. and Selkoe, D.J. (1992) Mutation of the β-amyloid precursor
       protein in familial Alzheimer's disease increases β-protein production. *Nature (London)*
       360, 672–674

56.   Cai, X.-D., Golde, T.E. and Younkin, S.G. (1993) Release of excess amyloid β protein from
       a mutant amyloid β protein precursor. *Science* **259**, 514–516

57.   Suzuki, N., Cheung, T.T., Cai, X.-D., Odaka, A., Otvos, Jr., L., Eckman, C., Golde, T.E.
       and Younkin, S.G. (1994) An increased percentage of long amyloid beta protein secreted by
       familial amyloid β protein precursor (βAPP717) mutants. *Science* **264**, 1336–1340

58.   Games, D., Adams, D., Alessandrini, R., Barbour, R., Berthelette, P., Blackwell, C., Carr,
       T., Clemens, J., Donaldson, T., Gillespie, F., et al. (1995) Alzheimer-type neuropathology in
       transgenic mice overexpressing V717F β-amyloid precursor protein. *Nature (London)* **373**,
       523–527

59.   Murphy, M.P., Hickman, L.J., Eckman, C.B., Uljon, S.N., Wang, R. and Golde, T.E. (1999)
       γ-secretase, evidence for multiple proteolytic activities and influence of membrane position-
       ing of substrate on generation of amyloid β peptides of varying length. *J. Biol. Chem.* **274**,
       11914–11923

60.   Kang, J., Lemaire, H.-G., Unterbeck, A., Salbaum, J.M., Masters, C.L., Grzeschik, K.-H.,
       Beyreuther, K. and Muller-Hill, B. (1987) The precursor of Alzheimer's disease amyloid A4
       protein resembles a cell-surface receptor. *Nature (London)* **325**, 733–736

61.   Simons, M., Ikonen, E., Tienari, P.J., Cid-Arregui, A., Monning, U., Beyreuther, K. and
       Dotti, C.G. (1995) Intracellular routing of human amyloid protein precursor: Axonal deliv-
       ery followed by transport to the dendrites. *J. Neurosci. Res.* **41**, 121–128

62.   Yamazaki, T., Selkoe, D.J. and Koo, E.H. (1995) Trafficking of cell surface β-amyloid pre-
       cursor protein: retrograde and transcytotic transport in cultured neurons. *J. Cell Biol.* **129**,
       432–442

63.   Allinquant, B., Moya, K.L., Bouillot, C. and Prochiantz, A. (1994) Amyloid precursor pro-
       tein in cortical neurons: coexistence of two pools differentially distributed in axons and
       dendrites and association with cytoskeleton. *J. Neurosci.* **14**, 6842–6854

64.   Luo, L., Tully, T. and White, K. (1992) Human amyloid precursor protein ameliorates
       behavioral deficit of flies deleted for *Appl* gene. *Neuron* **9**, 595–605

65.   Moya, K.L., Benowitz, L.I., Schneider, G.E. and Allinquant, B. (1994) The amyloid precur-
       sor protein is developmentally regulated and correlated with synaptogenesis. *Dev. Biol.* **171**,
       597–603

66.   Mucke, L., Masliah, E., Johnson, W.B., Ruppe, M.D., Alford, M., Rockenstein, E.M., Forss-
       Petter, S., Pietropaolo, M., Mallory, M. and Abraham, C.A. (1994) Synaptotrophic effects of
       human amyloid β protein precursors in the cortex of transgenic mice. *Brain. Res.* **666**,
       151–167

67.   Roch, J.-M., Masliah, E., Roch-Levecq, A.-C., Sundsmo, M.P., Otero, D.A., Veinbergs, I.
       and Saitoh, T. (1994) Increase of synaptic density and memory retention by a peptide repre-
       senting the trophic domain of the amyloid β/A4 protein precursor. *Proc. Natl. Acad. Sci.*
       U.S.A. **91**, 7450–7454

68.   Müller, U., Cristina, N., Li, A.-W., Wolfer, D.P., Lipp, H.-P., Rülick, T., Brandner, S.,
       Aguzzi, A. and Weissmann, C. (1994) Behavioral and anatomical deficits in mice homozy-
       gous for a modified β-amyloid precursor protein gene. *Cell* **79**, 755–765

69.   Qiu, W.Q., Ferreira, A., Miller, C., Koo, E.H. and Selkoe, D.J. (1995) Cell-surface β-amy-
       loid precursor protein stimulates neurite outgrowth of hippocampal neurons in an
       isoform-dependent manner. *J. Neurosci.* **15**, 2157–2167

70.   Storey, E., Spurck, T., Pickett-Heaps, J., Beyreuther, K. and Masters, C.L. (1996) The amy-
       loid precursor protein of Alzheimer's disease is found on the surface of static but not
       actively motile portions of neurites. *Brain Res.* **735**, 59–66

71. Yamazaki, T., Koo, E.H. and Selkoe, D.J. (1997) Cell surface amyloid β-protein precursor colocalizes with β integrins at substrate contact sites in neural cells. *J. Neurosci.* **17**, 1004–1010

72. Marquez-Sterling, N.R., Lo, A.C.Y., Sisodia, S.S. and Koo, E.H. (1997) Trafficking of cell-surface β-amyloid precursor protein: Evidence that a sorting intermediate participates in synaptic vesicle recycling. *J. Neurosci.* **17**, 140–151

73. Lang, J., Nishimoto, I., Okamoto, T., Regazzi, R., Kiraly, C., Weller, U. and Wollheim, C.B. (1995) Direct control of exocytosis by receptor-mediated activation of the heterotrimeric GAPases Gi and G(o) or by the expression of their active G alpha subunits. *EMBO J.* **14**, 3635–3644

74. Okamoto, T., Takeda, S., Murayama, Y., Ogata, E. and Nishimoto, I. (1995) Ligand-dependent G protein coupling function of amyloid transmembrane precursor. *J. Biol. Chem.* **270**, 4205–4208

75. Su, J.H., Anderson, A.J., Cummings, B.J. and Cotman, C.W. (1994) Immunohistochemical evidence for DNA fragmentation in neurons in the AD brain. *NeuroReport* **5**, 2529–2533

76. Tsang, S.Y., Tam, S.C., Bremner, I. and Burkitt, M.J. (1996) Copper-1,10-phenanthroline induces internucleosomal DNA fragmentation in HepG2 cells, resulting from direct oxidation by the hydroxyl radical. *Biochem. J.* **317**, 13–16

77. Stadelmann, C., Bruck, W., Bancher, C., Jellinger, K. and Lassmann, H. (1998) Alzheimer disease: DNA fragmentation indicates increased neuronal vulnerability, but not apoptosis. *J. Neuropathol. Exp. Neurol.* **57**, 456–464

78. Guo, Q., Fu, W., Xie, J., Luo, H., Sells, S.F., Geddes, J.W., Bondada, V., Rangnekar, V.M. and Mattson, M.P. (1998) Par-4 is a mediator of neuronal degeneration associated with the pathogenesis of Alzheimer disease. *Nat. Med. (N.Y.)* **4**, 957–962

79. Zhao, B., Chrest, F.J., Horton, Jr., W.E., Sisodia, S.S. and Kusiak, J.W. (1997) Expression of mutant amyloid precursor proteins induced apoptosis in PC12 cells. *J. Neurosci. Res.* **47**, 253–265

80. Barnes, N.Y., Li, L., Yoshikawa, K., Schwartz, L.M., Oppenheim, R.W. and Milligan, C.E. (1998) Increased production of amyloid precursor protein provides a substrate for caspase-3 in dying motoneurons. *J. Neurosci.* **18**, 5869–5880

81. Bursztajn, S., DeSouza, R., McPhie, D.L., Berman, S.A., Shioi, J., Robakis, N.K. and Neve, R.L. (1998) Overexpression in neurons of human presenilin-1 or a presenilin-1 familial Alzheimer disease mutant does not enhance apoptosis. *J. Neurosci.* **18**, 9790–9799

82. Nishimura, I., Uetsuki, T., Dani, S.U., Ohsawa, Y., Saito, I., Okamura, H., Uchiyama, Y. and Yoshikawa, K. (1998) Degeneration in vivo of rat hippocampal neurons by wild-type Alzheimer amyloid precursor protein overexpressed by adenovirus-mediated gene transfer. *J. Neurosci.* **18**, 2387–2398

83. Janicki, S. and Monteiro, M.J. (1997) Increased apoptosis arising from increased expression of Alzheimer's disease associated presenilin-2 mutation (N141I). *J. Cell Biol.* **139**, 485–495

84. Wolozin, B., Iwasaki, K., Vito, P., Ganjei, J.K., Lacana, E., Sunderland, T., Zhao, B., Kusiak, J.W., Wasco, W. and D'Adamio, L. (1996) Participation of presenilin 2 in apoptosis enhanced basal activity conferred by an Alzheimer mutation. *Science* **274**, 1710–1713

85. Guo, Q., Sopher, B.L., Furukawa, K., Pham, D.G., Robinson, N., Martin, G.M. and Mattson, M.P. (1997) Alzheimer's presenilin mutation sensitizes neural cells to apoptosis induced by trophic factor withdrawal and amyloid beta peptide: involvement of calcium and oxyradicals. *J. Neurosci.* **17**, 4212–4222

86. Deng, G., Pike, C.J. and Cotman, C.W. (1996) Alzheimer-associated presenilin-2 confers increased sensitivity to apoptosis in PC12 cells. *FEBS Lett.* **397**, 50–54

87. Elder, G.A., Tezapsidis, N., Carter, J., Shioi, J., Bouras, C., Li, H.C., Johnson, J.M., Efthimiopoulos, S., Friedrich, Jr., V.L. and Robakis, N.K. (1996) Identification and neuron specific expression of the PS-1/presenilin I protein in human and rodent brains. *J. Neurosci. Res.* **45**, 308–320

88.   Giannakopoulos, P., Bouras, C., Kovari, E., Shioi, J., Tezapsidis, N., Hof, P.R. and Robakis, N.K. (1997) Presenilin-1-immunoreactive neurons are preserved in late-onset Alzheimer's disease. *Am. J. Pathol.* **150**, 429–436

89.   Roperch, J.P., Alvaro, V., Prieur, S., Tuynder, M., Nemani, M., Lethrosne, F., Piouffre, L., Gendron, M.C., Israeli, D., Dausset, J., et al. (1998) Inhibition of presenilin 1 expression is promoted by p53 and p21WAF-1 and results in apoptosis and tumor suppression. *Nat. Med. (N.Y.)* **4**, 835–838

90.   Herrup, K. and Busser, J.C. (1995) The induction of multiple cell cycle events precedes target-related neuronal death. *Development* **121**, 2385–2395

91.   Heintz, N. (1993) Cell death and the cell cycle: a relationship between transformation and neurodegeneration? *Trends Biochem. Sci.* **18**, 157–159

92.   Freeman, R., Estus, S. and Johnson, E. (1994) Analysis of cell cycle-related gene expression in postmitotic neurons: selection induction of cyclin D1 during programmed cell death. *Neuron* **12**, 343–355

93.   Reference deleted

94.   Pope, W., Lambert, M., Leypole, B., Seupaul, R., Sletten, L., Krafft, G. and Klein, W. (1994) Microtubule-associated protein tau is hyperphosphorylated during mitosis in the human neuroblastoma cell line SH-SY5Y. *Exp. Neurol.* **126**, 185–194

95.   Liu, W.-K., Williams, R., Hall, F., Dickson, D. and Yen, S.-H. (1995) Detection of a cdc2-related kinase associated with Alzheimer paired helical filaments. *Am. J. Pathol.* **146**, 228–238

96.   Vincent, I., Rosado, M. and Davies, P. (1996) Mitotic mechanisms in Alzheimer's disease? *J. Cell Biol.* **132**, 413–425

97.   Vincent, I., Jicha, G., Rosado, M. and Dickson, D. (1997) Aberrant expression of mitotic cdc2/cyclin B1 kinase in degenerating neurons of Alzheimer's disease brain. *J. Neurosci.* **17**, 3588–3598

98.   Busser, J., Geldmacher, D.S. and Herrup, K. (1998) Ectopic cell cycle proteins predict the sites of neuronal cell death in Alzheimer's disease brain. *J. Neurosci.* **18**, 2801–2807

99.   Chow, N., Cox, C., Callahan, L.M., Weimer, J.M., Guo, L. and Coleman, P.D. (1998) Expression profiles of multiple genes in single neurons of Alzheimer's disease. *Proc. Natl. Acad. Sci. U.S.A.* **95**, 9620–9625

100. Illenberger, S., Zheng-Fischhofer, Q., Preuss, U., Stamer, K., Baumann, K., Trinczek, B., Biernat, J., Godemann, R., Mandelkow, E.-M. and Mandelkow, E. (1998) The endogenous and cell cycle-dependent phosphorylation of tau protein in living cells: Implications for Alzheimer's disease. *Mol. Biol. Cell* **9**, 1495–1512

101. Suzuki, T., Oishi, M., Marshak, D.R., Czernik, J., Nairn, A.C. and Greengard, P. (1994) Cell cycle-dependent regulation of the phosphorylation and metabolism of the Alzheimer amyloid precursor protein. *EMBO J.* **13**, 1114–1122

102. Oishi, M., Nairn, A.C., Czernik, A.J., Lim, G.S., Isohara, T., Gandy, S.E., Greengard, P. and Suzuki, T. (1997) The cytoplasmic domain of Alzheimer's amyloid precursor protein is phosphorylated at thr654, ser655, and thr668 in adult rat brain and cultured cells. *Mol. Med.* **3**, 111–123

Biochem. Soc. Symp. **67**, 51–57
(Printed in Great Britain)

5

Genetic dissection of primary neurodegenerative diseases

John Hardy

Mayo Clinic Jacksonville, 4500 San Pablo Road, Jacksonville, FL 32224, U.S.A.

Abstract

Neurodegenerative diseases have traditionally been defined as clinico-pathological entities. The clinician observes characteristic clusters of symptoms that relate to the anatomical distribution of the lesion. Typically, these symptoms progress in a characteristic sequence allowing the clinician to make a provisional diagnosis. At autopsy, the pathologist examines the nature and distribution of the lesions, reads the clinical report and makes a definitive diagnosis.

This structure is so deeply embedded in our concepts of neurodegenerative disease that we are hardly aware of it. It has become deeply embedded because it has been a useful construct that allows grouping of patients for research, especially in treatment trials. However this success has served to hide its limitations and molecular genetic analysis has clearly shown that there are other ways of thinking about neurodegenerative disease.

In this review, I will summarize the limitations of the clinicopathological approach, and discuss how molecular genetics offers an alternative way of thinking about neurodegeneration. My intention is not to suggest that we should replace the clinicopathological approach (Newtonian physics is a perfectly good way of thinking about the world on a day-to-day basis even though we know it is only an approximation to the truth) but rather, to suggest that future treatments for these most devastating diseases may come from a deeper understanding of their related pathogeneses.

The revealing myth of selective vulnerability

The major underlying factor in clinical diagnosis is that it reflects the loss and damage to a circumscribed set of neurons, leading to the idea of selective vulnerability. However, this selective vulnerability is never as clear-cut as it appears, and with closer study it has become clear that neuron loss is almost always more widespread than was originally suspected for any particular disease. Also, there is an element of circularity to the discussion of selective vulnerability. A stroke is recognized as a stroke irrespective of the brain region it strikes; however, if Lewy body disease occurs in the nigra it leads to 'Parkinson's disease', but if it strikes in cortical regions it leads to 'Lewy body dementia'.

In all probability, the appearance and documentation of selective vulnerability reflects the interplay of several factors. Firstly, there is undoubtedly an element of selectivity to any particular neurodegenerative process; secondly, neuronal domains are plastic, so as neurodegeneration eats away at any particular domain, this domain will continue to compensate until this is no longer possible. At this point a catastrophic loss of function will occur, presenting 'selective' vulnerability, which will overshadow the subtle defects in other clinical domains. As clinical care of the terminally ill has improved, it has become increasingly evident that 'selective' vulnerability is less selective than was thought.

The conundrum of multiple pathologies

The occurrence of multiple pathologies in a single individual is well recognized. For example, plaques, tangles and Lewy bodies frequently co-occur [1]. This co-occurrence has classically led to the question of whether an individual had both Parkinson's disease and Alzheimer's disease (AD). However, it has become clear more recently that this 'mixed pathology' occurs even in those relatively young cases of AD with β-amyloid precursor protein (APP) mutations [2], making the likelihood of independent processes extremely unlikely. A much more parsimonious explanation is that these are dependent processes and that one follows from the other (see below).

The conundrum of multiple aetiologies for a single pathology

An implicit assumption in disease definition was that each disease entity would be the outcome of a single aetiology. We now know that this is not the case and in both AD and Parkinson's disease, there are multiple simple genetic aetiologies [3,4]. Thus a given clinicopathological entity is not necessarily a result of a single aetiology.

The conundrum of multiple outcomes for a single aetiology

Even less well recognized than the occurrence of multiple aetiologies for a single outcome is the occurrence of multiple outcomes for a single aetiology. For example, the pathology in a single family with a prion mutation can vary enormously [5]. More subtly, the diseases can exhibit non-penetrance where some mutation carriers fail to develop the disease. This has been shown to be the case for both the chromosome 2p and chromosome 4p loci for Parkinson's disease [6,7].

Diseases as processes, rather than entities

The resolution of these conundrums comes from the recognition that these diseases are not static clinicopathological entities, but rather that they reflect the occurrence of detrimental biochemical pathways which can be instigated in diverse ways. When initiated, these pathways are subject to genetic and environmental influences. The clearest example of this comes from AD research. Autosomal-dominant AD can be caused by mutations in the *APP*, *presenilin 1* (*PS1*) or *presenilin 2* (*PS2*) genes [8–10]. It now seems clear that mutations in all of these genes lead to the disease through the common mechanism of increased production of the amyloidogenic peptide, Aβ42 (formed of the first 42 amino acids of the β-amyloid peptide) [11]; overproduction of this peptide seems to be one way of initiating the pathogenic cascade. The ε4 allele of *APOE* (the apolipoprotein E gene) is a risk factor locus for AD. The mechanism of action of apolipoprotein E (ApoE) is not clear, but it appears that it is involved in the clearance of β-amyloid (Aβ) [12]. Furthermore, genetic variability at the *APOE* locus clearly influences the age of onset of Alzheimer cases with APP mutations, with the APOE ε4 allele being associated with the earliest onset age [13]. Thus, it seems likely that ApoE's influence is on Aβ, but downstream of its production. This example gives a clear illustration of disease as a pathogenic process in which genetic factors play a role in initiating the process and, subsequent to initiation, in determining the rate of progression to disease state (this example is oversimplified herein since, unexpectedly, the *APOE* genotype does not influence the age of onset of Alzheimer cases with presenilin mutations [14]).

Neurodegenerative disease as overlapping processes

The pathology of various neurodegenerative diseases is shown in Table 1. A surprising observation is that there appear to be some rules which can be tentatively applied to these pathologies. Firstly, when there is an extracellular plaque pathology, pathogenic mutations occur in the genes for proteins which relate directly to that pathology (e.g. *APP*, or *PS1* or *PS2* for AD [3]); secondly, when there is only an intracellular pathology, the genetic lesion is in genes encoding that pathology (tau and α-synuclein [15–17]); and finally, these pathways seem to be alternatives to each other when there is extracellular pathology [1,2,17,18].

Sketching this series of data out (Figure 1) allows a tentative relationship to be drawn between the different diseases and the processes that occur during their pathogenesis. Of course, this diagram reveals how many gaps there are in our knowledge. Many pathogenic loci remain to be found for example, the genes on chromosomes 4p and 2p which lead to Lewy body disease are unknown. Perhaps the greatest gap, however, concerns our complete lack of understanding of how the two types of pathology, extracellular and intracellular, are related.

Despite the sketchiness and lack of detail of the pathways to neurodegeneration illustrated in Figure 1, some predictions follow from them. For

Table 1 The pathology and genetics of neurodegenerative disease

Disease	Extracellular pathology	Intracellular pathology	Genetic loci	Comments and references
AD	Aβ-containing plaques	Tangles consisting of three-and four-repeat tau (always) Lewy bodies consisting of α-synuclein (sometimes)	APP, PS1, PS2 and APOE	All penetrant mutations increase the production of Aβ42 [3]. ApoE seems to be associated with Aβ deposition [12]
Prion disease	Sometimes scrapies prion plaques	Tangles consisting of three-and four-repeat tau (sometimes) Lewy bodies consisting of α-synuclein (sometimes)	Prion	The pathology of prion diseases is highly variable [5,18,19]
Worster Drought syndrome (British dementia)	British Amyloid-containing plaques	Tangles consisting of three-and four-repeat tau Lewy bodies have not been looked for	APP	[20]
Frontotemporal dementia with Parkinsonism linked to chromosome 17	None	Tau pathology (actual form of pathology is dependent on tau mutation)	tau	[15,16]

(contd.) ☞

Table 1 (contd.)

Disease	Extracellular pathology	Intracellular pathology	Genetic loci	Comments and references
Lewy body diseases including Parkinson's disease	None	Lewy bodies	α-synuclein. At least two other loci yet to be found	In this review, I include Parkinson's disease with those dementias in which Lewy bodies are the only pathology [4,6,7,17]
Progressive supranuclear palsy	None	Tangles consisting of four-repeat tau only (slightly different in morphology to AD tangles)	tau haplotype	[21,22]
Multiple system atrophy	None	Synuclein-containing deposits in glia	Not yet known	[24]
Pick's disease	None	Pick bodies consisting of three-repeat tau only (slightly different in morphology to AD tangles)	Not yet known	[23]

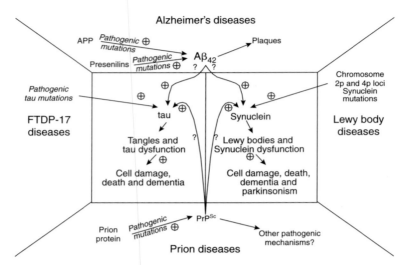

Figure 1 Figure demonstrating the aetiologic relationship between those neurodegenerative diseases in which tangles and Lewy bodies occur. FTDP-17, frontotemporal dementia with Parkinsonism linked to chromosome 17; PrP^{Sc}, scrapies prion.

example, while these pathways could suggest that inhibiting tangle formation may be a useful strategy for treating several disorders, they also suggest that in AD a side effect of this strategy would be to push neurons down a Lewy body pathway to cell death.

References

1. Hansen, L.A., Masliah, E., Galasko, D. and Terry, R.D. (1993) *J. Neuropathol. Exp. Neurol.* **52**, 648–654
2. Lantos, P., Ovenstone, I.M., Johnson, J., Clelland, C.A., Roques, P. and Rossor, M.N. (1994) *Neurosci. Lett.* **172**, 77–79
3. Hardy, J. (1997) *Trends Neurosci.* **20**, 154–159
4. Farrer, M., Gwinn-Hardy, K., Hutton, M. and Hardy, J. (1999) *Hum. Mol. Genet.* **8**, 1901–1905
5. Collinge, J., Owen, F., Poulter, M., Leach, M., Crow, T.J., Rossor, M.N., Hardy, J., Mullan, M.J., Janota, I. and Lantos, P.L. (1990) *Lancet* **336**, 7–9
6. Gasser, T., Muller-Myhsok, B., Wszolek, Z.K., Oehlmann, R., Calne, D.B., Bonifati, V., Bereznai, B., Fabrizio, E., Vieregge, P. and Horstmann, R. (1998) *Nat. Genet.* **18**, 262–265
7. Farrer, M., Gwinn-Hardy, K., Muenter, M., DeVrieze, F.W., Crook, R., Perez-Tur, J., Lincoln, S., Maraganore, D., Adler, C., Newman, S., et al. (1999) *Hum. Mol. Genet.* **8**, 81–85
8. Goate, A., Chartier-Harlin, M.C., Mullan, M., Brown, J., Crawford, F., Fidani, L., Giuffra, L., Haynes, A., Irving, N., James, L., et al. (1991) *Nature (London)* **349**, 704–706
9. Sherrington, R., Rogaev, E.I., Liang, Y., Rogaeva, E.A., Levesque, G., Ikeda, M., Chi, H., Lin, C., Li, G., Holman, K., et al. (1995) *Nature (London)* **375**, 754–760
10. Levey Lahad, E., Wasco, W., Poorkaj, P., Romano, D.M., Oshima, J., Pettingell, W.H., Yu, C.E., Jondro, P.D., Schmidt, S.D., Wang, K., et al. (1995) *Science* **269**, 970–973
11. Scheuner, D., Eckman, C., Jensen, M., Song, X., Citron, M., Suzuki, N., Bird, T.D., Hardy, J., Hutton, M., Kukull, W., et al. (1996) *Nat. Med. (N.Y.)* **2**, 864–870

12. Bales, K.R., Verina, T., Dodel, R.C., Du, Y., Altstiel, L., Bender, M., Hyslop, P., Johnstone, E.M., Little, S.P., Cummins, D.J., et al. (1997) *Nat. Genet.* **17**, 263–264

13. Houlden, H., Crook, R., Hardy, J., Roques, P., Collinge, J. and Rossor, M. (1994) *Neurosci. Lett.* **174**, 222–224

14. Van Broeckhoven, C., Backhovens, H., Cruts, M., Martin, J.J., Crook, R., Houlden, H. and Hardy, J. (1994) *Neurosci. Lett.* **169**, 179–180

15. Poorkaj, P., Bird, T.D., Wijsman, E., Nemens, E., Garruto, R.M., Anderson, L., Andreadis, A., Wiederholt, W.C., Raskind, M. and Schellenberg, G.D. (1998) *Ann. Neurol.* **43**, 815–825

16. Hutton, M., Lendon, C.L., Rizzu, P., Baker, M., Froelich, S., Houlden, H., Pickering-Brown, S., Chakraverty, S., Isaacs, A., Grover, A., et al. (1998) *Nature (London)* **393**, 702–705

17. Polymeropoulos, M.H., Lavedan, C., Leroy, E., Ide, S.E., Dehejia, A., Dutra, A., Pike, B., Root, H., Rubenstein, J., Boyer, R., et al. (1997) *Science* **276**, 2045–2047

18. Dlouhy, S.R., Hsiao, K., Farlow, M.R., Foroud, T., Conneally, P.M., Johnson, P., Prusiner, S.B., Hodes, M.E. and Ghetti, B. (1992) *Nat. Genet.* **1**, 64–67

19. Piccardo, P. and Ghetti, B. http://www.webcom.com/hag/alzh98/book/p724.htm

20. Vidal, R., Frangione, B., Rostagno, A., Mead, S., Revesz, T., Plant, G. and Ghiso, J. (1999) *Nature (London)* **399**, 776–781

21. Baker, M., Litvan, I., Houlden, H., Adamson, J., Dickson, D., Perez-Tur, J., Hardy, J., Lynch, T., Bigio, E. and Hutton, M. (1999) *Hum. Mol. Genet.* **8**, 711–715

22. Conrad, C., Andreadis, A., Trojanowski, J.Q., Dickson, D.W., Kang, D., Chen, X., Wiederholt, W., Hansen, L., Masliah, E., Thal, L.J., et al. (1997) *Ann. Neurol.* **41**, 277–281

23. Dickson, D.W. (1998) *Brain Pathol.* **8**, 339–354

24. Dickson, D.W., Liu, W., Hardy, J., Farrer, M., Mehta, N., Uitti, R., Mark, M., Zimmerman, T., Golbe, L., Sage, J., et al. (1999) *Am. J. Pathol.* **155**, 1241–1251

Biochem. Soc. Symp. **67**, 59–71
(Printed in Great Britain)

6

Tau gene mutations and neurodegeneration

Michel Goedert*[1] and Maria Grazia Spillantini†

*Medical Research Council Laboratory of Molecular Biology, Hills Road,
Cambridge CB2 2QH, U.K., and †Brain Repair Centre and Department of
Neurology, University of Cambridge, Robinson Way, Cambridge CB2 2PY, U.K.

Abstract

Abundant neurofibrillary lesions made of the microtubule-associated protein tau constitute a defining neuropathological characteristic of Alzheimer's disease. Filamentous tau protein deposits are also the defining neuropathological characteristic of other neurodegenerative diseases, many of which are frontotemporal dementias or movement disorders, such as Pick's disease, progressive supranuclear palsy and corticobasal degeneration. It is well established that the distribution of tau pathology correlates with the presence of symptoms of disease. However, until recently, there was no genetic evidence linking dysfunction of tau protein to neurodegeneration and dementia. This has now changed with the discovery of close to 20 mutations in the *tau* gene in frontotemporal dementia with Parkinsonism linked to chromosome 17. All cases with *tau* mutations examined to date have shown an abundant filamentous tau pathology in brain cells. Pathological heterogeneity is determined to a large extent by the location of mutations in *tau*. Known mutations are either coding region or intronic mutations located close to the splice-donor site of the intron downstream of exon 10. Most coding region mutations produce a reduced ability of tau to interact with microtubules. Several of these mutations also promote sulphated glycosaminoglycan-induced assembly of tau into filaments. Intronic mutations and some coding region mutations produce increased splicing in of exon 10, resulting in an overexpression of four-repeat tau isoforms. Thus a normal ratio of three-repeat to four-repeat tau isoforms is essential for preventing the development of tau pathology. The new work has shown that dysfunction of tau protein can cause neurodegeneration and dementia.

---

[1]To whom correspondence should be addressed.

Introduction

Arnold Pick provided the first clinical description of frontotemporal dementia in 1892 [1]. In 1911, Alois Alzheimer described the neuropathological lesions characteristic of Pick's disease [2]. In the 1960s, these so-called 'Pick bodies' were shown to contain abnormal filaments [3], which are now known to be made of the hyperphosphorylated, microtubule-associated protein tau [4,5]. The Pick bodies resemble the neurofibrillary lesions described by Alzheimer in 1907 in the disease subsequently named after him [6,7]. Filamentous inclusions made of tau protein are also a defining characteristic of other neurodegenerative diseases, such as progressive supranuclear palsy and corticobasal degeneration.

Frontotemporal dementias occur in familial forms and, more commonly, as sporadic diseases. Neuropathologically, they are characterized by a remarkably circumscribed atrophy of the frontal and temporal lobes of the cerebral cortex, often with additional, subcortical changes. In 1994, an autosomal-dominantly inherited familial form of frontotemporal dementia with Parkinsonism was linked to chromosome 17q21.2 [8]. This was followed by the identification of other familial forms of frontotemporal dementia that are linked to this region, resulting in this class of disease being given the denomination frontotemporal dementia with Parkinsonism linked to chromosome 17 (FTDP-17) [9]. A filamentous inclusion made of hyperphosphorylated tau protein is a major neuropathological characteristic of FTDP-17 [10]. Tau is a microtubule-associated protein that binds to microtubules and promotes microtubule assembly [7]. Tau filaments are space-occupying lesions that may interfere with a host of cellular processes, leading to the degeneration of affected nerve cells and glial cells. Importantly, the *tau* gene maps to the FTDP-17 locus on chromosome 17. Genetic linkage and neuropathology thus made *tau* a strong candidate gene for FTDP-17. The discovery of coding-region and intronic mutations in *tau* has shown that the FTDP-17 locus is indeed the *tau* gene [11–13].

Tau gene mutations

In the adult human brain, six tau isoforms are produced from a single gene by alternative mRNA splicing (Figure 1a, A–F) [14–18]. They differ from each other by the presence or absence of 29- or 58-amino-acid inserts located in the N-terminal half, and of a 31-amino-acid repeat located in the C-terminal half. Inclusion of the latter, which is encoded by exon 10 of the *tau* gene, gives rise to three tau isoforms (Figure 1a, D–F) with four repeats each. The other three isoforms (Figure 1a, A–C) have three repeats each. In normal cerebral cortex, similar levels of three-repeat and four-repeat tau isoforms are present. The repeats and some adjoining sequences constitute the microtubule-binding domains of tau [19,20].

Tau mutations in FTDP-17 are either missense, deletion or silent mutations in the coding region, or intronic mutations located close to the splice-donor site of the intron downstream of the alternatively spliced exon 10 (Figure 1) [11–13,21–40]. Missense mutations are located in the microtubule-binding

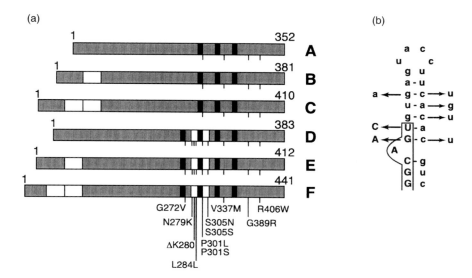

Figure 1 Mutations in the *tau* gene in frontotemporal dementia with Parkinsonism linked to chromosome 17 (FTDP-17). (a) Schematic diagram of the six tau isoforms (A–F) that are expressed in adult human brain. Alternatively spliced exons 2, 3 and 10 are shown in white. Black bars indicate the microtubule-binding repeats. Eight missense mutations, one deletion mutation and two silent mutations in the coding region are shown. Amino-acid numbering corresponds to the 441-amino-acid isoform of tau in the human brain. (b) Stem–loop structure in the pre-mRNA at the boundary between exon 10 and the intron downstream of exon 10. Seven mutations that reduce the stability of the stem–loop structure are shown. Exon sequences are shown in capital letters and intron sequences in lower-case letters.

repeat region or close to it. Mutations in exon 9 [Gly^{272}→Val (G272V)], exon 12 (V337M) and exon 13 (G389R and R406W) affect all six tau isoforms (Figure 1a). By contrast, mutations in exon 10 (N279K, ΔK280, L284L, P301L, P301S, S305N and S305S) only affect tau isoforms with four microtubule-binding repeats or their levels of expression (Figure 1a). Most missense mutations reduce the ability of the tau protein to interact with microtubules, as reflected by a reduction in the ability of mutant tau to promote microtubule assembly [23,30,38,41–44]. Mutations in exon 10 (ΔK280, P301L and P301S) produce the largest effects, with intermediate reductions for mutations in exon 9 (G272V) and exon 12 (V337M), and a smaller reduction for the G389R and R406W mutations in exon 13. Moreover, a number of missense mutations have a direct stimulatory effect on heparin-induced assembly of tau into filaments [45,46]. This effect is particularly marked for the P301L and P301S mutations, with smaller effects for the G272V and V337M mutations.

Intronic mutations are located in the intron downstream of exon 10 at positions +3, +12, +13, +14 and +16, with the first nucleotide of the splice-donor site taken as +1 (Figure 1b) [12,13,25,26,34,39]. Secondary-structure predictions have suggested the presence of an RNA stem–loop structure at the exon 10–intron boundary that is disrupted by the intronic mutations [12,13]. In addition, the +3 mutation is predicted to lead to increased binding of U1 snRNA to the 5' splice site [13]. Exon-trapping experiments have shown that intronic mutations increase splicing-in of exon 10 [12,26,29,32,39,47–49]. Increased production of transcripts encoding exon 10 has also been demonstrated in brain tissue from patients with intronic mutations of tau [12,39]. This increase is, in turn, reflected in a change in the ratio of three-repeat to four-repeat tau isoforms, resulting in a net overproduction of four-repeat isoforms [13,26,34,39,42].

The proposed existence of a stem–loop structure at the boundary between exon 10 and the downstream intron has received support from the determination by NMR spectroscopy of the three-dimensional structure of a 25-nucleotide-long strand of RNA (extending from positions −5 to +19) (Figure 1b) [47,50]. This sequence has been shown to form a stable, folded structure. The stem of the exon 10-splicing regulatory element of *tau* consists of a single G–C base-pair which is separated from a double helix of six base-pairs by an unpaired adenine. The apical loop consists of six nucleotides that adopt multiple conformations in rapid exchange. The structure differs in several respects from the two proposed representations of the stem–loop structure [12,13]. Known intronic mutations are located in the upper part of the stem of the exon 10-splicing regulatory element of *tau* (Figure 1b). All five mutations reduce the thermodynamic stability of the stem–loop structure, but do so to various extents [39,47]. The largest drop in melting temperature was observed for the +3 mutation. The +12 and +14 mutations also produced a large reduction in melting temperature, whereas the effects of the +13 and +16 mutations were smaller. The aminoglycoside antibiotic, neomycin, binds to the exon 10-splicing regulatory element of *tau* and markedly increases the thermodynamic stability of both wild-type and mutated elements [50]. The differential reductions in stem–loop stability resulting from the various intronic FTDP-17 mutations were reflected in the magnitude of increased splicing-in of exon 10, as revealed by exon trapping [12,29,39,47–49].

The emerging picture is one of missense mutations which lead to a reduced ability of tau to interact with microtubules and to a stimulatory effect on filament assembly, and of intronic mutations whose primary effects are at the RNA level, resulting in the overproduction of tau isoforms with four microtubule-binding repeats. However, two missense mutations in exon 10 (N279K and S305N) deviate from this rule: they do not lead to a reduction in the ability of tau to promote microtubule assembly [51]. Instead, they increase splicing-in of exon 10, as is the case with the intronic mutations. Mutation N279K (AAT to AAG) creates a purine-rich splice-enhancer sequence, which explains its effects on exon trapping and soluble four-repeat tau in the brain [22]. Similar findings have been obtained with the silent mutation L284L (CTT to CTC) in exon 10, which is believed to disrupt an exon 10-splicing silencer sequence [29]. This work has uncovered the presence of sequence elements within exon 10 that regulate its alternative splicing.

The S305N (AGT to AAT) mutation changes the last amino acid in exon 10 [24]. This sequence forms part of the stem–loop structure, where the mutation produces a G to A transition at position −1 (Figure 1b). It is, therefore, not surprising that the S305N mutation leads to a reduction in the thermodynamic stability of the stem–loop structure and to a marked increase in the splicing-in of exon 10 [47,51]. Like the +3 mutation, the −1 mutation is also expected to lead to increased binding of U1 snRNA to the 5′ splice site. The silent mutation S305S (AGT to AGC) produces a T to C transition at position 0 that disrupts the stem–loop structure, without a predicted effect on U1 snRNA binding (Figure 1b) [40]. As expected, it produced increased splicing-in of exon 10 by exon trapping. Besides mutations in the intron downstream of exon 10, additional pathogenic mutations may exist in other introns of the *tau* gene. A G to A transition at position +33 of the intron downstream of exon 9 has been described in a patient with familial frontotemporal dementia [23]. It disrupts one of several (A/T)GGG repeats that may play a role in the regulation of the alternative splicing of exon 10.

Neuropathology

All cases with *tau* gene mutations that have been examined to date have shown the presence of an abundance of filamentous lesions made of hyperphosphorylated tau protein. Strikingly, the morphologies of tau filaments and their isoform compositions appear to be determined by whether *tau* mutations affect mRNA splicing of exon 10, or whether they are missense mutations located inside or outside exon 10 [52].

Mutations that affect splicing-in of exon 10 lead to the formation of wide, twisted, ribbon-like filaments that only contain four-repeat tau isoforms. This has been shown in familial multiple system tauopathy with presenile dementia (MSTD) with the +3 intronic mutation [13,53], in FTD-Kumamoto with the +12 intronic mutation [39], as well as in familial progressive subcortical gliosis and Duke family 1684, both with the +16 intronic mutation [26,34]. Similar results have been obtained in pallido-ponto-nigral degeneration with the N279K mutation in exon 10 whose primary effect is at the RNA level [22,32,35]. The same may be true of families with the L284L, S305N and S305S mutations in exon 10 whose primary effects are also at the RNA level. In all these families, the tau pathology is widespread and present in both nerve cells and glial cells, with an abundant glial component.

Mutations in exon 10 that do not affect alternative mRNA splicing lead to the formation of narrow, twisted ribbons that contain four-repeat tau isoforms, with a small amount of the most abundant three-repeat isoform. This has been shown in Dutch family 1 and in an American family, both with the P301L mutation [27,54]. Based on electron microscopy of tissue sections, the same also appears to be true of the Italian family with the P301S mutation [30]. At present, no neuropathological information is available for patients with the ΔK280 mutation in exon 10. The P301L, P301S and ΔK280 mutations all lead to a markedly reduced ability of four-repeat tau to promote microtubule assembly [41]. Exon-trapping experiments have shown that the P301L and P301S mutations have no effect on the splicing-in of exon 10. In contrast, the ΔK280 mutation leads to reduced splicing-in of exon 10, suggesting that its primary effect might be the overproduction of three-repeat tau, and not the reduced ability of four-repeat tau to interact with microtubules [29]. Clarification of this issue must await the availability of frozen brain tissue from an individual with the ΔK280 mutation. In brain tissue from individuals with the P301L and P301S mutations, tau pathology is widespread and present in both nerve cells and glial cells; however, when compared with mutations that affect the splicing-in of exon 10, the glial component appears to be less pronounced.

Coding-region mutations located outside exon 10 lead to a tau pathology that is neuronal, without a significant glial component. Some of these mutations lead to the formation of paired helical and straight filaments that contain all six tau isoforms, like the tau filaments of Alzheimer's disease [55]. This has been shown for Seattle family A with the V337M mutation in exon 12 and for a family with the R406W mutation in exon 13 [36,56]. In both cases, the morphologies of tau filaments have been found to be indistinguishable from those of Alzheimer's disease. By contrast, the G389R mutation in exon 13 produces tau filament morphologies and a pattern of tau bands that resemble the characteristics of Pick's disease [38,57,58]. Based on light-microscopic staining, the G272V mutation in exon 9 leads to the formation of numerous Pick-body-like inclusions [54]. These findings indicate that, depending on the positions of missense mutations in exons 9, 12 and 13 of *tau*, and perhaps the nature of these mutations, a filamentous tau pathology ensues that resembles that of either Alzheimer's disease or Pick's disease.

Pathogenesis

The pathway leading from a mutation in the *tau* gene to neurodegeneration is unknown. The probable primary effect of most missense mutations is a reduced ability of mutant tau to interact with microtubules (Table 1). It may be equivalent to a partial loss of function, with resultant microtubule destabilization and deleterious effects on cellular processes, such as rapid axonal transport. However, in the case of the intronic mutations and the N279K, L284L, S305N and S305S mutations in exon 10, this appears unlikely. The net effect of these mutations is increased splicing-in of exon 10, leading to a change in the ratio of three- to four-repeat tau isoforms, and resulting in an overproduction of four-repeat tau. It is well known that four-repeat tau possesses a greater ability to interact with microtubules than three-repeat tau [17]. It is, therefore, possible that, in cases of FTDP-17 with intronic mutations and coding-region

Table 1 Proposed sequence of events leading from exonic and intronic mutations in the *tau* gene to neurodegeneration.

1. Reduced ability of tau protein to interact with microtubules.
2. Hyperphosphorylation of tau protein. Interaction with other factors (such as sulphated glycosaminoglycans)?
3. Ordered filamentous assemblies (gain of toxic function).
4. Degeneration of tau-filament-containing nerve cells and glial cells.

mutations that act at the RNA level, microtubules are more stable than in brain from control individuals. Moreover, missense mutations in exon 10 will only affect 20–25% of tau molecules, with 75–80% of tau being normal.

It is possible, however, that a correct ratio of wild-type three-repeat to four-repeat tau is essential for the normal function of tau in the human brain. An alternative hypothesis is that a partial loss of function of tau is necessary for setting in motion the mechanisms that will ultimately lead to filament assembly. Earlier work has suggested that three- and four-repeat tau isoforms may bind to different sites on microtubules [20]. Overproduction of tau isoforms with four repeats may result in an excess of tau over available binding sites on microtubules, thus creating a gain of toxic function similar to that of most missense mutations, with unbound excess tau available for assembly into filaments (Table 1).

Where studied, pathological tau from FTDP-17 brain is hyperphosphorylated [7,10]. Since known mutations in *tau* do not create additional phosphorylation sites (with the possible exception of the P301S mutation in exon 10), hyperphosphorylation of tau must be an event downstream of the primary effects of the mutation and may be a consequence of the partial loss of function (Table 1). However, some missense mutations may indirectly affect the phosphorylation state of tau. Thus, in transfected cells, tau protein with the R406W mutation displays only a little phosphorylation at T231, S396 and S404, in contrast with wild-type tau and tau with the P301L or V337M mutation [43,59]. Hyperphosphorylation of tau probably reinforces the primary effects of the mutations, since it is well established that hyperphosphorylated tau is unable to bind to microtubules and to promote microtubule assembly [60,61]. At present, there is no experimental evidence linking hyperphosphorylation of tau to filament assembly, and it is unclear whether hyperphosphorylation is either necessary or sufficient for assembly.

Sulphated glycosaminoglycans and RNA induce the bulk assembly of non-phosphorylated, recombinant tau protein into Alzheimer-like filaments *in vitro* [62–66]. This work has produced robust methods for the assembly of full-length tau into filaments. However, the mechanisms that lead to the assembly of tau into filaments in the brain remain to be discovered. It is possible that a reduced ability of tau to interact with microtubules, which could have several different causes, is a necessary step for filament formation (Table 1). Assembly is an energetically unfavourable, nucleation-dependent process that requires a critical concentration of tau [62,66]. Many cells may have levels of tau below the critical concentration. Other cells may have effective mechanisms for preventing the formation of tau nuclei, or may be able to degrade them once they have formed.

Insufficient protective mechanisms and high tau concentrations may underlie the selective degeneration of nerve cells and glial cells, which is especially striking in FTDP-17, with the characteristic, sometimes unilateral, razor-sharp demarcations between affected and unaffected areas in cerebral cortex. Similar factors may also underpin the late ages of onset of this and other diseases with filamentous tau protein deposits. Protective factors, such as proteases that degrade nucleation products, may be effective throughout much of life. However, as nerve cells age, these mechanisms may become less effective and the balance may shift in favour of filament formation.

The significance of the different filament morphologies observed in FTDP-17 is not clear. It is known that the repeat region of tau forms the densely packed core of paired helical and straight filaments of Alzheimer's disease, with the N- and C-terminal parts of the molecule forming a protease-sensitive coat [55,67]. Also, for filaments assembled *in vitro* in the presence of sulphated glycosaminoglycans, the morphology of the filaments depends on the number of repeats in the tau isoform used [62]. Thus, mutations in the repeat region or a change in the relative amounts of three- and four-repeat isoforms could well influence filament morphology. However, treatment of paired helical filaments, which contain all six tau isoforms, with acid leads to untwisted, ribbon-like filaments like those seen in cases of FTDP-17 with mutations in the intron downstream of exon 10, suggesting a close similarity in packing of tau molecules in the various structures [68]. The most important aspect may be the extended filamentous nature of the assemblies and the deleterious effects that this has on intracellular processes, rather than the detailed morphology of the different filaments.

Implications

The discovery of mutations in the *tau* gene has established that dysfunction of tau protein causes neurodegeneration. Most unexpectedly, it has shown that similar levels of three- and four-repeat tau isoforms are essential for preventing neurodegeneration and dementia.

The finding that overproduction of four-repeat tau leads to its assembly into twisted ribbons and causes disease may shed light on the pathogenesis of progressive supranuclear palsy (PSP) and corticobasal degeneration (CBD), two largely sporadic, neurodegenerative diseases. Neuropathologically they are characterized by an abundant filamentous pathology that is comprised predominantly of four-repeat tau isoforms [69–71]. A recent study has reported an increase in exon 10-containing transcripts in the brainstem in PSP [72]. It remains to be seen whether this is reflected in increased levels of soluble four-repeat tau isoforms. An association between PSP and homozygosity of a common allele at a dinucleotide repeat in the intron downstream of exon 9 of the *tau* gene has been described [73]. More recently, two common tau haplotypes that differ at the nucleotide level, but not at the level of the protein-coding sequence, have been reported [74]. Homozygosity of the more common allele H1 appears to predispose individuals to PSP. Taken together, this work suggests that PSP may be caused by an imbalance between three- and four-repeat tau isoforms, analogous to the FTDP-17 cases with mutations in the intron downstream of *tau* exon 10. It remains to be seen whether the same is true of CBD. It is noteworthy that a patient with the S305S mutation in *tau* presented with the symptoms of PSP [40], whereas a patient with the P301S mutation in *tau* showed the clinical signs of CBD [30].

The discovery that some mutations in *tau* exons 9 and 13 give rise to a clinical picture and a neuropathology similar to those of Pick's disease, indi-

References

1. Pick, A. (1892) *Prager Med. Wochenschr.* **16**, 765–767
2. Alzheimer, A. (1911) *Z. Gesamte Neurol. Psychiatr.* **4**, 356–385
3. Rewcastle, N.B. and Ball, M.J. (1968) *Neurology* **18**, 1205–1213
4. Pollock, N.J., Mirra, S.S., Binder, L.I., Hansen, L.A. and Wood, J.G. (1986) *Lancet* **ii**, 1211
5. Probst, A., Tolnay, M., Langui, D., Goedert, M. and Spillantini, M.G. (1996) *Acta Neuropathol.* **92**, 588–596
6. Alzheimer, A. (1907) *Allg. Z. Psychiatr. Psych. Gerichtl. Med.* **64**, 146–148
7. Spillantini, M.G. and Goedert, M. (1998) *Trends Neurosci.* **21**, 428–433
8. Wilhelmsen, K.C., Lynch, T., Pavlou, E., Higgins, M. and Nygaard, T.G. (1994) *Am. J. Hum. Genet.* **55**, 1159–1165
9. Foster, N.L., Wilhelmsen, K.C., Sima, A.A.F., Jones, M.Z., D'Amato, C., Gilman, S., Spillantini, M.G., Lynch, T., Mayeux, R.P., Gaskell, P.C., et al. (1997) *Ann. Neurol.* **41**, 706–715
10. Spillantini, M.G., Bird, T.D. and Ghetti, B. (1998) *Brain Pathol.* **8**, 387–402
11. Poorkaj, P., Bird, T.D., Wijsman, E., Nemens, E., Garruto, R.M., Anderson, L., Andreadis, A., Wiederholt, W.C., Raskind, M. and Schellenberg, G.D. (1998) *Ann. Neurol.* **43**, 815–825
12. Hutton, M., Lendon, C.L., Rizzu, P., Baker, M., Froelich, S., Houlden, H., Pickering-Brown, S., Chakraverty, S., Isaacs, A., Grover, A., et al. (1998) *Nature (London)* **393**, 702–705
13. Spillantini, M.G., Murrell, J.R., Goedert, M., Farlow, M.R., Klug, A. and Ghetti, B. (1998) *Proc. Natl. Acad. Sci. U.S.A.* **95**, 7737–7741
14. Goedert, M., Wischik, C.M., Crowther, R.A., Walker, J.E. and Klug, A. (1988) *Proc. Natl. Acad. Sci. U.S.A.* **85**, 4051–4055
15. Goedert, M., Spillantini, M.G., Potier, M.C., Ulrich, J. and Crowther, R.A. (1989) *EMBO J.* **8**, 393–399
16. Goedert, M., Spillantini, M.G., Jakes, R., Rutherford, D. and Crowther, R.A. (1989) *Neuron* **3**, 519–526
17. Goedert, M. and Jakes, R. (1990) *EMBO J.* **9**, 4225–4230
18. Andreadis, A., Brown, M.W. and Kosik, K.S. (1992) *Biochemistry* **31**, 10626–10633
19. Gustke, N., Trinczek, B., Biernat, J., Mandelkow, E.M. and Mandelkow, E. (1994) *Biochemistry* **33**, 9511–9522
20. Goode, B.L. and Feinstein, S.C. (1994) *J. Cell Biol.* **124**, 769–782
21. Dumanchin, C., Camuzat, A., Campion, D., Verpillat, P., Hannequin, D., Dubois, B., Saugier-Veber, P., Martin, C., Penet, C., Charbonnier, F., et al. (1998) *Hum. Mol. Genet.* **7**, 1825–1829
22. Clark, L.N., Poorkaj, P., Wszolek, Z., Geschwind, D.H., Nasreddine, Z.S., Miller, B., Li. D., Payami, H., Awert, F., Markopoulou, K., et al. (1998) *Proc. Natl. Acad. Sci. U.S.A.* **95**, 13103–13107
23. Rizzu, P., Van Swieten, J.C., Joosse, M., Hasegawa, M., Stevens, M., Tibben, A., Niermeijer, M.F., Hillebrand, M., Ravid, R., Oostra, B.A., et al. (1999) *Am. J. Hum. Genet.* **64**, 414–421
24. Iijima, M., Tabira, T., Poorkaj, P., Schellenberg, G.D., Trojanowski, J.Q., Lee, V.M.-Y., Schmidt, M.L., Takahashi, K., Nabika, T., Matsumoto, T., et al. (1999) *NeuroReport* **10**, 497–501
25. Morris, H.R., Perez-Tur, J., Janssen, J.C., Brown, J., Lees, A.J., Wood, N.W., Hardy, J., Hutton, M. and Rossor, M.N. (1999) *Ann. Neurol.* **45**, 270–271
26. Goedert, M., Spillantini, M.G., Crowther, R.A., Chen, S.G., Parchi, P., Tabaton, M., Lanska, D.J., Markesbery, W.R., Wilhelmsen, K.C., Dickson, D.W., et al. (1999) *Nat. Med. (N.Y.)* **5**, 454–457
27. Mirra, S.S., Murrell, J.R., Gearing, M., Spillantini, M.G., Goedert, M., Crowther, R.A., Levey, A.I., Jones, R., Green, J., Shoffner, J.M., et al. (1999) *J. Neuropathol. Exp. Neurol.* **58**, 333–345

28. Bird, T.D., Nochlin, D., Poorkaj, P., Cherrier, M., Kaye, J., Payami, H., Peskind, E., Lampe, T.H., Nemens, E., Boyer, P.J. and Schellenberg, G.D. (1999) *Brain* **122**, 741–756

29. D'Souza, I., Poorkaj, P., Hong, M., Nochlin, D., Lee, V.M.-Y., Bird, T. and Schellenberg, G.D. (1999) *Proc. Natl. Acad. Sci. U.S.A.* **96**, 5598–5603

30. Bugiani, O., Murrell, J.R., Giaccone, G., Hasegawa, M., Ghigo, G., Tabaton, M., Morbin, M., Primavera, A., Carella, F., Solaro, C., et al. (1999) *J. Neuropathol. Exp. Neurol.* **58**, 667–677

31. Nasreddine, Z.S., Loginov, M., Clark, L.N., Lamarche, J., Miller, B.L., Lamontagne, A., Zhukareva, V., Lee, V.M.-Y., Wilhelmsen, K.C. and Geschwind, D.H. (1999) *Ann. Neurol.* **45**, 704–715

32. Delisle, M.B., Murrell, J.R., Richardson, R., Trofatter, J.A., Rascol, O., Soulages, X., Mohr, M., Calvas, P. and Ghetti, B. (1999) *Acta Neuropathol.* **98**, 62–77

33. Houlden, H., Baker, M., Adamson, J., Grover, A., Waring, S., Dickson, D., Lynch, T., Boeve, B., Petersen, R.C., Pickering-Brown, S., et al. (1999) *Ann. Neurol.* **46**, 243–248

34. Hulette, C.M., Pericak-Vance, M.A., Roses, A.D., Schmechel, D.E., Yamaoka, L.H., Gaskell, P.C., Welsh-Bohmer, K.A., Crowther, R.A. and Spillantini, M.G. (1999) *J. Neuropathol. Exp. Neurol.* **58**, 859–866

35. Yasuda, M., Kawamata, T., Komure, O., Kuno, S., D'Souza, I., Poorkaj, P., Kawai, J., Tanimukai, S., Yamamoto, Y., Hasegawa, H., et al. (1999) *Neurology* **53**, 864–868

36. Van Swieten, J.C., Stevens, M., Rosso, S.M., Rizzu, P., Joosse, M., de Koning, I., Kamphorst, W., Ravid, R., Spillantini, M.G., Niermeijer, M.F. and Heutink, P. (1999) *Ann. Neurol.* **46**, 617–626

37. Sperfeld, A.D., Collatz, M.B., Baier, H., Palmbach, M., Storch, A., Schwarz, J., Tatsch, K., Reske, S., Joosse, M., Heutink, P. and Ludolph, A.C. (1999) *Ann. Neurol.* **46**, 708–715

38. Murrell, J.R., Spillantini, M.G., Zolo, P., Guazzelli, M., Smith, M.J., Hasegawa, M., Redi, F., Crowther, R.A., Pietrini, P., Ghetti, B. and Goedert, M. (1999) *J. Neuropathol. Exp. Neurol.* **58**, 1207–1226

39. Yasuda, M., Takamatsu, J., D'Souza, I., Crowther, R.A., Kawamata, T., Hasegawa, M., Hasegawa, H., Spillantini, M.G., Tanimukai, S., Poorkaj, P., et al. (2000) *Ann. Neurol.* **47**, 422–429

40. Stanford, P.M., Halliday, G.M., Brooks, W.S., Kwok, J.B.J., Storey, C.E., Creasey, H., Morris, J.G.L., Fulham, M.J. and Schofield, P.R. (2000) *Brain*, **123**, 880–893

41. Hasegawa, M., Smith, M.J. and Goedert, M. (1998) *FEBS Lett.* **437**, 207–210

42. Hong, M., Zhukareva, V., Vogelsberg-Ragaglia, V., Wszolek, Z., Reed, L., Miller, B.L., Geschwind, D.H., Bird, T.D., McKeel, D., Goate, A., et al. (1998) *Science* **282**, 1914–1917

43. Dayanandan, R., Van Slegtenhorst, M., Mack, T.G.A., Ko, L., Yen, S.-H., Leroy, K., Brion, J.P., Anderton, B.H., Hutton, M. and Lovestone, S. (1999) *FEBS Lett.* **446**, 228–232

44. DeTure, M., Ko, L.-W., Yen, S., Nacharaju, P., Easson, C., Lewis, J., Van Slegtenhorst, M., Hutton, M. and Yen, S.-H. (2000) *Brain Res.* **853**, 5–14

45. Nacharaju, P., Lewis, J., Easson, C., Yen, S., Hackett, J., Hutton, M. and Yen, S.-H. (1999) *FEBS Lett.* **447**, 195–199

46. Goedert, M., Jakes, R. and Crowther, R.A. (1999) *FEBS Lett.* **450**, 306–311

47. Varani, L., Hasegawa, M., Spillantini, M.G., Smith, M.J., Murrell, J.R., Ghetti, B., Klug, A., Goedert, M. and Varani, G. (1999) *Proc. Natl. Acad. Sci. U.S.A.* **96**, 8229–8234

48. Grover, A., Houlden, H., Baker, M., Adamson, J., Lewis, J., Prihar, G., Pickering-Brown, S., Duff, K. and Hutton, M. (1999) *J. Biol. Chem.* **274**, 15134–15143

49. Gao, Q.-S., Memmott, J., Lafyatis, R., Stamm, S., Screaton, G. and Andreadis, A. (2000) *J. Neurochem.* **74**, 490–500

50. Varani, L., Spillantini, M.G., Goedert, M. and Varani, G. (2000) *Nucl. Acid Res.* **28**, 710–719

51. Hasegawa, M., Smith, M.J., Iijima, M., Tabira, T. and Goedert, M. (1999) *FEBS Lett.* **443**, 93–96

52. Goedert, M., Crowther, R.A. and Spillantini, M.G. (1998) *Neuron* **21**, 955–958

53. Spillantini, M.G., Goedert, M., Crowther, R.A., Murrell, J.R., Farlow, M.J. and Ghetti, B. (1997) *Proc. Natl. Acad. Sci. U.S.A.* **94**, 4113–4118

54. Spillantini, M.G., Crowther, R.A., Kamphorst, W., Heutink, P. and Van Swieten, J.C. (1998) *Am. J. Pathol.* **153**, 1359–1363

55. Goedert, M., Spillantini, M.G., Cairns, N.J. and Crowther, R.A. (1992) *Neuron* **8**, 159–168

56. Spillantini, M.G., Crowther, R.A. and Goedert, M. (1996) *Acta Neuropathol.* **92**, 42–48

57. Kato, S. and Nakamura, H. (1990) *Acta Neuropathol.* **81**, 125–129

58. Murayama, S., Mori, H., Ihara, Y. and Tomonaga, M. (1990) *Ann. Neurol.* **27**, 394–404

59. Matsumura, N., Yamazaki, T. and Ihara, Y. (1999) *Am. J. Pathol.* **154**, 1649–1659

60. Bramblett, G.T., Goedert, M., Jakes, R., Merrick, S.E., Trojanowski, J.Q. and Lee, V.M.-Y. (1993) *Neuron* **19**, 1089–1099

61. Yoshida, H. and Ihara, Y. (1993) *J. Neurochem.* **61**, 1183–1186

62. Goedert, M., Jakes, R., Spillantini, M.G., Hasegawa, M., Smith, M.J. and Crowther, R.A. (1996) *Nature (London)* **383**, 550–553

63. Pérez, M., Valpuesta, J.M., Medina, M., Montejo de Garcini, E. and Avila, J. (1996) *J. Neurochem.* **67**, 1183–1190

64. Kampers, T., Friedhoff, P., Biernat, J., Mandelkow, E.M. and Mandelkow, E. (1996) *FEBS Lett.* **399**, 344–349

65. Hasegawa, M., Crowther, R.A., Jakes, R. and Goedert, M. (1997) *J. Biol. Chem.* **272**, 33118–33124

66. Friedhoff, P., von Bergen, M., Mandelkow, E.M., Davies, P. and Mandelkow, E. (1998) *Proc. Natl. Acad. Sci. U.S.A.* **95**, 15712–15717

67. Wischik, C.M., Novak, M., Thogersen, H.C., Edwards, P.C., Runswick, M.J., Jakes, R., Walker, J.E., Milstein, C., Roth, M. and Klug, A. (1988) *Proc. Natl. Acad. Sci. U.S.A.* **85**, 4506–4510

68. Crowther, R.A. (1991) *Biochim. Biophys. Acta* **1069**, 1–9

69. Flament, S., Delacourte, A., Vernay, M., Hauw, J.J. and Javoy-Agid, F. (1991) *Acta Neuropathol.* **81**, 591–596

70. Ksiezak-Reding, H., Morgan, K., Mattiace, L.A., Davies, P., Liu, W.-K., Yen, S.-H., Weidenheim, K. and Dickson, D.W. (1994) *Am. J. Pathol.* **145**, 1496–1508

71. Sergeant, N., Wattez, A. and Delacourte, A. (1999) *J. Neurochem.* **72**, 1243–1249

72. Chambers, C.B., Lee, J.M., Troncoso, J.C., Reich, S. and Muma, N.A. (1999) *Ann. Neurol.* **46**, 325–332

73. Conrad, C., Andreadis, A., Trojanowski, J.Q., Dickson, D.W., Kang, D., Chen, X., Wiederholt, W., Hansen, L., Masliah, E., Thal, L.J., et al. (1997) *Ann. Neurol.* **41**, 277–281

74. Baker, M., Litvan, I., Houlden, H., Adamson, J., Dickson, D., Perez-Tur, J., Hardy, J., Lynch, T., Bigio, E. and Hutton, M. (1999) *Hum. Mol. Genet.* **8**, 711–715

75. Delacourte, A., Robitaille, Y., Sergeant, N., Buée, L., Hof, P.R., Wattez, A., Laroche-Cholette, A., Mathieu, J., Chagnon, P. and Gauvreau, D. (1996) *J. Neuropathol. Exp. Neurol.* **55**, 159–168

76. Delacourte, A., Sergeant, N., Wattez, A., Gauvreau, D. and Robitaille, Y. (1998) *Ann. Neurol.* **43**, 193–204

77. Cohen, P. and Goedert, M. (1999) *Chem. Biol.* **5**, R161–R164

78. Thomas, G.M., Frame, S., Goedert, M., Nathke, I., Polakis, P. and Cohen, P. (1999) *FEBS Lett.* **458**, 247–251

79. Lu, P.-J., Wulf, G., Zhou, X.Z., Davies, P. and Lu, K.P. (1999) *Nature (London)* **399**, 784–788

80. Tseng, H.-C., Lu, Q., Henderson, E. and Graves, D.J. (1999) *Proc. Natl. Acad. Sci. U.S.A.* **96**, 9503–9508

81. Götz, J., Probst, A., Spillantini, M.G., Schäfer, T., Jakes, R., Bürki, K. and Goedert, M. (1995) *EMBO J.* **14**, 1304–1313

82. Brion, J.P., Tremp, G. and Octave, J.N. (1999) *Am. J. Pathol.* **154**, 255–270

83. Ishihara, T., Hong, M., Zhang, B., Nakagawa, Y., Lee, M.K., Trojanowski, J.Q. and Lee, V.M.-Y. (1999) *Neuron* **24**, 751–762
84. Spittaels, K., Van den Haute, C., Van Dorpe, J., Bruynseels, K., Vandezande, K., Laenen, I., Geerts, H., Mercken, M., Sciot, R., Van Lommel, A., et al. (1999) *Am. J. Pathol.* **155**, 2153–2165
85. Probst, A., Götz, J., Wiederhold, K.-H., Tolnay, M., Mistl, C., Jaton, A.L., Hong, M., Ishihara, T., Lee, V.M.-Y., Trojanowski, J.Q., et al. (2000) *Acta Neuropathol.* **99**, 469–481

Biochem. Soc. Symp. **67**, 73–80
(Printed in Great Britain)

7

Sites of phosphorylation in tau and factors affecting their regulation

Brian H. Anderton*[1], Joanna Betts†, Walter P. Blackstock†,

Jean-Pierre Brion‡, Sara Chapman*, James Connell*,

Rejith Dayanandan*, Jean-Marc Gallo*, Graham Gibb*,

Diane P. Hanger*, Mike Hutton§, Efterpi Kardalinou*,

Karell Leroy‡, Simon Lovestone*, Till Mack*,

C. Hugh Reynolds* and M. Van Slegtenhorst§

*Department of Neuroscience, Institute of Psychiatry, King's College London, De Crespigny Park, London SE5 8AF, U.K., †Biomolecular Structure Unit, Glaxo-Wellcome Research and Development, Gunnels Wood Road, Stevenage SG1 2NY, U.K., ‡Laboratory of Pathology and Electron Microscopy, Université Libre de Bruxelles, 808 Route de Lennik, Bldg C-10, 1070 Brussels, Belgium, and §The Birdsall Research Building, Mayo Clinic, 4500 San Pablo Road, Jacksonville, FL 32224, U.S.A.

Abstract

The microtubule-associated protein, tau, is the principal component of paired helical filaments (PHFs) in Alzheimer's disease. PHF-tau is highly phosphorylated and a total of 25 sites of phosphorylation have so far been identified. Many of these sites are serine or threonine residues that are immediately followed in the sequence by proline residues, and hence are candidate phosphorylation sites for proline-directed kinases. *In vitro*, glycogen synthase kinase-3 (GSK-3), extracellular signal-related kinase-1 and -2, and mitogen-activated protein kinases, p38 kinase and c-jun N-terminal kinase, all phosphorylate many of these sites, although with different efficiencies for particular sites. Phosphorylation studies in transfected cells and neurons show that GSK-3 phosphorylates tau more extensively than do these other proline-directed kinases. Mutations in *tau* have been shown to affect *in vitro* phosphorylation of

[1]To whom correspondence should be addressed.

73

tau by GSK-3. The Arg^{406}→Trp (R406W) *tau* mutation also affects tau phosphorylation in cells.

Identification of phosphorylation sites in paired helical filament (PHF)-tau

Perikaryal aggregates of PHFs form the classical neurofibrillary tangles of Alzheimer's disease. PHFs are also present in dystrophic senile plaque neurites and in neuropil threads. Isolation of PHF as dispersed structures and subsequent analysis with SDS-PAGE results in patterns of four bands of immunoreactive tau (three major and one minor, slower-migrating, band), usually referred to as PHF-tau, as well as a considerable amount of aggregated tau that is present as an immunoreactive smear at the top of the gel [1–3]. Identification of phosphorylation sites in tau has concentrated mainly on the discrete quadruplet of bands and, until recently, only 20 phosphorylation sites had been identified using mass spectrometry and Edman degradation [4]. However, to date, full sequence coverage of PHF-tau has not been achieved and hence there may be additional, unidentified, phosphorylated residues.

We have developed a modified method for isolating PHF-tau which partially separates the quadruplet of PHF-tau bands; the final product is approximately 50–70% pure. So far, we have subjected the total PHF-tau material to mass-spectrometric analysis. The PHF-tau (in polyacrylamide gel slices) was digested *in situ* with trypsin or endoproteinase Asp-N and the eluted phosphopeptides were enriched using iron-chelate chromatography. Phosphopeptides were sequenced by nanoelectrospray tandem MS/MS. Besides confirming the majority of previously reported phosphorylation sites, we identified five additional sites, bringing the total number of known sites to 25. These sites are listed in Table 1 (right-hand column).

In vitro phosphorylation of tau

Many residues that are phosphorylated in tau are serines or threonines immediately followed in the sequence by a proline [5]. This makes the sites candidates for proline-directed kinases. We have compared, *in vitro*, phosphorylation of recombinant 2N4R tau by glycogen synthase kinase (GSK)-3β, c-jun *N*-terminal kinase (JNK)-3, p38 mitogen-activated protein (MAP) kinase and extracellular signal-related kinase (ERK)-2.

All kinases phosphorylate tau *in vitro* to generate epitopes for several monoclonal antibodies that recognize PHF-tau by virtue of its phosphorylated state. These epitopes have been mapped with mutagenesis studies and, of several well-characterized sites in tau, we found that the AT8 epitope (Ser^{202} and Thr^{205}) was generated readily by JNK-3, p38 MAP kinase and ERK-2 but only feebly by GSK-3β [6,7].

We also used mass spectrometry to analyse the tau phosphorylated *in vitro* by these kinases and found that they phosphorylated the majority of the sites present in PHF-tau *in vitro* (Table 1).

Table 1 Phosphorylation sites identified on PHF-tau isolated from Alzheimer's disease brain and on tau phosphorylated *in vitro* by ERK-2, JNK-2, p38 MAP kinase and GSK-3β.

Sites were identified by chemical sequencing and/or by mass spectrometry [2,4,8] except where otherwise indicated. Heparin was required to give detectable phosphorylation on some of the GSK-3β sites, and on Ser[356] with ERK-2 (all *in vitro* data with all four protein kinases are from our own work [6–8]). Sites followed by prolines are shown in bold.

Site	ERK-2	JNK-3	p38 MAP kinase	GSK-3β	PHF-tau
Ser[46]	+		+		(+)[a]
Thr[175]	+	+	+	+	+
Thr[181]	+	+	+	+	+
Ser[184]					(+)[b]
Ser[185]			+		(+)[b]
Ser[195]				+	
Ser[198]					+
Ser[199]				+	+
Ser[202]	+	+	+		+
Thr[205]	+	+	+	+	(+)[a]
Ser[208]					+
Ser[210]					+
Thr[212]	+	+	+	+	+
Ser[214]					+
Thr[217]	+	+	+	+	+
Thr[231]	+	+	+	+	+
Ser[235]	+	+	+	+	+
Ser[237]					+
Ser[238]					+
Thr[245]			+		
Ser[262]				+	+
Ser[305]			+		
Ser[356]	+	+	+	+	+
Ser[396]	+	+	+	+	+
Ser[400]				+	+
Thr[403]					+
Ser[404]	+		+	+	+
Ser[409]					+
Ser[412]					+
Ser[413]				+	+
Ser[422]	(+)[a]	(+)[a]	(+)[a]		+

[a]Identified by phosphorylation-dependent antibodies.
[b] Ser184 or Ser185 is phosphorylated in PHF-tau.

In vitro phosphorylation of mutant tau

The discovery of mutations in the *tau* gene in cases of frontotemporal dementia with Parkinsonism linked to chromosome 17 (FTDP-17) has demonstrated the primary pathogenic potential for abnormalities in tau leading to neurodegeneration [10,11]. Although several studies have demonstrated differences both in microtubule-binding properties and in the ability to promote microtubule assembly of some mutant forms of tau, it is not yet established how mutations in tau exert their pathogenic effects. We have investigated whether the phosphorylation of several mutants is different from wild-type tau.

Wild-type 2N4R tau and P301L, V337M and R406W mutants on this isoform background were phosphorylated *in vitro* with GSK-3β using [γ-^{32}P]ATP.

Comparison of the two-dimensional phosphopeptide maps of wild-type tau with those of the mutants revealed that the R406W, but not the P301L or V337M, mutations affected the phosphorylation of tau even though residue 406 is not a phosphorylation site (Figure 1). Two phosphopeptide spots were absent in the R406W peptide map: one phosphopeptide contains residue 406, which in wild-type tau is a trypsin cleavage site; the other spot represents phosphorylated Thr^{231} and Ser^{235} residues which are remote from the site of mutation. Thus this mutation appears to have a marked effect on tau structure, presumably via a conformational change that affects phosphorylation at distant sites.

Phosphorylation of tau in transfected cells and neurons

Since several proline-directed kinases are capable of phosphorylating tau *in vitro* at many sites shown to be pathophysiologically relevant, it is important to identify which, if any, of these kinases phosphorylates tau *in vivo*. We therefore undertook a study of tau phosphorylation in transfected cells and in neurons.

HEK-293 cells were stably transfected with GSK-3β in the Tet-on system, such that expression of GSK-3β occurred when the cells were exposed to doxycycline. On induction the level of GSK-3β protein increased and, in the most responsive clones, was increased by ten-fold. GSK-3β activity was assayed and also found to increase by six-fold (results not shown). When tau cDNA was transfected into these cells and GSK-3β induced, the phosphorylation of tau was modestly increased, as indicated by a small reduction in the mobility of the transfected tau (Figure 2a), demonstrating that GSK-3β phosphorylates tau in a cellular environment.

In a further series of experiments, COS-7 cells were transiently transfected with tau and co-transfected with GSK-3β, ERK-2, JNK-3 or p38 MAP kinase. Transient transfection results in a greater elevation of kinase protein and, hence, activity compared with the stably transfected cells described earlier. Transfected cells were additionally treated to activate maximally the appropriate transfected kinase [i.e. epidermal growth factor (EGF) for ERK-2, anisomycin for JNK-3 or sorbitol for p38 MAP kinase]. Cells were also triple-transfected to investigate whether there was synergism between these kinases. The phosphory-

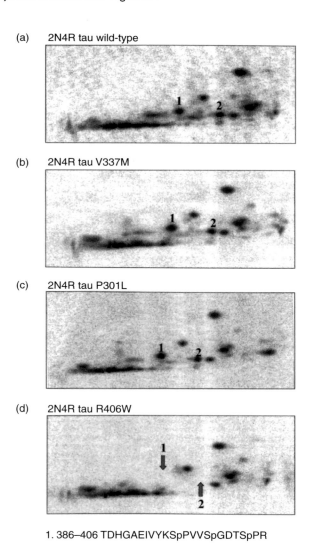

(a) 2N4R tau wild-type

(b) 2N4R tau V337M

(c) 2N4R tau P301L

(d) 2N4R tau R406W

1. 386–406 TDHGAEIVYKSpPVVSpGDTSpPR

2. 231–240 TpPPKSpPSSAK

Figure 1 Phosphopeptide maps of GSK-3β-phosphorylated recombinant tau showing the differences in phosphorylation patterns between wild-type and three mutant forms of tau. Purified recombinant wild-type and the three mutant forms of tau indicated (longest human isoforms) were phosphorylated *in vitro* with GSK-3β using [γ-^{32}P]ATP. The tau protein was separated by SDS-PAGE and transferred to nitrocellulose membrane on which the protein was digested with trypsin. The eluted peptides were separated by two-dimensional thin-layer electrophoresis and chromatography and exposed in a phosphorimager to reveal the positions of the phosphopeptides. Two phosphopeptides in the R406W mutant tau were absent and these were sequenced by mass spectrometry and are given below the two-dimensional map of this mutant.

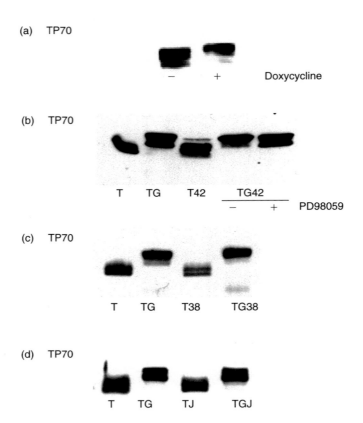

(a)   TP70

                                              −   +   Doxycycline

(b)   TP70

                        T   TG   T42   TG42
                                           −   +   PD98059

(c)   TP70

                        T   TG   T38   TG38

(d)   TP70

                        T   TG   TJ   TGJ

Figure 2 GSK-3β, ERK-2, p38 MAP kinase and JNK-3 phosphoryla-tion of tau after co-expression in HEK-293 or COS-7 cells. Western blots are shown using the polyclonal tau antibody TP70, which recognizes phosphorylated and non-phosphorylated tau. The slower-migrating tau bands represent increasingly phosphorylated tau forms. (A) HEK-293 cells stably expressing GSK-3β under the Tet-on inducible promoter system and tran-siently transfected with tau; induction of GSK-3β expression by doxycycline leads to a modest decrease in tau mobility, indicating an increase in phosphory-lation. (B) The effects on mobility of tau transfected alone (T), in combination with GSK-3β (TG) or ERK-2 (T42), or triple transient transfections (TG42) in COS-7 cells; PD98059 inhibits activation of ERK-2. (C) The effects of p38 MAP kinase, alone (T38) or in combination with GSK-3β (TG38), on tau mobility. (D) The effects of JNK-3 alone (TJ) or in combination with GSK-3β (TGJ), on tau mobility.

lation state of tau was assessed by its reduced mobility in SDS-PAGE and reac-tivity with certain phosphorylation-dependent tau monoclonal antibodies.

We confirmed that GSK-3β markedly phosphorylated tau in co-trans-fected cells (Figures 2b–2d) [12]. ERK-2 also phosphorylated tau but to a lesser extent than GSK-3β, whereas p38 MAP kinase weakly phosphorylated tau and JNK-3 apparently failed to phosphorylate tau. In triple-transfection experiments, ERK-2 and p38 MAP kinase synergized with GSK-3 but JNK-3 had no such effect (Figures 2b–2d). The inhibitor of ERK-2 activation, PD98059, also inhibited the synergistic effect of ERK-2 with GSK-3β.

In primary cultures of rat brain cortical neurons, tau is endogenously heavily phosphorylated; this phosphorylation can be reduced by lithium treatment to inhibit GSK-3 [13]. Therefore, we treated such cultures with lithium and EGF to activate MAP kinases maximally. There was a modest increase in phosphorylation in response to EGF compared with the control lithium-treated cells (results not shown).

We conclude that GSK-3β is the strongest candidate as a physiological tau kinase; however, ERK-1/ERK-2 are also probably physiological kinases. JNK-3 appears not to be a tau kinase and it remains unclear whether p38 MAP kinase phosphorylates tau *in vivo*.

Phosphorylation of mutant tau in cells

Since phosphorylation of tau by GSK-3β *in vitro* is affected by the R406W mutation, we investigated whether mutations in tau might affect its ability to be phosphorylated in cells [14]. CHO cells were transfected with wild-type and mutant 0N4R tau isoforms, either alone or co-transfected with GSK-3β. Western blots of heat-stable proteins were probed with antibodies to determine the phosphorylation state of the tau.

Wild-type tau and V337M, and P301L mutants were all indistinguishable in terms of their SDS-PAGE mobility and their reactivity with TP70, Tau.1, AT8 and PHF-1 antibodies. However, in cells transfected with R406W mutant tau, the tau migrated almost exclusively as a single band, rather than a triplet, due to partial phosphorylation by endogenous kinases. Co-transfection of R406W tau with GSK-3β resulted in increased phosphorylation similar to wild-type tau. Thus, certainly with physiologically normal levels of protein kinases, the R406W mutation affects the phosphorylation state of tau [14].

Work in our laboratory is supported by MRC, The Wellcome Trust, The Alzheimer's Disease Society, Action Research and Research into Ageing.

References

1. Greenberg, S.G. and Davies, P. (1990) *Proc. Natl. Acad. Sci. U.S.A.* **87**, 5827–5831
2. Hanger, D.P., Betts, J.C., Loviny, T.L., Blackstock, W.P. and Anderton, B.H. (1998) *J. Neurochem.* **71**, 2465–2476
3. Watanabe, A., Takio, K. and Ihara, Y. (1999) *J. Biol. Chem.* **274**, 7368–7378
4. Morishima-Kawashima, M., Hasegawa, M., Takio, K., Suzuki, M., Yoshida, H., Titani, K., and Ihara, Y. (1995) *J. Biol. Chem.* **270**, 823–829
5. Lovestone, S. and Reynolds, C.H. (1997) *Neuroscience* **78**, 309–324
6. Reynolds, C.H., Utton, M.A., Gibb, G.M., Yates, A. and Anderton, B.H. (1997) *J. Neurochem.* **68**, 1736–1744
7. Reynolds, C.H., Nebreda, A.R., Gibb, G.M., Utton, M.A. and Anderton, B.H. (1997) *J. Neurochem.* **69**, 191–198

8.   Reynolds, C.H., Betts, J.C., Blackstock, W.P., Nebveda, A.R. and Anderton, B.H. (2000)
      J. Neurochem. **74**, 1587–1595
9.   Spillantini, M.G. and Goedert, M. (1998) *Trends Neurosci.* **21**, 428–433
10.   Hong, M., Zhukareva, V., Vogelsberg-Ragaglia, V., Wszolek, Z., Reed, L., Miller, B.I.,
      Geschwind, D.H., Bird, T.D., McKeel, D., Goate, A., et al. (1998) *Science* **282**, 1914–1917
11.   Frappier, T., Liang, N.S., Brown, K., Leung, C.L., Lynch, T., Liem, R.H.K. and Shelanski,
      M.L. (1999) *FEBS Lett.* **455**, 262–266
12.   Lovestone, S., Reynolds, C.H., Latimer, D., Davis, D.R., Anderton, B.H., Gallo, J.-M.,
      Hanger, D., Mulot, S., Marquardt, B., Stabel, S., et al. (1994) *Curr. Biol.* **4**, 1077–1086
13.   Lovestone, S., Davis, D.R., Webster, M.T., Kaech, S., Brion, J.P., Matus, A. and Anderton,
      B.H. (1999) *Biol. Psychiatry* **45**, 995–1003
14.   Dayanandan, R., Van Slegtenhorst, M., Mack, T.G., Ko, L., Yen, S.H., Leroy, K., Brion,
      J.P., Anderton, B.H., Hutton, M. and Lovestone, S. (1999) *FEBS Lett.* **446**, 228–232

Biochem. Soc. Symp. **67**, 81–88
(Printed in Great Britain)

8

Neurofibrillary tangles and tau phosphorylation

Jean-Pierre Brion[*1]**, Brian H. Anderton**[†]**, Michéle Authelet**[*]**,
Rejith Dayanandan**[†]**, Karelle Leroy**[*]**, Simon Lovestone**[†]**,
Jean-Noël Octave**[‡]**, Laurent Pradier**[§]**, Nicole Touchet**[§] **and
Günter Tremp**[§]

[*]Laboratory of Histology, Neuroanatomy and Neuropathology, Université Libre de
Bruxelles, 808 Route de Lennik, 1070 Brussels, Belgium, [†]Department of
Neuroscience, Institute of Psychiatry, King's College London, De Crespigny Park,
London SE5 8AF, U.K., [‡]Laboratory of Pharmacology, Université Catholique de
Louvain, Brussels, Belgium, and [§]Rhône-Poulenc-Rorer, Centre de Recherches de
Vitry-Alfortville, Vitry, France

Abstract

Neurofibrillary tangles (NFTs) are a characteristic neuropathological
lesion of Alzheimer's disease (AD). They are composed of a highly-phospho-
rylated form of the microtubule-associated protein tau. We are investigating
the relationship betweeen NFTs and microtubule stability and how tau phosphorylation and function is affected in transgenic models and by co-expression
with β-amyloid precursor protein and presenilins. In most NFT-bearing
neurons, we observed a strong reduction in acetylated α-tubulin immunoreactivity (a marker of stable microtubules) and a reduction of the *in situ* hybridization signal for tubulin mRNA. In transfected cells, mutated tau forms
(corresponding to tau mutations identified in familial forms of frontotemporal
dementias linked to chromosome 17) were less efficient in their ability to sustain microtubule growth. These observations are consistent with the hypothesis that destabilization of the microtubule network is an important mechanism
of cell dysfunction in Alzheimer's disease. The glycogen synthase kinase-3β
(GSK-3β) generates many phosphorylated sites on tau. We performed a
neuroanatomical study of GSK-3β distribution showing that developmental
evolution of GSK-3β compartmentalization in neurons paralleled that of phosphorylated tau. Studies on transfected cells and on cultured neurons showed
that GSK-3β activity controls tau phosophorylation and tau functional interac-

[1]To whom correspondence should be addressed.

cates their relevance for an understanding of the aetiology and pathogenesis of Pick's disease. These mutations affect all six tau isoforms, and in cases with the G389R mutation in exon 13, the tau filaments contain three- and four-repeat isoforms [38]. This is in apparent contrast to sporadic Pick's disease, which is characterized by the assembly of three-repeat, but not four-repeat, tau into filaments [75,76].

All cases of FTDP-17 examined to date are characterized by an abundant filamentous tau pathology. The V337M and R406W mutations lead to a tau pathology that is identical to that of Alzheimer's disease in its biochemical and morphological characteristics [36,56]. It follows that in Alzheimer's disease nerve cells may also degenerate as a direct result of the development of tau filaments. Unlike in Alzheimer's disease, abundant neuritic plaques are not a general characteristic of FTDP-17; however, isolated cases of FTDP-17 with abundant amyloid deposits have been described [29,36]. Although one cannot exclude associated Alzheimer's disease pathology in these patients, future work may uncover mechanisms by which the development of tau pathology can lead to deposition of β-amyloid.

Prevention or reduction of tau pathology is likely to be beneficial therapeutically. Current evidence suggests that binding of tau to microtubules and self-assembly of tau into filaments are mutually exclusive. Therefore, increasing the ability of abnormally hyperphosphorylated tau to interact with microtubules may be of benefit. This could, in principle, be achieved by using specific protein kinase inhibitors, proteins that bind to protein kinases and inactivate them or a *cis–trans* prolyl isomerase, such as Pin1 [77–79]. The latter has been shown to bind to hyperphosphorylated tau protein *in vitro* and restore its ability to interact with microtubules [79]. Naturally occurring osmolytes, such as trimethylamine *N*-oxide, have also been shown to restore the ability of phosphorylated tau to interact with microtubules [80]. Assembly of tau into filaments is a nucleation-dependent process that is strongly concentration dependent. Therefore, a reduction in the cellular levels of tau protein must be a therapeutic target. This is especially true of *tau* mutations whose primary effect is at the RNA level. Small organic compounds that specifically stabilize the stem–loop structure at the boundary between *tau* exon 10 and the intron downstream of exon 10 may be able to restore the disturbed ratio between three- and four-repeat tau isoforms [50]. Compounds that prevent the assembly of tau protein into filaments can be identified using existing methods for filament formation *in vitro*. Validation of their usefulness will require the development of experimental animal models of tau filament formation. Although current transgenic mouse models have exhibited some signs of neurodegeneration as a result of the overexpression of human tau protein, they have so far failed to show abundant tau filaments [81–85]. The hope is that expression of mutant human tau isoforms in transgenic mice will result in the formation of tau filaments in nerve cells and glial cells. This is not only important for the study of FTDP-17, but also constitutes a necessary prerequisite for a true animal model of Alzheimer's disease.

tion with microtubules. Tau phosphorylation was not affected in neurons over-expressing β-amyloid precursor protein. Transgenic mice expressing a human tau isoform and double transgenic animals for tau and mutated presenilin 1 have been generated; a somatodendritic accumulation of phosphorylated trans-genic tau proteins, as observed in the pretangle stage in AD, has been observed but NFTs were not found, suggesting that additional factors might be necessary to induce their formation.

Introduction

The characteristic neuropathological lesions of Alzheimer's disease (AD) — senile plaques and neurofibrillary tangles (NFTs) — are present both in sporadic cases and in familial forms of the disease, indicating that they constitute a 'final common pathway' responsible for the clinical expression of the disease. Particularly, the formation of NFTs is thought to be linked closely to neuronal dysfunction and dementia in AD. In addition, mutations of the *tau* gene, whose product is the molecular component of NFTs, have recently been identified in familial forms of frontotemporal dementia with Parkinsonism linked to chromosome 17 (FTDP-17). Some of these cases and other neurodegenerative diseases exhibit neuronal and/or glial tau-positive inclusions and have been regrouped under the term 'tauopathies' [1]. The study of the molecular composition and the mechanisms of formation of NFTs, and their effects on neuronal function, is thus believed to be essential for our understanding of the pathogenesis of AD and the other tauopathies.

NFTs are composed of bundles of abnormal filaments accumulating in neuronal perikarya, dendrites and axons. Ultrastructurally, these filaments show regular constrictions or appear straight and have been described as two filaments twisted around each other in a helical fashion, hence their name 'paired helical filaments' (PHFs). In AD, PHFs have been demonstrated to be composed of the microtubule-associated protein tau [2–4]; self-assembly of tau proteins into PHF-like filaments has been performed *in vitro* [5]. The tau proteins that PHFs are composed of are generally referred to as PHF-tau proteins and differ from normal tau by several post-translational modifications, the best documented being a high state of phosphorylation [2–4].

Since tau plays an important role in the stabilization of the microtubule network, we have investigated the relationship between NFT microtubule stability and tubulin expression in AD. Many of the phosphorylated sites identified in PHF-tau can be generated by the protein kinase glycogen synthase kinase-3β (GSK-3β). We have investigated the distribution of GSK-3β in AD and in normal rat brain, and we have studied how GSK-3β can modulate tau function in cellular models. We have also started to investigate how the phosphorylation, and some aspects of the function, of tau can be affected by overexpression in transgenic models and by co-expression with β-amyloid precursor protein (APP) and presenilins.

Microtubules in AD

Tau proteins play an important role in the nucleation and stabilization of microtubules by their ability to bind to tubulin through semi-homologous repeats localized in the half-carboxyl domain of tau. Transfection or micro-injection of tau into cells induces its binding to microtubules and the formation of thick bundles of microtubules, which it stabilizes against depolymerizing agents.

Highly phosphorylated tau proteins are less efficient at promoting microtubule polymerization and stabilization, and differential effects of phosphorylation on selected sites have been identified. The high state of phosphorylation of PHF-tau is believed to play a critical role in AD, by affecting the stability of the microtubule network in affected neurons. This in turn would lead to disturbances in the cellular functions performed by microtubules, such as axoplasmic transport [6]. In ultrastructural studies, it was reported that NFT-bearing neurons are devoid of normal microtubules [7,8] and show accumulation of membranous organelles, consistent with disturbances in axoplasmic flow [9–11]. PHF-tau is highly inefficient at promoting microtubule assembly [12] and can bind to normal tau, possibly sequestering the latter in a non-functional form [13].

To explore further the hypothesis that microtubule stability is decreased in AD, we studied the relative content of stable microtubules in neurons containing NFT, using double-immunolabelling with antibodies to tau and to acetylated α-tubulin (as a marker of stable microtubules) [14]. We observed a strong reduction in the immunoreactivity of acetylated α-tubulin in most NFT-bearing neurons, including the neuronal population with a lower tau-immunoreactivity, suggesting that reduction in acetylated α-tubulin immunoreactivity, and hence reduction in microtubule stability, could be an early event in these cells. In familial forms of FTDP-17 that are due to tau mutations, destabilization of microtubules might be favoured further by the reduced ability of mutated tau forms to sustain microtubule growth [15]. The distribution of α-tubulin mRNA in the human hippocampus of normal subjects and those with AD was also investigated by *in situ* hybridization [16]. A significant reduction in the hybridization signal was observed in areas rich in NFTs; neurons containing NFTs exhibited a weaker hybridization signal than adjacent neurons devoid of NFTs. This result suggests that tubulin transcription is reduced in NFT-bearing neurons, a reduction which might play a role in the decreased amount of microtubules in these cells.

GSK-3β: a link between tau, presenilins and APP metabolism?

Many protein kinases can phosphorylate tau *in vitro*. GSK-3β, however, is a strong candidate for a physiological kinase for tau. GSK-3β phosphorylates tau *in vitro* [17,18] and in transfected cells [19–21], and tau proteins phosphorylated by GSK-3β acquire the electrophoretic mobilities of PHF-tau proteins [22]. GSK-3β is able to modulate the activity of tau *in vitro*, rendering it less efficient in nucleating microtubule assembly [23], and thereby reducing the stability of the microtubule network in transfected cells [24]. We observed that GSK-3β is expressed in human neurons, including those containing NFT [17]. We have performed a neuroanatomical study of the distribution of GSK-3β in both the adult and the developing rat brain [25]. GSK-3β was widely expressed in neurons in most brain areas but not in glial cells. The highest expression was observed in late-embryonic and early-postnatal life. The developmental evolution of GSK-3β compartmentalization in neurons paralleled that of phosphorylated tau [26].

The mechanism by which GSK-3β can affect tau function was studied in CHO cells that had been double-transfected with tau and GSK-3β and treated with cytochalasin B. Transfection with tau induces the formation of bundles of microtubules in these cells. The weakening of the actin network by cytochalasin, as shown in other cell types [27], led to the formation of straight cell extensions containing microtubule bundles in tau-transfected CHO cells. Measurements of the length of these extensions and of the proportion of extension-bearing cells was used as a functional assay for the ability of tau to drive microtubule assembly. After double-transfection with tau and GSK-3β, the proportion of cells with extensions was strongly reduced, although their mean length was not significantly affected. This suggests that GSK-3β affects the initial nucleation step of microtubule assembly and bundling rather than the growth of microtubule bundles. This effect of GSK-3β was reversed in a dose-dependent manner by lithium, an inhibitor of GSK-3β activity [28]. We have observed that inhibition of GSK-3β activity by lithium induces a tau dephosphorylation in transfected non-neuronal cells and in cultured neurons [29].

An additional potential role for GSK-3β in the pathophysiological mechanisms of AD has been suggested by its connections with presenilins and the wingless/wnt pathway. GSK-3β is negatively regulated by the wingless/wnt pathway, a signal transduction cascade involved in developmental patterning. Inactivation of GSK-3β induces stabilization of β-catenin, which mediates wingless/wnt signalling by regulating gene expression. Presenilin 1, which is known to affect Aβ peptide formation, forms a complex with GSK-3β and β-catenin [30] that is associated with stabilization of β-catenin. Mutant presenilin 1 induces degradation of β-catenin in transgenic mice and also potentiates neuronal apoptosis. Furthermore, a reduction in β-catenin levels is observed in the brains of individuals with AD with presenilin mutations, and these mutations have been shown to cause defective trafficking of β-catenin [31]. Presenilin 1 was also observed to form a complex with GSK-3β and tau [32] and mutant presenilin 1 induced a phosphorylation of tau. If these effects are mediated by increased activity of GSK-3β, it follows that the metabolisms of tau, presenilin 1 and APP may be linked.

A molecular interaction between tau and APP has also been reported in several studies [33]. In a previous study we characterized a monoclonal antibody to tau that was generated using recombinant APP, and suggested that this might be an anti-idiotypic antibody generated against a motif involved in a binding domain between tau and APP [34]. To assess further the potential effect of APP on tau function, we studied the impact on process formation in CHO cells double-transfected with tau and wild-type APP_{695}. However, the

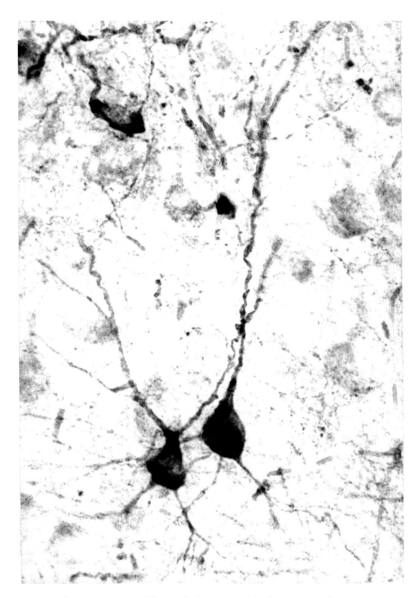

Figure 1 Immunolabelling of the entorhinal cortex of a tau transgenic mouse with the AT180 anti-tau antibody (a phosphorylation-dependent monoclonal antibody). A few neurons show a strong immunoreactivity to phosphorylated tau in their cell bodies and dendrites. Magnification × 700.

length of extensions in double-transfected cells was found not to be affected. Preliminary results using a recombinant adenovirus for the expression of human APP [35] in cultured rat neurons indicate that overexpression of APP in these neurons does not massively affect tau phosphorylation. The phosphorylation state of tau in these embryonic neurons is, however, already high [36], and might mask minor changes induced by expression of human APP.

Tau transgenic mice

PHF-like filaments can be generated *in vitro* using truncated [5] or full-length tau molecules in the presence of glycosaminoglycans or RNA [37,38]. In an attempt to develop a cellular model for PHF formation, we have generated transgenic mice expressing the shortest human tau isoform [39]. Transgenic tau proteins were expressed in neurons in the developing and adult brain of these mice and, using electron microscopy, the transgenic tau was detected in microtubules in axons and dendrites but not in cell bodies. NFTs were not detected in transgenic animals examined up to the age of 24 months. In contrast to the endogenous tau that progressively disappeared from neuronal cell bodies during development, the human transgenic tau remained abundant in the cell bodies and dendrites of a subset of neurons in the adult. This somatodendritic transgenic tau was immunoreactive with some antibodies to phosphorylated tau (Figure 1). It is not known whether phosphorylation of tau itself is needed for PHF formation, although phosphorylation of tau *in vitro* promotes the formation of tau dimers and is suggested to be a key step in the assembly of PHFs [40]. In addition, the accumulation of phosphorylated tau in neurons at the pretangle stage, before the formation of NFTs, is an early event [41,42]. A similar somatodendritic localization of transgenic tau proteins has been reported in another transgenic line expressing the longest tau isoform [43]. In animals transgenic for both tau and presenilin 1 [44], we observed a similar somatodendritic accumulation of the transgenic tau, but with no NFT formation up to the age of 13 months.

Conclusions

In summary, early accumulation of phosphorylated tau proteins in neuronal cell bodies observed at the pretangle stage in AD might be a consequence of changes in transduction pathways involving GSK-3β as a key step. Resulting changes in the phosphorylation state of tau would then lead to disturbances in the microtubule network. Transgenic manipulation of tau expression appears to be sufficient to affect tau compartmentalization and phosphorylation, partly as it has been observed at the pretangle stage in AD, but additional factors might be necessary to induce PHF formation.

This study was supported by grants from the Belgian FRSM (no. 3.4509.99), the International Alzheimer Research Foundation, the European Neuroscience Foundation and the Wellcome Trust. K. Leroy is a recipient of the Belgian FRIA.

References

1.   Spillantini, M.G. and Goedert, M. (1998) *Trends Neurosci.* **21**, 428–433
2.   Goedert, M. (1993) *Trends Neurosci.* **16**, 460–465

3. Delacourte, A. and Buée, L. (1997) *Int. Rev. Cytol.* **171**, 167–224
4. Brion, J.P. (1998) *Eur. Neurol.* **40**, 130–140
5. Wille, H., Drewes, G., Biernat, J., Mandelkow, E.-M. and Mandelkow, E. (1992) *J. Cell Biol.* **118**, 573–584
6. Terry, R.D. (1996) *J. Neuropathol. Exp. Neurol.* **55**, 1023–1025
7. Flament-Durand, J. and Couck, A.M. (1979) *Acta Neuropathol.* **46**, 159–162
8. Gray, E.G., Paula-Barbosa, M. and Roher, A. (1987) *Neuropathol. Appl. Neurobiol.* **13**, 91–110
9. Terry, R.D., Gonatas, N.K. and Weiss, M. (1964) *Am. J. Pathol.* **44**, 669–697
10. Dustin, P. and Flament-Durand, J. (1982) in *Axoplasmic Transport in Physiology and Pathology* (Weiss, D.G. and Gorio, A., eds.), pp. 131–136, Springer, Berlin
11. Richard, S., Brion, J.P., Couck, A.M. and Flament-Durand, J. (1989) *J. Submicrosc. Cytol.* **21**, 461–467
12. Lu, Q. and Wood, J.G. (1993) *J. Neurosci.* **13**, 508–515
13. Alonso, A.D., Grundke-Iqbal, I. and Iqbal, K. (1996) *Nat. Med. (N.Y.)* **2**, 783–787
14. Hempen, B.J. and Brion, J.P. (1996) *J. Neuropathol. Exp. Neurol.* **55**, 964–972
15. Dayanandan, R., Van Slegtenhorst, M., Mack, T.G.A., Ko, L., Yen, S.H., Leroy, K., Brion, J.P., Anderton, B.H., Hutton, M. and Lovestone, S. (1999) *FEBS Lett.* **446**, 228–232
16. Brion, J.P. and Flament-Durand, J. (1995) *Pathol. Res. Pract.* **191**, 490–498
17. Hanger, D.P., Hughes, K., Woodgett, J.R., Brion, J.P. and Anderton, B.H. (1992) *Neurosci. Lett.* **147**, 58–62
18. Mandelkow, E.-M., Drewes, G., Biernat, J., Gustke, N., Van Lint, J., Vandenheede, J.R. and Mandelkow, E. (1992) *FEBS Lett.* **314**, 315–321
19. Anderton, B.H., Brion, J.P., Couck, A.M., Davis, D.R., Gallo, J.M., Hanger, D.P., Ladhani, K., Latimer, D., Lewis, C., Lovestone, S., et al. (1995) *Neurobiol. Aging* **16**, 389–402
20. Sperber, B.R., Leight, S., Goedert, M. and Lee, V.M.Y. (1995) *Neurosci. Lett.* **197**, 149–153
21. Wagner, U., Utton, M., Gallo, J.M. and Miller, C.C.J. (1996) *J. Cell Sci.* **109**, 1537–1543
22. Mulot, S.F.C., Hughes, K., Woodgett, J.R., Anderton, B.H. and Hanger, D.P. (1994) *FEBS Lett.* **349**, 359–364
23. Utton, M.A., Vandecandelaere, A., Wagner, U., Reynolds, C.H., Gibb, G.M., Miller, C.C.J., Bayley, P.M. and Anderton, B.H. (1997) *Biochem. J.* **323**, 741–747
24. Lovestone, S., Hartley, C.L., Pearce, J. and Anderton, B.H. (1996) *Neuroscience* **73**, 1145–1157
25. Leroy, K. and Brion, J.P. (1999) *J. Chem. Neuroanat.* **16**, 279–293
26. Brion, J.P., Octave, J.N. and Couck, A.M. (1994) *Neuroscience* **63**, 895–909
27. Edson, K., Weisshaar, B. and Matus, A. (1993) *Development* **117**, 689–700
28. Stambolic, V., Ruel, L. and Woodgett, J.R. (1996) *Curr. Biol.* **6**, 1664–1668
29. Lovestone, S., Davis, D.R., Webster, M.T., Kaech, S., Brion, J.P., Matus, A. and Anderton, B.H. (1999) *Biol. Psychiatry* **45**, 995–1003
30. Zhang, Z.H., Hartmann, H., Do, V.M., Abramowski, D., Sturchler-Pierrat, C., Staufenbiel, M., Sommer, B., Van de Wetering, M., Clevers, H., Saftig, P., et al. (1998) *Nature (London)* **395**, 698–702
31. Nishimura, M., Yu, G., Levesque, G., Zhang, D.M., Ruel, L., Chen, F., Milman, P., Holmes, E., Liang, Y., Kawarai, T., et al. (1999) *Nat. Med. (N.Y.)* **5**, 164–169
32. Takashima, A., Murayama, M., Murayama, O., Kohno, T., Honda, T., Yasutake, K., Nihonmatsu, N., Mercken, M., Yamaguchi, H., Sugihara, S. and Wolozin, B. (1998) *Proc. Natl. Acad. Sci. U.S.A.* **95**, 9637–9641
33. Caputo, C.B., Sobel, I.R.E., Scott, C.W., Brunner, W.F., Barth, P.T. and Blowers, D.P. (1992) *Biochem. Biophys. Res. Commun.* **185**, 1034–1040
34. Philippe, B., Brion, J.P. and Octave, J.N. (1996) *J. Neurosci. Res.* **46**, 709–719
35. Macq, A.F., Czech, C., Essalmani, R., Brion, J.P., Maron, A., Mercken, L., Pradier, L. and Octave, J.N. (1998) *J. Biol. Chem.* **273**, 28931–28936

36.   Brion, J.P., Smith, C., Couck, A.M., Gallo, J.M. and Anderton, B.H. (1993) *J. Neurochem.* **61**, 2071–2080

37.   Goedert, M., Jakes, R., Spillantini, M.G., Hasegawa, M., Smith, M.J. and Crowther, R.A. (1996) *Nature (London)* **383**, 550–553

38.   Kampers, T., Friedhoff, P., Biernat, J. and Mandelkow, E.M. (1996) *FEBS Lett.* **399**, 344–349

39.   Brion, J.P., Tremp, G. and Octave, J.N. (1999) *Am. J. Pathol.* **154**, 255–270.

40.   Schweers, O., Mandelkow, E.M., Biernat, J. and Mandelkow, E. (1995) *Proc. Natl. Acad. Sci. U.S.A.* **92**, 8463–8467

41.   Bancher, C., Brunner, C., Lassmann, H., Budka, H., Jellinger, K., Wiche, G., Seitelberger, F., Grundke-Iqbal, I., Iqbal, K. and Wisniewski, H.M. (1989) *Brain Res.* **477**, 90–99

42.   Braak, E., Braak, H. and Mandelkow, E.-M. (1994) *Acta Neuropathol.* **87**, 554–567

43.   Götz, J., Probst, A., Spillantini, M.G., Schäfer, T., Jakes, R., Bürki, K. and Goedert, M. (1995) *EMBO J.* **14**, 1304–1313

44.   Pradier, L., Czech, C., Mercken, L., Moussaoui, S., Reibaud, M., Delaère, P. and Tremp, G. (1998) in *Progress in Alzheimer's and Parkinson's Diseases* (Fisher, A., ed.), pp. 25–30, Plenum Press, New York

Biochem. Soc. Symp. **67**, 89–100
(Printed in Great Britain)

9

Presenilin function: connections to Alzheimer's disease and signal transduction

Paul E. Fraser*†[1], Gang Yu*, Lyne Lévesque*, Masaki Nishimura*, Dun-Sheng Yang*, Howard T.J. Mount*‡, David Westaway*§ and Peter H. St George-Hyslop*‡

Departments of *Medicine, †Medical Biophysics, ‡Medicine (Neurology), and §Laboratory of Medicine and Pathobiology,Centre for Research in Neurodegenerative Diseases, University of Toronto, Toronto, Ontario M5S 3H2, Canada

Abstract

Missense mutations in presenilin 1 (PS1) and presenilin 2 (PS2) are associated with early-onset familial Alzheimer's disease which displays an accelerated deposition of amyloid plaques and neurofibrillary tangles. Presenilins are multi-spanning transmembrane proteins which localize primarily to the endoplasmic reticulum and the Golgi compartments. We have previously demonstrated that PS1 exists as a high-molecular-mass complex that is likely to contain several functional ligands. Potential binding proteins were screened by the yeast two-hybrid system using the cytoplasmically orientated PS1 loop domain which was shown to interact strongly with members of the armadillo family of proteins, including β-catenin, p0071 and a novel neuron-specific plakophilin-related armadillo protein (NPRAP). Armadillo proteins can have dual functions that encompass the stabilization of cellular junctions/synapses and the mediation of signal transduction pathways. Our observations suggest that PS1 may contribute to both aspects of armadillo-related pathways involving neurite outgrowth and nuclear translocation of β-catenin upon activation of the wingless (Wnt) pathway. Alzheimer's disease (AD)-related presenilin mutations exhibit a dominant gain of aberrant function resulting in the prevention of β-catenin translocation following Wnt signalling. These findings indicate a functional role for PS1 in signalling and suggest that

---

[1]To whom correspondence should be addressed.

mistrafficking of selected presenilin ligands may be a potential mechanism in the genesis of AD.

Introduction

The pathogenesis of Alzheimer's disease (AD) is complex [1] and the common clinical and neuropathological features can arise from several different genetic and non-genetic causes. Nevertheless, a certain proportion of AD cases (~10%) appear to be transmitted as a pure autosomal-dominant trait with age-dependent but high penetrance. Molecular genetic analysis of these pedigrees has led to the discovery of four causative elements: β-amyloid precursor protein (APP), apolipoprotein E (ApoE), presenilin 1 (PS1) and prensenilin 2 (PS2). In this chapter, we will focus on studies on presenilin biology, how it relates to signal transduction and its association with AD pathogenesis.

AD and pathological mutations of PS1

Following the discovery that APP missense mutations and the ApoE polymorphisms failed to account for all cases of familial AD, a series of poly-morphic markers on chromosome 14q24.3 was revealed to be linked to a particularly aggressive early-onset form of familial AD. PS1 was then cloned as a causative gene in this locus [2], leading to the subsequent discovery of the homologous PS2. PS1 is highly conserved in evolution, also being present in *Caenorhabditis elegans* and *Drosophila*. Hydrophobicity analysis reveals that PS1 contains between five and ten transmembrane (TM) domains, an aqueous

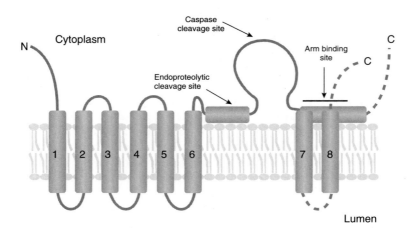

Figure 1 Topology of presenilin proteins. Alternative models with six and eight transmembrane domains, endoproteolytic cleavage sites as well as the putative armadillo (arm)/catenin binding sequence are shown. Orientation of the N-terminal and Loop domains towards the cytoplasmic space are also indicated.

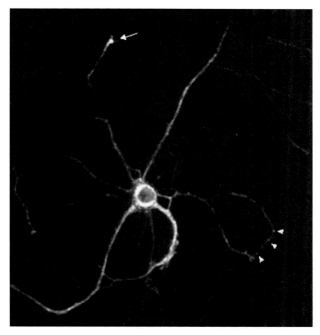

Figure 2 Immunofluorescence of PS1 in fully differentiated mouse hippocampal neuron. PS1 is localized to the cell body within the Golgi/ER compartments, extending growth cones (arrow) and as punctate, possibly vesicular, structures within the processes (arrowheads).

N-terminus and a loop domain, between the putative 6th and 7th TM (TM6–TM7) helices, which contains an acidic apex and two flanking hydrophobic sequences (Figure 1).

Full-length PS1 is approximately 50 kDa in size and is located predominantly in intracellular membranous organelles such as the endoplasmic reticulum (ER), nuclear envelope and Golgi apparatus [3]. Studies of the topology of PS1 suggest that both the N-terminus and the residues in the TM6–TM7 loop are orientated to the cytoplasm [3–5]. Although the orientation of the C-terminus is not yet completely resolved, a line of evidence suggests that it is also located in the cytoplasm and that the preceding hydrophobic residues are either membrane-associated or represent two additional TM domains – TM7 and TM8 (Figure 1) [3–5].

PS1 is transcribed at low levels in many tissues, both within the central nervous system (CNS) and in non-neuronal organs. In the CNS, PS1 transcripts can be detected in the neocortex (especially in layers II and IV), in the CA1–CA3 fields, dentate gyrus and subiculum of the hippocampus and in the cerebellar cortex and deep nuclei, as well as in lesser amounts in the olfactory bulb, striatum, thalamus and some brainstem nuclei. PS1 is an important developmental protein whose expression is regulated in differentiating hippocampal neurons [6]. *In vitro*, PS1 is localized to both the cell body and extending growth cones and may be contained within vesicular structures as indicated by punctate staining in neuronal processes (Figure 2).

To date, more than 40 different pathological mutations of PS1 have been reported. The majority are missense mutations and are predominantly located in highly conserved TM domains, at/near putative membrane interfaces, or in the large hydrophilic loop. Additionally, two splicing defect mutations have been identified. One involves a point mutation in the splice acceptor site at the 5' end of exon 10 (the numbering of exon is followed by [6a]), and allows exon 9 to be fused in-frame with exon 11, thereby removing a series of charged residues at the apex of the large hydrophilic loop domain. Interestingly, this mutation removes residues near the endoproteolytic cleavage site at or near residue Met[290] and results in an increase of uncleaved holoprotein. The second splice site mutation arises from the deletion of a G nucleotide from the splice donor site at the 3' end of exon 5.

Structure and endoproteolytic processing of the presenilins

Analysis of the PS1 transcript suggests the presence of some splicing variants. Thus there is a variably present four-amino-acid VRQS insert which arises from the use of an alternate splice donor site at the 3' end of exon 4. In some tissues (especially leukocytes), there is also alternate splicing of exon 9, which encodes a series of hydrophobic residues at the C-terminus of TM6 and the beginning of the TM6–TM7 loop domain. As a result, this splicing event is predicted to significantly alter the functional properties of the TM6–TM7 loop and, along with physiological endoproteolytic cleavage of this loop, is one of the arguments that suggests that this large hydrophilic loop is an important functional domain.

Studies of the PS1 protein in brain tissue, as well as many other peripheral tissues, reveal that very small amounts of the PS1 holoprotein exist within the cell at any given time [7,8]. Instead, the holoprotein is actively catabolized, possibly by at least two different proteolytic mechanisms, one of which appears to involve the proteasome [9]. Another mechanism involves a series of heterogeneous endoproteolytic cleavage near residue 290 within the TM6–TM7 loop domain [7,8]. This cleavage by 'presenilase' generates N- and C-terminal fragments of approximately 35 kDa and 20 kDa, respectively. A series of endoproteolytically processed fragments specific to the CNS have also been observed and may reflect heterogeneous cleavage of PS1 [10]. Remarkably, the stoichiometry of the N- and C-terminal fragments is maintained on a 1:1 ratio and their absolute abundance is also tightly regulated, such that artificial overexpression of PS1 results in only a modest increase in these fragments [7]. This has led to the suggestion that this physiological proteolytic cleavage involves a tightly regulated saturable process [10]. A third mechanism involves members of the caspase 3 family. Activation of apoptotic pathways, which culminate in activation of caspase 3, results in cleavage of PS1 near residue Asp[345] [11–13]. It is currently unclear whether caspase cleavage of the presenilins is actively involved in the regulation of apoptosis, or whether presenilins simply represent innocent bystanders, although preliminary data suggest an anti-apoptotic effect for the C-terminal derivative by caspase [14]. Certainly, caspase-mediated cleavage is not required for the effects on amyloidogenesis and Notch signalling [13].

High-molecular-mass membrane-bound presenilin complexes

Whether the holoprotein or the physiological proteolytic fragments, or both, have biological activities is currently unclear. However, it is clear that the holoprotein and its endoproteolytic fragments are components of high-molecular-mass protein complexes. Thus the holoprotein appears to be a component of a ~180 kDa complex which is predominantly resident in the rough ER [15–17]. The N- and C-terminal fragments appear to associate with each other as heterodimeric components of a larger (~250 kDa) multimeric protein complex that appears to be resident in the ER, Golgi, and some additional membranous domains whose identity has not been clarified [15–17]. The latter may include detergent-insoluble glycosphingolipid-rich domains [18]. The incorporation of presenilin proteins into a larger complex represents a rate-limiting step in the presenilin-processing pathway [19,20]. Thus once incorporated into these high-molecular-mass complexes, the endoproteolytic fragments remain together with a stable 1:1 stoichiometry and with very long half-lives. Holoprotein monomers that do not become incorporated into these complexes are rapidly degraded via a proteasome-dependent mechanism and have a half-life of less than 1 hour [19]. Recent data has suggested that this incorporation into protein complexes is necessary for biological activity in APP processing [21]. In addition, there is evidence from some laboratories that presenilins may also directly interact with APP [21a,21b] but this finding remains controversial as evidenced by conflicting data from other groups [15].

To identify PS1- and PS2-binding proteins, we used two complementary approaches. Initially, sequences encoding the PS1 cytoplasmic loop (residues 266–409) were used as bait in a yeast two-hybrid interaction trap to screen a human cDNA library. The cytoplasmic loop domain of the presenilins was chosen as a putative functional domain because it undergoes physiological endoproteolytic cleavage near residue 299, is the site of physiological tissue-specific alternative splicing, undergoes physiological post-translational phosphorylation, is abnormally cleaved by caspases during apoptosis, and is the site of several missense mutations and one splicing mutation associated with AD. We identified several independent His$^+$, β-gal$^+$ clones. Six of these clones, generated with independent bait sequences, were identified as being derived from the same transcript which encoded a novel, neuron-specific armadillo protein termed neuronal plakophilin-related armadillo protein (NPRAP). NPRAP was simultaneously and independently identified by other groups searching for plakophilin-related proteins, as well as PS1 ligands, and has also been called δ-catenin [17,22,23]. NPRAP is exclusively expressed in the brain as a 3.9–5.0 kb transcript which encodes a protein of 1084 residues with a unique N-terminus and 10 armadillo (arm) repeats at the C-terminus. The interaction was confirmed by reciprocal co-immunoprecipitation from transfected cells and from native mammalian brain; by affinity chromatography with a recombinant PS1 loop peptide, which demonstrated specific binding; and by co-localization on immunofluorescence and *in situ* hybridization studies. NPRAP also interacts with PS2.

The interaction of the presenilins with armadillo proteins appears to be specific to a subset of armadillo proteins since NPRAP/δ-catenin and β-catenin both interacted with PS1, while γ-catenin did not bind either presenilin. An additional protein termed p0071 was also isolated by the yeast two-hybrid screen. It is a member of the plakophilin family of proteins and shares homology with NPRAP. A potential binding site on PS1 was identified by a candidate arm-protein-binding domain contained within residues 372–399 in the large TM6–TM7 loop of PS1 (Figure 1) [23]. This domain is a single pseudo-arm repeat which is highly conserved in PS2 and also in the invertebrate homologues. Peptides to this region have been shown to displace the binding of NPRAP to the PS1 loop *in vitro*, suggesting this region may be the primary site of interaction. The biological effects of NPRAP/δ-catenin are not currently known but in association with PS1 it may be involved in stabilization of synaptic junctions and/or mediation of intracellular signalling. A possible connection of NPRAP with cytoskeletal organization has been reported by the induction of an unusual cell morphology with high levels of expression of this armadillo protein [24]. Further investigations into the effects of NPRAP will help to uncover its potential links to AD pathology.

Cellular roles of presenilin

The physiological function of PS1 has not yet been defined. However, functional analogies have been made to a nematode homologue, Spe-4, which is involved in the maintenance of a Golgi-derived membranous organelle. It is considered to be important in trafficking protein and cell membrane products in the maturing spermatocyte [25]. This has led to speculation that PS1 might subserve a similar role in protein and vesicle sorting. This hypothesis is supported by two different lines of experimental evidence. Firstly, ablation of functional PS1 expression causes aberrant processing of APP with the failure of γ-secretase cleavage, which results in the accumulation of uncleaved α-secretase or β-secretase stubs in a variety of intracellular loci including ER, Golgi, and lysosomes [26,27]. Similar findings were observed for an APP homologue, APLP1, which has a limited sequence identity in the TM region including the γ-secretase sites. This fact supports the hypothesis that PS deficiency alters trafficking of proteolytic C-terminal fragments of APP and APLP1 to specific subcellular compartments which contain γ-secretase activity, rather than the alternative speculation that presenilins play a direct role in APP processing by γ-secretase [28]. Secondly, the presenilins form multimeric complexes with β-catenin and missense mutations in PS1 and PS2 cause perturbation of nuclear translocation of this PS ligand [29].

Other putative roles for PS1 have included the regulation of signal transduction during development, in apoptosis and possibly in cellular calcium ion homoeostasis. The former suggestion arose because null mutations in a second *C. elegans* presenilin orthologue termed, Sel-12, exert a suppressor effect on abnormalities in vulva progenitor cell fate decisions induced by activated Notch mutants [30]. Notch is involved in intercellular signalling during development. Nematode Sel-12 shows stronger amino-acid-sequence identity to the human presenilins than does Spe-4. The effect of PS on Notch signalling is further supported by the fact that targeted disruption of the murine *PS1* gene causes embryonic lethality around day E13 and is associated with severe developmental defects in somite formation and axial skeleton formation; the occurrence of cerebral haemorrhage; and reduced Notch1 and Dll1 transcription in selected cell types [31,32]. Similar phenotypes have been observed in knockout mice for Notch1 and Dll1, also supporting this hypothesis. More recent data has also revealed that PS1 is directly involved in Notch processing and may therefore play a key part in this signal transduction pathway [33–35]. Studies in transfected cells have also suggested a role in the suppression of apoptosis. Overexpression of full-length wild-type PS1 or PS2 can induce apoptosis in transfected cells and mutations further sensitize these cells to apoptosis, possibly through a mechanism involving heterotrimeric G-proteins [36].

PS1 mutations and alterations in cellular function

The dominant inheritance mode and wide scattering of missense mutations has led to speculation that the effect of the familial AD-related mutations is a gain-of-function effect. This is partially borne out by two observations in PS1-knockout mice. Firstly, these mice have a phenotype of perinatal lethality without evidence of AD [31,32]. This loss-of-function phenotype can be completely rescued not only by wild-type but also by mutant *PS1* transgenes [37,38]. Secondly, PS1-deficient mice have a defect in APP processing manifested through the failure of γ-secretase cleavage, leading to an abnormal accumulation of the APP C-terminal fragment [26]. This defect is completely reversed by both wild-type and mutant *PS1* transgenes. A gain-of-function is imparted by the mutant transgenes because it also induces an increase in the more amyloidogenic Aβ residues 1–42 (Aβ42), which is a biochemical marker of PS1 mutations [37,38]. However, a very different perspective is provided by complementation assays of mutant Sel-12 in *C. elegans*. The wild-type human PS1, but not mutant human protein are able to complement the loss-of-function Sel-12 mutants [39,40]. This suggests that the human PS1 mutants may not be fully functional in the nematode system.

One definitive effect of PS1 (and PS2) mutations is to alter the processing of APP by preferentially favouring the production of potentially toxic Aβ peptides terminating at either residue 42 or 43 (Aβ42 or Aβ43). These peptides are more fibrillogenic and have been shown to comprise the earliest deposits in the brains of affected individuals [41–45]. In addition, fibroblasts from heterozygous carriers of mutant PS1, APP-transfected cell lines stably expressing PS1 mutations as well as mutant PS1-transgenic mice all contain or secrete increased quantities of Aβ42 with only a variable but minor increase in shorter Aβ peptides terminating at residue 40 (Aβ40). These findings are supported by direct measurements of Aβ in the *post mortem* brain tissue of patients with PS1-linked familial AD, who display similar increases in the amount of Aβ42 compared to control brain tissue and to brain tissue from subjects with sporadic AD [46]. This effect of mutant PS1 appears to represent a gain-of-function mode.

β-catenin signalling pathways and the effects of presenilins

The functional significance of the interactions between the presenilins and armadillo proteins is not entirely clear, because the armadillo proteins have diverse functions ranging from a structural role in stabilization of intercellular junctions (including synapses), a role in signal transduction of Wingless (Wnt) and certain growth factors and also in apoptotic pathways. Our findings suggest that the physiological and mutational effects of the presenilins are linked to the β-catenin signalling pathway (Figure 3). In response to activation of the Wnt/β-catenin signal transduction pathway and certain other stimuli, β-catenin undergoes translocation to the nucleus via a transport mechanism that is independent of nuclear localization signals and importin/karyopherin 19. Wnt signal transduction is mediated in part by inhibition of glycogen synthase kinase-3 (GSK-3), which regulates the stability of β-catenin which can be mimicked by low concentrations of lithium ions [47–49]. This activity specifically arises from the inhibition of GSK-3 by lithium, and has been widely used to dissect the biochemistry of downstream elements in the Wnt signalling pathway [48,49]. To examine the effects of presenilin mutations on nuclear translocation of β-catenin, we used lithium to activate the Wnt/β-catenin signal transduction pathway in cells expressing mutant or wild-type presenilin proteins. Under these conditions, we observed a reduction of 50–80% of β-catenin translocation in fibroblasts expressing a variety of PS1 mutations [29]. A similar but less dramatic effect was observed with the PS2 Met[239]→Val mutation. Cumulatively, these observations reveal that mutant presenilin proteins influence the intracellular trafficking of β-catenin – a proven presenilin ligand. This gain-of-aberrant-function effect probably reflects functional compromise of the presenilin–β-catenin protein complexes.

Additional studies [50] have demonstrated that the formation of PS1–β-catenin complex leads to increased stability of β-catenin. Furthermore, pathogenic mutant PS1 loses this stabilization effect, causing suppression of β-catenin signalling. In contrast, our data indicated that the function of PS in this pathway is not clear under physiological conditions [29]. A recent report has indicated that the ability of PS1 to bind β-catenin is abolished by caspase cleavage, suggesting that these alternately cleaved fragments are not incorporated into PS complexes and could be non-functional [51]. Additionally, PS1 has been observed to have the ability to bind microtubule-associated protein tau and GSK-3β [52]. This may result in a mutant PS1-facilitated phosphorylation of tau via GSK-3. The precise details of this potentially direct link to AD-related pathology remain to be clarified as some conflicting data have been reported [53]. However, the possibility that these mutational effects are related to AD pathogenesis is an important future issue.

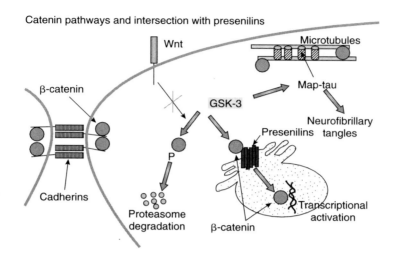

Figure 3 Putative presenilin effects in the β-catenin signalling pathway. The major intracellular pool of β-catenin is in a cadherin-bound form. A cytoplasmic-free form is rather minor but mediates important signal transduction such as the Wnt pathway. Without stimulation by Wnt ligand, free β-catenin is phosphorylated by GSK-3β, then ubiquitinated and rapidly degraded by proteasome. Upon activation of the Wnt pathway, the GSK-3β activity is inhibited and free β-catenins increase and translocate into the nucleus to activate the downstream genes. Mutations in PS1 and PS2 significantly reduce β-catenin translocation to the nucleus. GSK-3β also phosphorylates tau, and the hyperphosphorylation of tau could lead to formation of neurofibrillary tangles in AD brains.

Conclusions

AD research seems to be standing at the turning point. Recently an intriguing hypothesis has been proposed, raised mainly from the research on inherited diseases with trinucleotide repeats. This hypothesis proposes that the majority of adult-onset neurodegenerative disorders might be commonly caused by progressive precipitation of proteolysis-resistant proteins specific for each disease [54]. In the case of AD, the causative precipitates are composed of Aβ peptides (cores of senile plaques) or hyperphosphorylated tau proteins (neurofibrillary tangles). Given that this hypothesis is true, a key role for presenilins in leading to AD development could be solely an overproduction of long-tailed Aβ peptides whatever the physiological functions or the other mutational effects of the presenilins. Since both homologous molecules PS1 and PS2 cause AD, the research on presenilins could be a powerful clue to resolve this issue.

References
1. St George-Hyslop, P.H., Haines, J.L. Farrer, L.A., Polinsky, R., Van Broeckhoven, C., Goate, A., McLachlan, D.R., Orr, H., Bruni, A.C., Sorbi, S., et al. (1990) *Nature (London)* **347**, 194–197
2. Sherrington, R., Rogaev, E.I., Liang, Y., Rogaeva, E.A., Levesque, G., Ikeda, M., Chi, H., Lin, C., Li, G., Holman, K., et al. (1995) *Nature (London)* **375**, 754–760
3. De Strooper, B., Beulens, M., Contreras, B., Craessaerts, K., Moechars, D., Bollen, M., Fraser, P., St George-Hyslop, P. and Van Leuven, F. (1997) *J. Biol. Chem.* **272**, 3590–3598
4. Lehmann, S., Chiesa, R. and Harris, D.A. (1997) *J. Biol. Chem.* **272**, 12047–12051
5. Doan, A., Thinakaran, G., Borchelt, D.R., Slunt, H.H., Ratovitsky, T., Podlisny, M., Selkoe, D.J., Seeger, M., Gandy, S.E., Price, D.L. and Sisodia, S.S. (1996) *Neuron* **17**, 1023–1030
6. Lévesque, L., Annaert, W., Craessaets, K., Mathews, P., Seeger, M., Nixon, R.A., Gandy, S., Westaway, D., Van Leuven, F., St George-Hyslop, P., De Strooper, B. and Fraser, P.E. (1999) *Mol. Med.* **5**, 542–554
6a. Rogaev, E.I., Sherrington, R., Wu, C., Lévesque, G., Chi, H., Liang, Y., Rogaeva, E.A., Chi, H., Ikeda, M., Holman, K., et al. (1997) *Genomics* **40**, 415–424
7. Thinakaran, G., Borchelt, D.R., Lee, M.K., Slunt, H.H., Spitzer, L., Kim, G., Ratovitsky, T., Davenport, F., Nordstedt, C., Seeger, M., et al. (1996) *Neuron* **17**, 181–190
8. Podlisny, M.B., Citron, M., Amarante, P., Sherrington, R., Xia, W., Zhang, J., Diehl, T., Levesque, G., Fraser, P., Haass, C., et al. (1997) *Neurobiol. Dis.* **3**, 325–337
9. Fraser, P.E., Lévesque, G., Yu, G., Mills, L.R., Thirwell, J., Frantseva, M., Carlen, P. and St George-Hyslop, P. (1998) *Neurobiol. Aging* **19**, S19–S21
10. Hartmann, H., Busciglio, J., Baumann, K.H., Staufenbiel, M. and Yankner, B.A. (1997) *J. Biol. Chem.* **272**, 14505–14508
11. Kim, T.W., Pettingell, W.H., Jung, Y.K., Kovacs, D.M. and Tanzi, R.E. (1997) *Science* **277**, 373–376
12. Grunberg, J., Walter, J., Loetscher, H., Deuschle, U., Jacobsen, H. and Haass, C. (1998) *Biochemistry* **37**, 2263–2270
13. Brockhaus, M., Grunberg, J., Rohrig, S., Loetscher, H., Wittenburg, N., Baumeister, R., Jacobsen, H. and Haass, C. (1998) *NeuroReport* **9**, 1481–1486
14. Vito, P., Ghayur, T. and D'Adamio, L. (1997) *J. Biol. Chem.* **272**, 28315–28320
15. Thinakaran, G., Regard, J.B., Bouton, C.M., Harris, C.L., Price, D.L., Borchelt, D.R. and Sisodia, S.S. (1998) *Neurobiol. Dis.* **4**, 438–453
16. Capell, A., Grunberg, J., Pesold, B., Diehlmann, A., Citron, M., Nixon, R., Beyreuther, K., Selkoe, D.J. and Haass, C. (1998) *J. Biol. Chem.* **273**, 3205–3211
17. Yu, G., Chen, F., Levesque, G., Nishimura, M., Zhang, D.-M., Levesque, L., Rogaeva, E., Xu, D., Liang, Y., Duthie, M., St George-Hyslop, P. and Fraser, P.E. (1998) *J. Biol. Chem.* **273**, 16470–16475
18. Lee, S.J., Liyanage, U., Bickel, P.E., Xia, W., Lansbury, Jr, P.T. and Kosik, K.S. (1998) *Nat. Med. (N.Y.)* **4**, 730–734
19. Steiner, H., Capell, A., Pesold, B., Citron, M., Kloetzel, P.M., Selkoe, D.J., Romig, H., Mendla, K. and Haass, C. (1998) *J. Biol. Chem.* **273**, 32322–32331
20. Thinakaran, G., Harris, C.L., Ratovitski, T., Davenport, F., Slunt, H.H., Price, D.L., Borchelt, D.R. and Sisodia, S.S. (1997) *J. Biol. Chem.* **272**, 28415–28422
21. Tomita, T., Tokuhiro, S., Hashimoto, T., Aiba, K., Saido, T.C., Maruyama, K. and Iwatsubo, T. (1998) *J. Biol. Chem.* **273**, 21153–21160
21a. Weidemann, A., Paliga, K., Durrwang, U., Czech, C., Evin, G., Masters, C.L. and Beyreuther, K. (1997) *Nat. Med. (N.Y.)* **3**, 328–332
21b. Xia, W., Zhang, J., Perez, R., Koo, E.H. and Selkoe, D.J. (1997) *Proc. Natl. Acad. Sci. U.S.A.* **94**, 8208–8213

22. Zhou, J., Liyanage, U., Medina, M., Ho, C., Simmons, A.D., Lovett, M. and Kosik, K.S. (1997) *NeuroReport* **8**, 2085–2090

23. Levesque, G., Yu, G., Nishimura, M., Zhang, D.-M., Levesque, L., Yu, H., Xu, D., Liang, Y., Rogaeva, E., Ikeda, M., et al. (1998) *J. Neurochem.* **72**, 999–1008

24. Lu, Q., Paredes, M., Medina, M., Zhou, J., Cavallo, R., Peifer, M., Orecchio, L. and Kosik, K.S. (1999) *J. Cell Biol.* **144**, 519–532

25. L'Hernault, S.W. and Arduengo, P.M. (1992) *J. Cell. Biol.* **119**, 55–68

26. De Strooper, B., Saftig, P., Craessaerts, K., Vanderstichele, H., Guhde, G., Annaert, W., Von Figura, K. and Van Leuven, F. (1998) *Nature (London)* **391**, 387–390

27. Xia, W., Zhang, J., Ostaszewski, B.L., Kimberly, W.T., Seubert, P., Koo, E.H., Shen, J. and Selkoe, D.J. (1998) *Biochemistry* **37**, 16465–16471

28. Naruse, S., Thinakaran, G., Luo, J.J., Kusiak, J.W., Tomita, T., Iwatsubo, T., Qian, X., Ginty, D.D., Price, D.L., Borchelt, D.R., et al. (1998) *Neuron* **21**, 1213–1221

29. Nishimura, M., Yu, G., Levesque, G., Zhang, D.M., Ruel, L., Chen, F., Levesque, L., Millman, P., Holmes, E., Liang, Y., et al. (1999) *Nat. Med. (N.Y.)* **5**, 164–169

30. Levitan, D. and Greenwald, I. (1995) *Nature (London)* **377**, 351–354

31. Shen, J., Bronson, R.T., Chen, D.F., Xia, W., Selkoe, D.J. and Tonegawa, S. (1997) *Cell* **89**, 629–639

32. Wong, P.C., Zheng, H., Chen, H., Becher, M.W., Sirinathsinghji, D.J., Trumbauer, M.E., Chen, H.Y., Price, D.L., Van der Ploeg, L.H. and Sisodia, S.S. (1997) *Nature (London)* **387**, 288–292

33. De Strooper, B., Annaert, W., Cupers, P., Saftig, P., Craessaerts, K., Mumm, J.S., Schroeter, E.H., Schrijvers, V., Wolfe, M.S., Ray, W.J., Goate, A. and Kopan, R. (1999) *Nature (London)* **398**, 518–522

34. Struhl, G. and Greenwald, I. (1999) *Nature (London)* **398**, 522–526

35. Ye, Y., Lukinova, N. and Fortini, M.E. (1999) *Nature (London)* **398**, 525–529

36. Wolozin, B., Iwasaki, K., Vito, P., Ganjei, J.K., Lacana, E., Sunderland, T., Zhao, B., Kusiak, J.W., Wasco, W. and D'Adamio, L. (1996) *Science* **274**, 1710–1713

37. Davis, J.A., Naruse, S., Chen, H., Eckman, C., Younkin, S., Price, D.L., Borchelt, D.R., Sisodia, S.S. and Wong, P.C. (1998) *Neuron* **20**, 603–609

38. Qian, S., Jiang, P., Guan, X.M., Singh, G., Trumbauer, M.E., Yu, H., Chen, H.Y., Van de Ploeg, L.H. and Zheng, H. (1998) *Neuron* **20**, 611–617

39. Levitan, D., Doyle, T.G., Brousseau, D., Lee, M.K., Thinakaran, G., Slunt, H.H., Sisodia, S.S. and Greenwald, I. (1996) *Proc. Natl. Acad. Sci. U.S.A.* **93**, 14940–14944

40. Baumeister, R., Leimer, U., Zweckbronner, I., Jakubek, C., Grunberg, J. and Haass, C. (1997) *Genes Funct.* **1**, 149-159

41. Martins, R.N., Turner, B.A., Carroll, R.T., Sweeney, D., Kim, K.S., Wisniewski, H.M., Blass, J.P., Gibson, G.E. and Gandy, S. (1995) NeuroReport **7**, 217–220

42. Scheuner, D., Eckman, C., Jensen, M., Song, X., Citron, M., Suzuki, N., Bird, T.D., Hardy, J., Hutton, M., Kukull, W., et al. (1996) *Nat. Med. (N.Y.)* **2**, 864–870

43. Duff, K., Eckman, C., Zehr, C., Yu, X., Prada, C.M., Perez-tur, J., Hutton, M., Buee, L., Harigaya, Y., Yager, D., et al. (1996) *Nature (London)* **383**, 710–713

44. Borchelt, D.R., Thinakaran, G., Eckman, C.B., Lee, M.K., Davenport, F., Ratovitsky, T., Prada, C.M., Kim, G., Seekins, S., Yager D., et al. (1996) *Neuron* **17**, 1005–1013

45. Citron, M., Westaway, D., Xia, W., Carlson, G., Diehl, T., Levesque, G., Johnson-Wood, K., Lee, M., Seubert, P., Davis, A., et al. (1997) *Nat. Med. (N.Y.)* **3**, 67–72

46. Tamaoka, A., Fraser, P., Ishii, K., Sahara, N., Ozawa, K., Ikeda, M., Saunders, A., Komatsuzaki, Y., Sherrington, R., Levesque, G., et al. (1998) *Brain Res. Mol. Brain Res.* **56**, 178–185

47. Kao, K.R., Masui, Y. and Elinson, R.P. (1986) *Nature (London)* **322**, 371–373

48. Klein, P. and Melton, D.A. (1996) *Proc. Natl. Acad. Sci. U.S.A.* **93**, 8455–8459

49. Stambolic, V., Ruel, L. and Woodgett, J.R. (1996) *Curr. Biol.* **6**, 1664–1668

50. Zhang, Z., Hartmann, H., Do, V.M., Abramowski, D., Sturchler-Pierrat, C., Staufenbiel, M., Sommer, B., van de Wetering, M., Clevers, H., Saftig, P., et al. (1998) *Nature (London)* **395**, 698–702

51. Tesco, G., Kim, T.W., Diehlmann, A., Beyreuther, K. and Tanzi, R.E. (1998) *J. Biol. Chem.* **273**, 33909–33914

52. Takashima, A., Murayama, M., Murayama, O., Kohno, T., Honda, T., Yasutake, K., Nihonmatsu, N., Mercken, M., Yamaguchi, H., Sugihara, S. and Wolozin, B. (1998) *Proc. Natl. Acad. Sci. U.S.A.* **95**, 9637–9641

53. Irving, N.G. and Miller, C.C.J. (1997) *Neurosci. Lett.* **222**, 71–74

54. Kakizuka, A. (1998) *Trends Genet.* **14**, 396–402

Biochem. Soc. Symp. **67**, 101–109
(Printed in Great Britain)

10

Apolipoprotein E and Alzheimer's disease: signal transduction mechanisms

Warren J. Strittmatter

Division of Neurology, Duke University Medical Center, Durham, NC 27710, U.S.A.

Abstract

The three common apolipoprotein E (ApoE) alleles differentially contribute to the risk of Alzheimer's disease (AD). While the *APOE* genotype alters susceptibility to disease expression, individuals with APOE ϵ4 alleles have the highest risk of developing AD; the APOE ϵ4 allele is neither essential nor sufficient on its own to cause AD. Since the discovery, in 1992, of the involvement of *APOE* in AD, many scientists have explored the role of the ApoE isoforms in the central nervous system in an effort to elucidate their roles in the pathophysiological mechanism of this disease. While many hypotheses have been proposed, none has been proven. ApoE was discovered through investigations into cholesterol metabolism. In serum and in cerebrospinal fluid ApoE binds lipoprotein particles, which contain cholesterol esters, and is critical in the shuttling of cholesterol from cell to cell. Trafficking of ApoE is mediated by specific interactions with cell-surface receptors. As described later, several families of ApoE receptors with diverse functions have been discovered. The roles of these receptors are proving increasingly complex since additional interactions with other ligands and with other intracellular proteins are rapidly being identified. It was once thought that these receptors only shuttle ApoE-containing phospholipid particles from the extracellular environment into the cell, but they also transduce a number of additional intracellular signals and interactions. Molecular signalling cascades initiated by the various ApoE receptors modulate a number of critical cellular processes. To date, two functional classes of ApoE receptors have been identified. The first is the low-density lipoprotein receptor family and the second the scavenger receptor families.

The low-density lipoprotein (LDL) receptor family

The most extensively investigated ApoE receptors are a family of seven receptors in the LDL receptor gene family. These receptors share common molecular features critical for their roles in binding and internalizing ApoE-lipoprotein particles and regulating intracellular cholesterol metabolism. Receptors in this class are the LDL receptor, the very-low-density lipoprotein (VLDL) receptor, neuro-ApoE receptor (LR8B), vitellogenin (two related receptors), LDL receptor-related protein (LRP) and megalin (gp330) [1].

Functional domains of the LDL receptor family

ApoE receptors in this family share functional motifs. Two representative LDL receptors, LRP and LR8B are shown in Figure 1. All receptors in this family are single transmembrane-spanning receptors with their C-terminus in the cytoplasmic compartment. The extracellular N-terminus of these receptors includes ligand binding domains. Each of these ligand binding domains is approximately 40 amino acids long. The LDL receptor contains six of these domains, and the largest ApoE receptor, megalin, contains 36. These individual ligand binding domains share amino acid sequences, with approximately 50% homology both within and among these receptors. All receptors in this class recognize and bind ApoE, but details of the kinetics and the specificity for interactions with the various isoforms of ApoE have only been extensively studied for the LDL receptor [1].

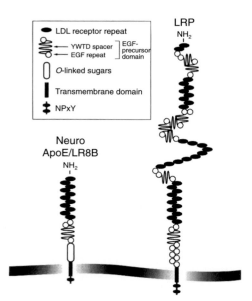

Figure 1 Two prototypic members of the LDL receptor family, LRP and LR8B. YWTD, tyrosine, tryptophan, threonine, aspartic acid. Reprinted with permisstion from *Nature* [1]. © (1997) Macmillan Magazines Limited.

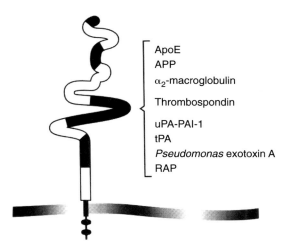

ApoE
APP
α₂-macroglobulin
Thrombospondin
uPA-PAI-1
tPA
Pseudomonas exotoxin A
RAP

Figure 2 The LRP receptor is a multi-ligand receptor.

Several of these receptors interact with other ligands in addition to ApoE (see Figure 2). The LDL receptor appears to interact only with ApoE and ApoB. In contrast, the LRP receptor also binds α_2-macroglobulin, the β-amyloid precursor protein (APP), thrombospondin, plasminogen activators and *Pseudomonas* exotoxin A [2]. The receptor-associated protein (RAP) is a 39 kDa protein which associates with the nascent receptor as it is translated in the endoplasmic reticulum. It appears to play an important role in ensuring that the correct tertiary structure of the receptor is reached and in preventing indiscriminate association of the receptor with other molecules. It also competitively inhibits ApoE from interacting with this class of receptors, and has therefore been used as a pharmacological tool to determine whether an effect of ApoE is mediated by interaction with this class of receptors.

In addition to the ApoE ligand binding domains, the extracellular domain of these receptors contains an epidermal growth factor (EGF)-precursor domain. Deletion of this EGF-precursor domain prevents these receptors from binding to LDL, but has no effect on their binding to ApoE. The EGF-precursor domain appears necessary for mediating the pH-dependent dissociation of ligand from receptor [1].

The third functional domain of the LDL receptor family is within the cytoplasmic domain of the receptor and is necessary for interactions between the receptor protein and other proteins in the cytoplasm. Neuronal ApoE receptors contain the consensus sequence NPxY (found twice in the cytoplasmic domain of LRP and megalin). This sequence was initially identified as the domain necessary for the localization of the receptors in coated pits; this occurs through its interaction with the adaptor protein AP-2 which in turn binds clathrin. The role of this protein–protein interaction in receptor-mediated endocytosis is described in the next section. Additional interactions of the cytoplasmic domain of these receptors, recently identified by Joachim Herz

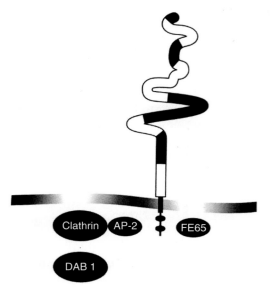

Figure 3 Intracytoplasmic interactions of the LDL receptor family important in signal transduction.

and colleagues, present additional signalling transduction pathways for these receptors. Using yeast two-hybrid and protein co-immunoprecipitation techniques he demonstrated that the cytoplasmic domains of these proteins interact with the neuronal adaptor proteins FE65 and mammalian Disabled (DAB), as shown in Figure 3 [3]. These proteins in turn interact with other cytoplasmic proteins, discussed later. Intriguingly, APP also contains an NPxY consensus sequence and interacts with FE65 [3] and DAB [4].

Cellular trafficking of the LDL receptor family

With a turnover time of approximately 10 minutes, the LDL family of receptors bind ApoE-containing lipoprotein particles, and internalize them within the cell (Figure 4) [2]. These receptors locate in the coated pits of the plasma membrane through interactions with the cytoplasmic protein clathrin, which are mediated by the adaptor protein AP-2. After invagination of the coated pit, the newly formed coated vesicle fuses to form an acid endosome. The decrease in pH dissociates the receptor from the ligand, and the receptor is recycled to the plasma membrane. Acid hydrolases free the cholesterol from the ApoE-containing lipoprotein particles and the cholesterol then enters the cytoplasmic compartment.

Receptor transduction through DAB

The binding of the cytoplasmic tail of the LDL receptor family to DAB presents additional opportunities for signal transduction [3]. DAB is primarily a neuronal protein which contains a single protein-interaction domain. DAB is tyrosine phosphorylated by the non-receptor tyrosine kinases SRC and ABL

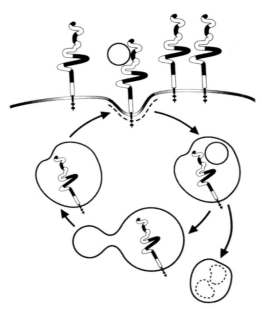

Figure 4 Receptor-mediated endocytosis. Reproduced from Herz, J. The LDL-receptor-related protein — portrait of a multifunctional receptor. Curr. Opin. Lipidol. **4**, 107–113 with permission. © (1993) Lippincott, Williams & Wilkins.

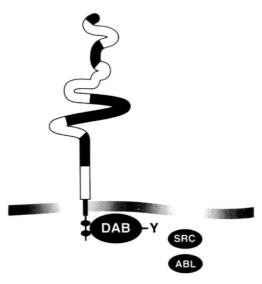

Figure 5 Interaction of the LDL family of receptors with DAB.

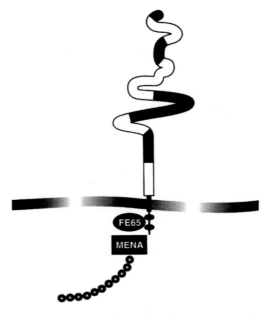

Figure 6 Interaction of the LDL family of receptors with FE65.

(Figure 5). Knockout of the *DAB* gene produces a lethal neurological pheno-type characterized by abnormal cortical cell-layering.

Receptor transduction through FE65

FE65 is another protein which binds to the cytoplasmic tail of these receptors [3]. Unlike DAB, FE65 contains three protein binding domains, pre-senting the opportunity for molecular scaffolding. FE65 contains two distinct binding domains that bind both the LDL family of receptors and also APP, suggesting a mechanism by which the metabolism of these receptors may be linked. FE65 also contains a WW domain capable of binding mammalian enabled (MENA). MENA in turn is implicated in the control of microfilament dynamics by enhancing the formation of f-actin filaments through interactions with its binding partner profilin (Figure 6) [5].

Calcium transients induced by ApoE

ApoE transiently increases intraneuronal calcium. Müller and colleagues demonstrated that ApoE increases free calcium concentrations in hippocampal neurons, with ApoE4>ApoE3>ApoE2 [6]. This calcium transient is inhibited by agatoxin-IVa, suggesting a P/Q type calcium channel. The ApoE receptor mediating this effect was not determined. In a more recent study Tolar demon-strated that ApoE peptides, or truncated ApoE, also increase calcium concentrations in rat hippocampal neurons [7]. This effect of ApoE was inhib-ited by RAP, suggesting that interaction occurs through an LDL receptor family member.

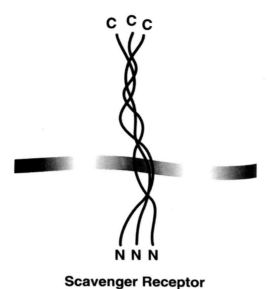

Scavenger Receptor

Figure 7 Class A Scavenger receptor. With permission, from the *Annual Review of Biochemistry*, Volume 63 © 1994 by Annual Reviews www.Annual Reviews.org.

ApoE scavenger receptors

Scavenger receptors of ApoE-containing LDL were initially identified on macrophages and have been extensively studied for their role in the binding and subsequent metabolism of chemically modified LDL particles. Scavenger receptors bind oxidized LDL, acetylated LDL and maleylated LDL, but do not bind native, unmodified LDL. Similar to the LRP receptor described previously, scavenger receptors are multi-ligand receptors. After binding scavenger receptors, these modified LDL particles are subsequently internalized and degraded in lysosomes. These receptors are thought to be critical in the conversion of the macrophage to the cholesterol-laden foam cell and are critical in the pathophysiology of atherosclerosis.

Class A scavenger receptors

Class A scavenger receptors are homotrimeric proteins (Figure 7), with six functional domains: an N-terminus cytoplasmic domain, a single transmembrane-spanning domain, a spacer domain, an α-helical coiled coil domain, a collagen-like repeat and a cysteine-rich domain (found on one type of scavenger receptor) [8].

Class B scavenger receptor SR-B1

In contrast to the Class A scavenger receptors, which contain a charged collagenous receptor domain, Class B receptors are a more heterogeneous

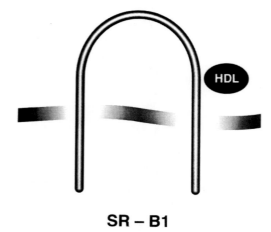

SR – B1

Figure 8 The SR-BI receptor. Modified from High-density lipoprotein receptors, binding proteins, and ligands by Noel H. Fidge. J. Lipid Res. **40**, 187–201, 1999. © (1999) Lipid Research Inc.

group of receptors containing an immunodominant ligand binding domain. The dominant ligand for this class of receptors is the high-density lipoprotein particle (HDL) which does not contain ApoE. However, one of these receptors, SR-B1, also binds both LDL and modified LDL, which contain ApoE. SR-B1 appears to have both its N- and C- termini in the cytoplasm (Figure 8) [9]. The SR-B1 receptor appears concentrated in the caveoli of the plasma membrane and co-purifies with caveolin. Although SR-B1 binds HDL and LDL, and internalizes cholesterol, the apolipoproteins themselves are not internalized. This observation generates the hypothesis that this receptor is involved in the non-endocytotic internalization of cholesterol esters, and also in reverse cholesterol transport.

Lectin-like oxidized-LDL receptor (LOX-1)

LOX-1 is another receptor for oxidized LDL. Unlike the Class A receptors described above, which are found primarily on macrophages, LOX-1 is highly expressed in endothelial cells and in the brain [10]. The *LOX-1* gene is closely related to C-type lectin receptor genes expressed in natural killer cells, and the receptor proteins share common structural and functional motifs.

Conclusion

Although ApoE has been extensively studied for its role in cholesterol metabolism through its ability to bind phospholipid particles, and is a ligand for cell-surface receptors which undergo endocytosis, ApoE metabolism is far more complex. Of relevance to roles in the central nervous system, ApoE binds other molecules including growth factors, basement membrane proteins, and the β-amyloid peptide. It is oxidatively modified in the central nervous system, altering the complement of cell-surface receptors it recognizes and binds. ApoE receptors are involved not only in conventional endocytotic shuttling, but also directly mediate an expanding repertoire of transduction pathways. Intriguing hypotheses of the role of the various ApoE isoforms in the variable risk of AD can be developed, and tested, for each of these receptor-mediated transduction pathways.

References

1. Brown, M.S., Herz, J. and Goldstein, L. (1997) *Nature (London)* **388**, 629–630
2. Herz, J. (1993) *Curr. Opin. Lipidol.* **4**, 107–113
3. Trommsdorff, M., Borg, J.-P., Margolis, B. and Herz, J. (1998) *J. Biol. Chem.* **273**, 33556–33560
4. Homayouni, R., Rice, D.S., Sheldon, M. and Curran, T. (1999) *J. Neurosci.* **19**, 7507–7515
5. Gertler, F.B., Niebuhr, K., Reinhard, M., Wehland, J. and Soriano, P. (1996) *Cell* **87**, 227–239
6. Müller, S., Meske, V., Berlin, K., Scharnagi, H., März, W. and Ohm, T.G. (1998) *Brain Pathol.* **8**, 641–653
7. Tolar, M., Keller, J.N., Chan, S., Mattson, M.P., Marques, M.A. and Crutcher, K.A. (1999) *J. Neurosci.* **19**, 7100–7110
8. Krieger, M. and Herz, J. (1994) *Annu. Rev. Biochem.* **63**, 601–637
9. Fidge, H.H. (1999) *J. Lipid Res.* **40**, 187–201
10. Yamanaka, S., Zhang, X.-Y., Miura, K., Kim, S. and Iwao, H. (1998) *Genomics* **54**, 191–199

Biochem. Soc. Symp. **67**, 111–120
(Printed in Great Britain)

11

Apolipoprotein E gene and Alzheimer's disease: is tau the link?

Simon Lovestone[1], Brian Anderton, Joanna Betts, Rejith Dayanandan, Graham Gibb, Cecilia Ljungberg and Janice Pearce

Department of Neuroscience, Institute of Psychiatry, King's College London, De Crespigny Park, London SE5 8AF, U.K.

Abstract

The finding that *APOE* (the gene encoding apolipoprotein E) polymorphic variation was associated with an altered risk of developing Alzheimer's disease (AD) was a significant advance and immediately prompted a search for the mechanisms responsible for this alteration. Some 6 years later, a number of different hypotheses remain that might account for this influence on pathogenesis with no single mechanism being unequivocally accepted. The different approaches to understanding these mechanisms can be broadly categorized as: those suggesting a remote effect, such as different rates of vascular risk factors in those with the different APOE alleles; those proposing altered neuronal vulnerability, perhaps due to apolipoprotein E (ApoE)-isoform-specific differences in local cholesterol transport; and those hypotheses postulating an ApoE interaction with the two key lesions of AD, plaques and tangles. In this chapter we will review the evidence for and against an interaction between ApoE and the neuronal cytoskeleton, in particular with the microtubule-associated protein tau.

Introduction

The first proposal that such an interaction might underlie the observed association came soon after the association was first reported when it was shown that apolipoprotein E (ApoE)3, in contrast to ApoE4, bound to tau avidly *in vitro* [1]. Subsequently it was shown that another microtubule-associ-

---

[1]To whom correspondence should be addressed.

ated protein MAP2c also bound ApoE, again with a similar isoform-specific affinity [2]. These findings led to the hypothesis that the strong binding of ApoE3 to tau would reduce the amount of tau available for phosphorylation [3]. As reviewed elsewhere, in Alzheimer's disease (AD), highly phosphory-lated tau aggregates in neurofibrillary tangles (NFTs); this phosphorylation reduces the ability of tau to bind to, and hence stabilize, microtubules. If, there-fore, ApoE3 reduced the degree of phosphorylation of tau even by a modest amount, then, over an extended period, this might increase the stability of microtubules and reduce the availability of tau for self-aggregation into paired helical filaments. Hence a hypothesis was born.

Evidence from neuropathology

Refuting this hypothesis has not proved easy. A number of studies have attempted to correlate the pathological lesions of AD with the *APOE* genotype in the hope that an association between an APOE allele and one particular pathological lesion would suggest a mechanistic link. However the data is far from consistent and the results correspondingly inconclusive. With respect to cytoskeletal pathology, increased NFT pathology has been correlated in late-onset AD with possession of the APOE ε4 allele [4,5], although in both of these studies there was a similar association with amyloid pathology. In a single early-onset, chromosome 14-linked family it did appear that the pathological features varied between individuals with different *APOE* genotypes. An APOE ε3 homozygote, for example, had a high amyloid load, whereas tau-related pathologies – NFTs and neuritic plaques – were greater in the individual with an APOE ε4 allele [6]. Other studies fail to find any association between NFT pathology and AD [7–10]. Studies of intraneuronal ApoE have also been inconsistent: one study suggested that intraneuronal ApoE occurs following cytoskeletal pathology [11] whereas another found intraneuronal ApoE pre-ceding tau pathology [12], although in this latter study there was a correlation between the distribution of ApoE immunoreactivity and tau pathology in the more advanced stages of the disease.

In AD, the levels of tau increase in the cerebrospinal fluid (CSF); a possi-ble biological marker and potential diagnostic test [13]. This increase in tau protein correlates positively with the number of APOE ε4 alleles [14–16]. These results have received varying interpretation. Most commonly, the find-ing is assumed to represent accelerated neurodegeneration in individuals with APOE ε4, and hence more tau in the CSF. However longitudinal studies do not support the contention that there is an accelerated neurological decline in individuals with APOE ε4 [17] and, as Golombowski and colleagues [14] point out, the correlation may represent increased binding of tau to ApoE3 in the CSF.

An alternative approach using neuropathological data is to compare dis-orders which do and do not present with cytoskeletal pathology. Vascular dementia, a dementia without cytoskeletal pathology, has been reported to be associated with *APOE* variation in some studies [18–22] but not in others [23,24]. However, vascular dementia generally occurs as a mixed disorder which may make it meaningless to compare subjects with clinically diagnosed AD to those with clinically diagnosed vascular dementia since most of these subjects will have some evidence of AD pathology *post mortem* whether the primary post-mortem diagnosis agrees or not with the clinical diagnosis [25]. Even in post-mortem studies, the diagnosis matters less than the presence and degree of the different pathologies. In our clinical series using strict clinical criteria for vascular dementia, we found allele frequency for APOE2 and 4 in vascular dementia to be the same as that for the controls but different from that for AD; we aimed to repeat this in a post-mortem confirmed study of 'pure' vascular dementia but were unable to find sufficient cases from a large brain bank.

For dementias with tau pathology, Guamanian amyotrophic lateral sclerosis Parkinsonism dementia complex provides some evidence for an interaction between ApoE and cytoskeletal pathology. This disorder is characterized by the presence of NFTs in the relative absence of amyloid. The putative neuroprotective allele APOE ε2 is decreased in this condition and those few cases examined with plaques did not have any APOE ε4 alleles, as would be expected if APOE ε4 enhances amyloid deposition [26]. Another group of disorders with neuronal cytoskeletal pathology, the frontotemporal dementias, show an age-of-onset effect for *APOE* in some studies [27,28], although once again, other studies have failed to confirm this finding [29,30]. These attempts to correlate *APOE* with pathology have reached their nemesis in dementia with Lewy bodies (DLB). In groups of subjects diagnosed clinically, it is clear that the *APOE* frequency is higher than in controls [31–33]. However, as for vascular dementia most cases have co-existing AD. Three studies have examined cases of DLB without co-existing AD, two with biochemical confirmation of the absence of highly phosphorylated tau. These cases are rare and the studies are small. One study found an increase of APOE ε4 in these AD-free DLB cases [34], another found no increase in APOE ε4 in PHF-tau-free DLB cases [35] and a third showed an increase in APOE ε4 in AD-free DLB cases with neuritic degeneration [36]. Such studies with precise definition and even quantification of pathology may be necessary but may be difficult to pursue for DLB because the condition, in pure form, is rare.

These neuropathological studies of diverse conditions have been comprehensive but ultimately inconclusive as to whether *APOE* influences either NFTs or other neuropathological lesions in AD. Observational studies such as these have been compounded by problems of diagnostic criteria, differences between the level of severity of subjects between studies and, importantly, by mixed disease.

The effects of ApoE on neuronal morphology in culture

The most convincing evidence that ApoE might alter neuronal cytoskeletal properties came from Nathan and colleagues [37] who demonstrated that purified human ApoE3 increased neuritic extension and decreased branching in rabbit dorsal root ganglions whilst ApoE4 decreased both extension and branching. It is possible that such changes in morphology might be due to an interaction between ApoE and the matrix on which neurons are cultured [38]; however, it was subsequently shown that in a neuroblastoma cell line, ApoE4 induced microtubule collapse alongside neurite morphology changes [39]. In a human neuronal-like cell line this effect of ApoE was blocked by antibodies to the low-density lipoprotein receptor-related protein (LRP) [40]; and in a mouse neuroblastoma cell line stably expressing human ApoE isoforms, the addition of lipid to the culture medium was a necessary prerequisite to obtaining an isoform differential effect on neurite outgrowth [41]. Together, these data suggest that ApoE4 induces microtubule collapse or that ApoE3 protects microtubules (the two are not mutually incompatible), and that this effect is mediated via ApoE bound to lipid taken up into the cell via LRP. It is possible that the effects on neurite outgrowth might be mediated by extracellular mechanisms as in other experiments. ApoE3 was found to induce neurite outgrowth in the absence of addition of lipids [42], although in this model ApoE was expressed at very high levels. Neurons grown on astrocytes from transgenic mice expressing only human ApoE isoforms showed longer neurites when cultured on ApoE3-expressing astrocytes than when grown in the presence of ApoE4 astrocytes or knockout astrocytes, an effect mediated through LRP [43].

The effects of ApoE on microtubules and associated proteins *in vitro*

These data indicate that there is an ApoE isoform-specific effect on neurite outgrowth and microtubule stability in cells. *In vitro*, ApoE accelerates microtubule assembly in a specific manner but without isoform differences [44]. The mechanism whereby ApoE exerts not only a specific but isoform-different effect on microtubules remains uncertain. Since ApoE binds to tau but does not bind to tau phosphorylated at certain sites [45], we have examined the ability of ApoE to regulate, or at least interfere with, the phosphorylation of tau. The microtubule-binding properties of tau are regulated, to a large part, by phosphorylation [46] and in turn tau phosphorylation is regulated by a number of different kinases and phosphatases. We, and others, have previously demonstrated that glycogen synthase kinase-3β (GSK-3β) phosphorylates tau *in vitro* in cells and in so doing alters its microtubule-stabilizing properties [47–49].

We have therefore addressed whether ApoE alters the ability of GSK-3β to phosphorylate tau using mass spectrometry. Tau was phosphorylated *in vitro* by GSK-3β in the absence or presence of ApoE2, ApoE3 or ApoE4. Phosphopeptide maps were analysed and most spots identified by mass spectrometry. We have found that the overall migration patterns of phosphopeptide spots were very similar on the two-dimensional maps of tau alone, of tau with ApoE3 and of tau with ApoE4. When ApoE2 was present a further four spots were evident. Of the 15 peptides phosphorylated in the presence or absence of ApoE, subtle yet consistent differences, some isoform specific, in the relative amounts of phosphorylation were observed. Ser^{262} was consistently more phosphorylated in the presence of any ApoE isoform. Compared to either ApoE2 or ApoE3, ApoE4 resulted in less phosphorylation of Thr^{231} but more of Thr^{212} and of a peptide containing both Thr^{231} and Ser^{235}. Control proteins did not alter the phosphorylation of tau indicating that these changes in tau phosphorylation are not only ApoE-isoform different but also ApoE-protein specific. Flaherty and colleagues have also examined the phosphorylation of tau *in vitro* using bovine microtubule fractions [50]. This study also found a specific phosphorylation change in tau induced by ApoE but not by ApoA. No isoform differences were observed in line with our mass spectrometry results, demonstrating that such isoform specificity is subtle and unlikely to be identified by western blotting.

Can ApoE alter tau phosphorylation in cells?

The finding that ApoE can alter the phosphorylation of tau by GSK-3 is in line with the findings that ApoE4 destabilizes and ApoE3 protects the microtubule network in cells. Two studies have examined the ability of ApoE to alter the phosphorylation of tau in cells. We found no change in phosphorylation in COS cells expressing both tau and the low-density lipoprotein (LDL) receptor when incubated with CSF [51] and Caillet-Boudin and colleagues [52] found no difference in tau phosphorylation when they compared different neuroblastoma cell lines which express different ApoE isoforms. However, both of these studies used western blotting at restricted epitopes and it is clear from our *in vitro* experiments that if there is any change in tau phosphorylation it is subtle and may not affect some of the epitopes examined in these studies. In mice, the absence of ApoE has been found to result in increased tau phosphorylation in one study but not in another [53,54]. If ApoE does alter tau phosphorylation it must do so either through a signalling mechanism or through a direct interaction with tau, in which case ApoE must be present in the same compartment of the cell as tau. Some evidence may suggest that signalling to GSK-3 is possibly the way ApoE alters phosphorylation of tau. For example, ApoE isoforms induce a differential increase in intracellular calcium [55] and transient increases in intracellular calcium induce tau phosphorylation, a process that can be inhibited by the GSK-3 inhibitor lithium [56].

However, our data indicate that it would be possible for ApoE to have a direct effect on the phosphorylation of tau by GSK-3 if tau was in the same compartment as ApoE. Whether ApoE is expressed by neurons is not clear. *In situ* hybridization studies suggested that the ApoE message was restricted to astrocytes [57–59]. If this is the case then in order to reach tau, ApoE must bind to one or more of its many receptors, be taken up into the endosomal/lysosomal system and from there escape to the cytoplasm. Although surprising, such mechanisms of 'reverse trafficking' of peptides do occur – a fact first recognized from study of bacterial protein toxins that are endocytosed and have been shown to pass through the Golgi to the endoplasmic reticulum and from there to the cytosol [60,61]. Immunocytochemical and electron microscopy studies of human neurons do indicate that ApoE reaches an intracellular and cytosolic location [12,62,63]. However, it remains uncertain whether this ApoE has been taken up by the cell or is expressed in the cell, as some recent evidence suggests that human-specific elements of that ApoE promoter induce neuronal expression of ApoE [64]. In order to examine whether ApoE can be taken up by cells and distributed to the cytoplasm, we expressed the LDL receptor in a non-neuronal cell line and exposed the cells to CSF from APOE ε3 or APOE ε4 homozygous individuals. We found that both isoforms were taken up by cells and remained in a vesicular compartment [51]. More recent work has demonstrated that the majority of these vesicles are in endosomes although some evidence suggests that a small proportion may reach the Golgi. However, when tau is present in the cells ApoE3, but not ApoE4, appeared to have a different distribution appearing diffuse or even co-localizing with tau [51]. An identical observation – that ApoE3 but not ApoE4 distributes to cytosol in tau-expressing cells – was also reported using an entirely different system by Bellosta and colleagues [41].

In an important recent challenge to these findings DeMattos and colleagues [65] generated a construct in which a nuclear localization signal (NLS) was tagged to ApoE. Neuro-2a (neuroblastoma) cells were incubated with lipidated ApoE-NLS derived from transiently transfected cells. This ApoE was taken up into a vesicular compartment as previously observed in other cell models. If ApoE were to escape from this compartment and enter the cytosol then it would be transferred to the nucleus. As nuclear fractions contained no ApoE it was concluded that ApoE remains within the vesicles and does not reach the cytoplasm. The authors also emphasize that previous studies reporting intracellular ApoE have not fully clarified whether the ApoE is truly cytoplasmic. Furthermore, in initial studies, transfection of cells with ApoE3 lacking the normal signal peptide, and therefore cytosolic on expression, resulted in low expression and few clones in attempts to generate cell lines. The authors interpret this as excitotoxicity. However, despite the findings of this important study the cytosolic hypothesis of the mechanism of action of ApoE cannot be entirely rejected. Firstly, the intracellular fate of ApoE is clearly both cell and ApoE-type dependent. We reported that ApoE from CSF remains, even visually, restricted to a vesicular compartment in the absence of tau. It was only when tau was massively overexpressed in COS cells (when the tau becomes one of the major proteins produced by the cell) that a redistribution of ApoE, occurs. Neuro-2a cells, a neuroblastoma cell line, express tau, at relatively low levels. As we found no redistribution of ApoE, even in COS cells expressing low amounts of tau, it is not surprising that DeMattos and colleagues failed to find ApoE entering a cytosolic compartment. Secondly, in ongoing studies we find that the intracellular fate of ApoE is highly dependent upon ApoE type. We have compared different recombinant ApoEs combined with different lipid preparations to CSF and to ApoE derived from different cell lines stably expressing ApoE. It is apparent from these experiments that the fate of recombinant, lipidated ApoE, on incubation with cells expressing the LDL receptor, is entirely different from that of CSF ApoE. ApoE from cell lines is taken up by cells but less effectively than ApoE from CSF. It may be that there are important differences between the entirely physiological ApoE in CSF and the ApoE used in the experiments of DeMattos and colleagues. Finally, the finding that there was a reduced transfection efficiency for ApoE3 directed to the cytosol cannot be accepted as evidence for cell toxicity. Indeed the generation of cell lines stably expressing tau is difficult and neuroblastoma cell lines tend to express low levels of tau (and even less before differentiation). One plausible explanation of these observations is that the expression of tau stabilizes the microtubule network and that, therefore, cell division is inhibited, rendering the generation of stable cell lines expressing high levels of tau difficult. If the cytosolic tau-interaction hypothesis of the ApoE mechanism is correct then this is exactly what would be expected if ApoE3 were expressed in the cytosol of cells expressing some tau – that the tau would be relatively less phosphorylated, that it would be more effective in stabilizing microtubules, that cell division would be inhibited and that, therefore, the generation of high-expressing cell lines would be prevented.

In order to clarify the intracellular localization of tau further we have generated cell lines expressing and secreting ApoE–GFP (green fluorescent protein) and are using a combination of living-cell and co-localization confocal studies to determine the fate of tau after endocytosis. The important question is: does exogenous ApoE enter the cytosol, as suggested by some studies [51,41] but not others [65]. Initial studies suggest that the majority of ApoE taken up following binding to the LDL receptor remains in a vesicular compartment, which co-localization studies suggest is early endosomes. However, treatment of such cells with brefeldin A, which causes a redistribution of the Golgi, demonstrated a change in distribution of ApoE suggesting that a proportion of ApoE might be in this compartment. It may be that the fate of ApoE is dependent upon the expression of neuronal microtubule-associated proteins as it has been demonstrated that tau influences Golgi architecture. For example, in neurons, dispersal of the Golgi apparatus by brefeldin A induces apoptosis, a process dependent upon the phosphorylation state of tau [66]. Lightly phosphorylated tau renders neurons more susceptible to apoptosis and as lightly phosphorylated tau binds microtubules more strongly this suggests that the stable microtubules normally found in neurons result in a highly sensitive Golgi, and indeed Golgi fragmentation is a feature of other neurodegenerative conditions [67,68]. Retrograde transport from endosomes to the trans-Golgi network is inhibited by microtubule-associated proteins [69].

Further work is needed to clarify whether ApoE does indeed pass from endosomes into Golgi, endoplasmic reticulum and thence to the cytosol. However, even if exogenous ApoE does not enter the cytosol, the finding that human ApoE message is present in neurons [64], suggests that a tau–ApoE interaction within the cytosol is plausible. In summary, evidence has accumulated for isoform-specific effects of ApoE in binding to microtubule-associated proteins, influencing neurite outgrowth, inducing microtubule depolymerization and influencing the phosphorylation of tau. The hypothesis first debated soon after the association between AD and *APOE*, that ApoE4 induces or ApoE3 or 2 protect the neuronal cytoskeleton, still stands. The answer to the question regarding whether tau is the link between *APOE* and AD is that it might be.

Work in our laboratory is funded by the Alzheimer's Disease Society, The Wellcome Trust, The Medical Research Council and the European Union. Some aspects of the work reported here were part of a EU funded Biomed II collaboration including the laboratory of Winfried Maerz, Freiburg, Germany.

References

1. Strittmatter, W.J., Saunders, A.M., Goedert, M., Weisgraber, K.H., Dong, L.M., Jakes, R., Huang, D.Y., Pericak-Vance, M., Schmechel, D. and Roses, A.D. (1994) *Proc. Natl. Acad. Sci. U.S.A.* **91**, 11183–11186

2. Huang, D.Y., Goedert, M., Jakes, R., Weisgraber, K.H., Garner, C.C., Saunders, A.M., Pericak-Vance, M.A., Schmechel, D.E., Roses, A.D. and Strittmatter, W.J. (1994) *Neurosci. Lett.* **182**, 55–58

3. Strittmatter, W.J., Weisgraber, K.H., Goedert, M., Saunders, A.M., Huang, D., Corder, E.H., Dong, L.–M., Jakes, R., Alberts, M.J., Gilbert, J.R., et al. (1994) *Exp. Neurol.* **125**, 163–171

4. Ohm, T.G., Kirca, M., Bohl, J., Scharnagl, H., Gross, W. and März, W. (1995) *Neuroscience* **66**, 583–587

5. Nagy, Z., Esiri, M.M., Jobst, K.A., Johnston, C., Litchfield, S., Sim, E. and Smith, A.D. (1995) *Neuroscience* **69**, 757–761

6. Egensperger, R., Kösel, S., Schnabel, R., Mehraein, P. and Graeber, M.B. (1995) *Acta Neuropathol.* **90**, 257–265

7. Gomez-Isla, T., West, H.L., Rebeck, G.W., Harr, S.D., Growdon, J.H., Locascio, J.J., Perls, T.T., Lipsitz, L.A. and Hyman, B.T. (1996) *Ann. Neurol.* **39**, 62–70

8. Zubenko, G.S., Stiffler, S., Stabler, S., Kopp, U., Hughes, H.B., Cohen, B.M. and Moossy, J. (1994) *Am. J. Med. Genet.* **54**, 199–205

9. Mukaetova-Ladinska, E.B., Harrington, C.R., Roth, M. and Wischik, C.M. (1997) *Dementia* **8**, 288–295

10. Salehi, A., Martinez, V.G. and Swaab, D.F. (1998) *Neurobiol. Aging* **19**, 505–510

11. Benzing, W.C. and Mufson, E.J. (1995) *Exp. Neurol.* **132**, 162–171

12. Einstein, G., Patel, V., Bautista, P., Kenna, M., Melone, L., Fader, R., Karson, K., Mann, S., Saunders, A.M., Hulette, C., et al. (1998) *J. Neuropathol. Exp. Neurol.* **57**, 1190–1201

13. Bancher, C., Jellinger, K. and Wichart, I. (1998) *J. Neural Transm.* **105** (Suppl. 53), 185–197

14. Golombowski, S., Müller-Spahn, F., Romig, H., Mendla, K. and Hock, C. (1997) *Neurosci. Lett.* **225**, 213–215

15. Kanai, M., Shizuka, M., Urakami, K., Matsubara, E., Harigaya, Y., Okamoto, K. and Shoji, M. (1999) *Neurosci. Lett.* **267**, 65–68

16. Tapiola, T., Lehtovirta, M., Ramberg, J., Helisalmi, S., Linnaranta, K., Riekkinen, Sr., P. and Soininen, H. (1998) *Neurology* **50**, 169–174

17. Holmes, C., Levy, R., McLoughlin, D.M., Powell, J.F. and Lovestone, S. (1996) *J. Neurol. Neurosurg. Psychiatry* **61**, 580–583

18. Chapman, J., Wang, N.S., Treves, T.A., Korczyn, A.D. and Bornstein, N.M. (1998) *Stroke* **29**, 1401–1404

19. Frisoni, G.B., Calabresi, L., Geroldi, C., Bianchetti, A., D'Acquarica, A.L., Govoni, S., Sirtori, C.R., Trabucchi, M. and Franceschini, G. (1994) *Dementia* **5**, 240–242

20. Helisalmi, S., Linnaranta, K., Lehtovirta, M., Mannermaa, A., Heinonen, O., Ryynänen, M., Riekkinen, Sr., P. and Soininen, H. (1996) *Neurosci. Lett.* **205**, 61–64

21. Ji, Y., Urakami, K., Adachi, Y., Maeda, M., Isoe, K. and Nakashima, K. (1998) *Dementia* **9**, 243–245

22. Marin, D.B., Breuer, B., Marin, M.L., Silverman, J., Schmeidler, J., Greenberg, D., Flynn, S., Mare, M., Lantz, M., Libow, L., et al. (1998) *Atherosclerosis* **140**, 173–180

23. Betard, C., Robitaille, Y., Gee, M., Tiberghien, D., Larrivee, D., Roy, P., Mortimer, J.A. and Gauvreau, D. (1994) *NeuroReport* **5**, 1893–1896

24. Kawamata, J., Tanaka, S., Shimohama, S., Ueda, K. and Kimura, J. (1994) *J. Neurol. Neurosurg. Psychiatry* **57**, 1414–1416

25. Holmes, C., Cairns, N., Lantos, P. and Mann, A. (1999) *Br. J. Psychiatry* **174**, 45–50

26. Buée, L., Pérez-Tur, J., Leveugle, B., Buée-Scherrer, V., Mufson, E.J., Loerzel, A.J., Chartier-Harlin, M.C., Perl, D.P., Delacourte, A. and Hof, P.R. (1996) *Acta Neuropathol.* **91**, 247–253

27. Farrer, L.A., Abraham, C.R., Volicer, L., Foley, E.J., Kowall, N.W., McKee, A.C. and Wells, J.M. (1995) *Exp. Neurol.* **136**, 162–170

28. Minthon, L., Hesse, C., Sjögren, M., Englund, E., Gustafson, L. and Blennow, K. (1997) *Neurosci. Lett.* **226**, 65–67

29. Bird, T.D., Nochlin, D., Poorkaj, P., Cherrier, M., Kaye, J., Payami, H., Peskind, E., Lampe, T.H., Nemens, E., Boyer, P.J. and Schellenberg, G.D. (1999) *Brain* **122**, 741–756

30. Houlden, H., Rizzu, P., Stevens, M., de Knijff, P., van Duijn, C.M., Van Swieten, J.C., Heutink, P., Perez-Tur, J., Thomas, V., Baker, M., et al. (1999) *Neurosci. Lett.* **260**, 193–195

31. Galasko, D., Saitoh, T., Xia, Y., Thal, L.J., Katzman, R., Hill, L.R. and Hansen, L. (1994) *Neurology* **44**, 1950–1951

32. Martinoli, M.G., Trojanowski, J.Q., Schmidt, M.L., Arnold, S.E., Fujiwara, T.M., Lee, V.M.Y., Hurtig, H., Julien, J.P. and Clark, C. (1995) *Acta Neuropathol.* **90**, 239–243

33. St Clair, D., Norrman, J., Perry, R., Yates, C., Wilcock, G. and Brookes, A. (1994) *Neurosci. Lett.* **176**, 45–46

34. Harrington, C.R., Louwagie, J., Rossau, R., Vanmechelen, E., Perry, R.H., Perry, E.K., Xuereb, J.H., Roth, M. and Wischik, C.M. (1994) *Am. J. Pathol.* **145**, 1472–1484

35. Carter, J., Hanger, D. and Lovestone, S. (1996) in *Lewy Body Dementias* (Perry, R., Perry, E.K. and McKeith, I., eds.), Cambridge University Press, Cambridge

36. Lippa, C.F., Smith, T.W., Saunders, A.M., Crook, R., Pulaski Salo, D., Davies, P., Hardy, J., Roses, A.D. and Dickson, D. (1995) *Neurology* **45**, 97–103

37. Nathan, B.P., Bellosta, S., Sanan, D.A., Weisgraber, K.H., Mahley, R.W. and Pitas, R.E. (1994) *Science* **264**, 850–852

38. Huang, D.Y., Weisgraber, K.H., Strittmatter, W.J. and Matthew, W.D. (1995) *Exp. Neurol.* **136**, 251–257

39. Nathan, B.P., Chang, K.C., Bellosta, S., Brisch, E., Ge, N.F., Mahley, R.W. and Pitas, R.E. (1995) *J. Biol. Chem.* **270**, 19791–19799

40. Holtzman, D.M., Pitas, R.E., Kilbridge, J., Nathan, B., Mahley, R.W., Bu, G.J. and Schwartz, A.L. (1995) *Proc. Natl. Acad. Sci. U.S.A.* **92**, 9480–9484

41. Bellosta, S., Nathan, B.P., Orth, M., Dong, L.-M., Mahley, R.W. and Pitas, R.E. (1995) *J. Biol. Chem.* **270**, 27063–27071

42. De Mattos, R.B., Curtiss, L.K. and Williams, D.L. (1998) *J. Biol. Chem.* **273**, 4206–4212

43. Sun, Y., Wu, S., Bu, G., Onifade, M.K., Patel, S.N., LaDu, M.J., Fagan, A.M. and Holtzman, D.M. (1998) *J. Neurosci.* **18**, 3261–3272

44. Scott, B.L., Welch, K., DeSerrano, V., Moss, N.C., Roses, A.D. and Strittmatter, W.J. (1998) *Neurosci. Lett.* **245**, 105–108

45. Huang, D.Y., Weisgraber, K.H., Goedert, M., Saunders, A.M., Roses, A.D. and Strittmatter, W.J. (1995) *Neurosci. Lett.* **192**, 209–212

46. Lovestone, S. and Reynolds, C.H. (1997) *Neuroscience* **78**, 309–324

47. Hanger, D.P., Hughes, K., Woodgett, J.R., Brion, J.-P. and Anderton, B.H. (1992) *Neurosci. Lett.* **147**, 58–62

48. Lovestone, S., Hartley, C.L., Pearce, J. and Anderton, B.H. (1996) *Neuroscience* **73**, 1145–1157

49. Lovestone, S., Reynolds, C.H., Latimer, D., Davis, D.R., Anderton, B.H., Gallo, J.-M., Hanger, D., Mulot, S., Marquardt, B., Stabel, S., Woodgett, J.R. and Miller, C.C.J. (1994) *Curr. Biol.* **4**, 1077–1086

50. Flaherty, D., Lu, Q., Soria, J. and Wood, J.G. (1999) *J. Neurosci. Res.* **56**, 271–274

51. Lovestone, S., Anderton, B.H., Hartley, C., Jensen, T.G. and Jorgensen, A.L. (1996) *NeuroReport* **7**, 1005–1008

52. Caillet-Boudin, M.L., Dupont-Wallois, L., Soulié, C. and Delacourte, A. (1998) *Neurosci. Lett.* **250**, 83–86

53. Genis, I., Gordon, I., Sehayek, E. and Michaelson, D.M. (1995) *Neurosci. Lett.* **199**, 5–8

54. Mercken, L. and Brion, J.P. (1995) *NeuroReport* **6**, 2381–2384

55. Muller, W., Meske, V., Berlin, K., Scharnagl, H., Marz, W. and Ohm, T.G. (1998) *Brain Pathol.* **8**, 641–653

56. Hartigan, J.A. and Johnson, G.V. (1999) *J. Biol. Chem.* **274**, 21395–21401

57. Elshourbagy, N.A., Liao, W.S., Mahley, R.W. and Taylor, J.M. (1985) *Proc. Natl. Acad. Sci. U.S.A.* **82**, 203–207

58. Poirier, J., Hess, M., May, P.C. and Finch, C.E. (1991) *Brain Res. Mol. Brain Res.* **11**, 97–106

59. Nakai, M., Kawamata, T., Taniguchi, T., Maeda, K. and Tanaka, C. (1996) *Neurosci. Lett.* **211**, 41–44

60. Lord, J.M. and Roberts, L.M. (1998) *J. Cell Biol.* **140**, 733–736

61. Johannes, L. and Goud, B. (1998) *Trends Cell Biol.* **8**, 158–162

62. Han, S.-H., Hulette, C., Saunders, A.M., Einstein, G., Pericak-Vance, M., Strittmatter, W.J., Roses, A.D. and Schmechel, D.E. (1994) *Exp. Neurol.* **128**, 13–26

63. Han, S.-H., Einstein, G., Weisgraber, K.H., Strittmatter, W.J., Saunders, A.M., Pericak-Vance, M., Roses, A.D. and Schmechel, D.E. (1994) *J. Neuropathol. Exp. Neurol.* **53**, 535–544

64. Roses, A.D., Gilbert, J., Xu, P.T., Sullivan, P., Popko, B., Burkhart, D.S., Christian-Rothrock, T., Saunders, A.M., Maeda, N. and Schmechel, D.E. (1998) *Neurobiol. Aging* **19** (Suppl.), S53–S58

65. DeMattos, R.B., Thorngate, F.E. and Williams, D.L. (1999) *J. Neurosci.* **19**, 2464–2473

66. Yardin, C., Terro, F., Esclaire, F., Rigaud, M. and Hugon, J. (1998) *Neurosci. Lett.* **250**, 1–4

67. Gonatas, N.K., Stieber, A., Mourelatos, Z., Chen, Y., Gonatas, J.O., Appel, S.H., Hays, A.P., Hickey, W.F. and Hauw, J.J. (1992) *Am. J. Pathol.* **140**, 731–737

68. Gonatas, N.K., Gonatas, J.O. and Stieber, A. (1998) *Histochem. Cell Biol.* **109**, 591–600

69. Itin, C., Ulitzur, N., Muhlbauer, B. and Pfeffer, S.R. (1999) *Mol. Biol. Cell* **10**, 2191–2197

Biochem. Soc. Symp. **67**, 121–129
(Printed in Great Britain)

12

Apolipoprotein E and βA4-amyloid: signals and effects

Thomas G. Ohm[*1], **Ulrike Hamker**[*],
Angel Cedazo-Minguez[†], **Wolfgang Röckl**[*],
Hubert Scharnagl[‡], **Winfried März**[‡], **Richard Cowburn**[†],
Wolfgang Müller[§] and **Volker Meske**[*]

[*]Institute fur Anatomie, University Klinikum Charité, D-10098 Berlin, Germany,
[†]Department of Clinical Neuroscience, Div. Geriatric Medicine, Karolinska, 14186
Huddinge, Sweden, [‡]Department of Clinical Chemistry, Albert-Ludwigs-University,
D-79106 Freiburg, Germany, and [§]Institute of Physiology, University Klinikum
Charité, D-10098 Berlin, Germany

Abstract

In humans, the apolipoprotein E gene (*APOE*) is polymorphic with the alleles APOE ε2, 3 and 4 coding for apolipoproteins (Apo) E2, 3 and 4. Apart from age, the APOE ε4 allele represents the most important risk factor in sporadic Alzheimer's disease (AD). Compared to APOE ε3 homozygotes, the histopathological onset of tau pathology is found 1–2 decades earlier but progresses with the same speed. ApoE dose-dependently and specifically increases free intraneuronal calcium levels in the order ApoE4>ApoE3>ApoE2. This effect is amplified in the presence of βA4-peptide. The ApoE effects on calcium are not affected by the blockade of action potentials with tetrodotoxin, or by inhibition of common ApoE binding sites. The calcium channel involved has been identified as a P/Q-type-like channel. Brain tissue ApoE levels differ with respect to APOE alleles and Braak-stage for Alzheimer-histopathology. The production of ApoE in astrocytes is controlled by several receptor/effector systems such as adrenoceptors and cAMP. In the presence of βA4-peptide fragments, astrocytes stop their synthesis of ApoE resulting in a massive reduction in the bioavailability of ApoE. In the periphery, ApoE directs cholesterol transport and thereby influences its cellular concentrations. In neurons, changes in the concentration of cholesterol influence the phosphorylation status of the microtubule-associated protein tau at sites known to be altered in AD.

[1]To whom correspondence should be addressed.

Introduction

Alois Alzheimer's precedental case description of presenile and progressive dementia in a middle-aged woman initially aroused little interest [1]. Today, it is essential to recognize the disease he described as a source of tremendous social and economic burden for modern industrial society. At the age of 60, the relative risk of having first intraneuronal cytoskeletal changes is 0.5 [2]. Over the age of 65, the relative risk for the disease to present itself with overt clinical signs increases dramatically. At an age of 78 years, the average life expectancy in Germany, the estimates for the prevalence of Alzheimer's disease (AD) range between 10 and 20%. In Alzheimer's time only 5% of German society reached an age over 65; by 2020, this group will represent 30% of the population.

At present, four major proteins have been closely associated with the pathogenesis of AD: β-amyloid precursor protein (APP), the presenilins (PS) 1 and 2, microtubule-associated protein tau and apolipoprotein (Apo)E [3–11]. Though relatively rare, various mutations in the *APP* or *PS* genes are predictive for AD, whereas the different alleles of the APOE polymorphism are differentially related to the risk of developing the disease. The relatively common APOE є4 allele, which codes for the ApoE4 isoform, is associated with an onset of both the clinical features of AD and its histopathology up to 15 years earlier than in non-carriers [12–16]. Although mutations in the *tau* gene itself are yet to be implicated in AD, it may be linked to the cause of other forms of dementia. Moreover, tau retains importance as a central element in the histopathology of AD [8].

The diagnostic hallmarks of fully developed AD are sufficiently high numbers of so-called neurofibrillary tangles and senile plaques [17,18]. The tangles, formed in neurons, are made up of filamentous aggregates of tau, which is otherwise highly soluble [19,20]. In addition to straight filaments, these aggregates also form paired helical filaments (PHFs) [21]. PHF-tau is phosphorylated at several identified motifs [22,23] and can be demarcated selectively with highly sensitive silver stains or with antibodies [24–26], some of which are sensitive to the phosphorylation state of the relevant motifs [27]. Along with the formation of PHF-tau, there is a loss of tau's functional stabilization of microtubules [28]. Consequently, functions of the neuron's structure which depend on microtubules, the transport of synaptic vesicles for example, are disturbed by these changes [29–31]. The resulting disorganization and disintegration of the neuronal cytoskeleton eventually leads to the death of the cell. The degree of synaptic pathology and neuronal loss correlates strongly with changes in the individual's cognitive performance [32,33]. The other histopathological hallmark, the senile plaque, is located in the extracellular space. It consists mainly of βA4-peptide, a 39–43 mer fragment of APP, partly taken from the ectodomain and partly from the transmembrane spanning domain of APP [34,35]. When the Aβ-peptide forms β-sheet aggregates, the resulting βA4-amyloid can be demonstrated with Congo Red or, more specifically, with silver stains or antibodies [25,26,36]. Among various other molecules, ApoE, APP and PS are found co-localized with the Aβ-peptide plaque [37,38]. Around a core of βA4-amyloid, a halo of dystrophic cell processes forms, the 'neuritic' part of a senile plaque. In spite of strong evidence implicating each of these four major molecules in the development of AD, the detailed mechanisms behind these changes remain unresolved.

Although the APOE ε4 allele is not predictive for AD, it represents a major risk as it is found among the vast majority of AD patients. It is present in up to 20–25% of our population [12]. This paper deals with putative mechanisms by which ApoE isoforms might influence neuronal and glial signalling as well as with the possible interactions of ApoE with other molecules relevant to AD such as βA4-peptide and tau.

ApoE's role in cellular metabolism has been mainly studied in non-nervous tissue, i.e. in liver, fibroblasts, smooth muscle cells etc. [39]. Here, ApoE was found to have a major role in directing lipid transport, with its selective interaction with lipid particles and with ApoE receptors guiding these processes [40]. The binding of ApoE to an appropriate receptor induces internalization via clathrin-coated pits, delivery of complexes to the endosome, processing of the complex, return of the receptor to the cell membrane and subsequent routing of the lipids to different intracellular compartments. During this process, ApoE is not found in the cytosol, where tau and microtubules are located. The possession of the APOE ε4 allele is, however, associated with an earlier onset of PHF-tau formation [12,16]. Together, these facts suggest that ApoE isoforms influence tau indirectly rather than through direct interaction of the molecules themselves [41,42]. In addition, PHF-tau is phosphorylated at distinct motifs, possibly indicating that changes in cellular signalling are responsible for its formation, and that ApoE isoforms participate differentially in the process [43,44]. Among the major signalling systems, the cAMP-mediated and the calcium-associated pathways have been shown to be altered early in the development of AD [45–48]. Both second messengers are also known to be involved in the phosphorylation of motifs seen in PHF-tau [49,50].

Following the idea that ApoE might induce or modify intracellular signals [51], the monitoring of free intracellular calcium in cultured, rat primary hippocampal neurons was used to trace ApoE isoform-dependent changes [52]. Recombinant ApoE was applied to fura-2-acetoxymethyl-ester-loaded neurons by adding the respective ApoE isoform to the buffer used to superfuse the neurons in the examination chamber. After a brief incubation time, during which the superfusion flow was stopped, the cells were washed using the same buffer without ApoE. Throughout the whole procedure, the cells were monitored in close-meshed intervals by a calcium imaging system and intracellular free calcium concentrations were determined in the nanomolar range. In order to avoid bias arising from the effects of different ApoE isoforms on putative preconditioning when the same cells were used for testing, the order of application was systematically varied. Cells were always allowed to reach resting levels of free intracellular calcium before subsequent compounds were applied. The analysis of several hundred neurons (as subsequently controlled by microtubule-associated protein 2-immunocytochemistry) showed a clear rank order. Although all three examined isoforms increased the concentration of free intracellular calcium (up to 2.5-fold), the effects were differentially expressed, with

ApoE2<ApoE3<ApoE4. The observed increases in free intraneuronal calcium were dose- and time-dependent. ApoE concentrations as low as 20 nM resulted in measurable, non-permanent changes. Even when the levels of ApoE were maintained for longer periods of time, the neurons consistently returned to normal resting levels of free intracellular calcium after 12 minutes. A blockade of ion channels with tetrodotoxin indicated that the observed effects did not result from action potential activity. Further trials with the calcium chelator EGTA showed that the effects do require extracellular calcium, at least at the beginning of the cellular response. The effects persisted despite the addition of low-density lipoprotein (LDL), activated α_2-macroglobulin, lactoferrin and receptor-associated protein (RAP) to the cells. This argues against the involvement of the typical ApoE binding sites in the observed mechanism.

Of the different types of calcium channels, only the P/Q-type variant was shown to be involved, not the L-type, T-type or N-type channel. Initial attempts were made to identify the putative domain(s) of ApoE that influences this channel. At the same concentration, a synthetic peptide sequence identical to the receptor binding domain of ApoE was shown to have no measurable effect on this channel, as opposed to those attained with recombinant, full-length ApoE. However, attempts to mimic the co-operation of two ApoE molecules by using a repetitive sequence of the binding domain did increase the free intracellular calcium concentration (V. Meske, F. Albert, W. März and T.G. Ohm, unpublished work). It should be noted that the observed changes in free intraneuronal calcium levels were transient and not strong enough to cause cell death. Small but repetitive changes, however, especially those presented as regular oscillations, could produce an additive effect over time, inducing changes not only in cell signalling, but also at the level of gene transcription [53].

Several previous studies have suggested that βA4-peptide induces an increase in free intraneuronal calcium, raising cells' vulnerability to excitotoxicity [54,55]. Interestingly, the effects induced by ApoE isoforms were amplified significantly when ApoE and βA4-peptide were applied together (following joint incubation at 37°C overnight) [52]. The changes remained dependent on the presence of the ApoE isoform. The reversed sequence of βA4-peptide did not show the same amplification effect. In this context, one should keep in mind that ApoE and βA4 are found co-localized in senile plaques surrounding neuronal cell processes, a necessity for any physiological relevance of these mechanisms. Another factor amplifying the effect of ApoE on the concentration of calcium is the activation of G-proteins. Overnight incubation of cells with cholera toxin prior to application of ApoE resulted in a statistically significant increase in the induced changes in calcium levels. Pre-incubations with pertussis toxin have shown no effect as yet (V. Meske, F. Albert and T.G. Ohm, unpublished work).

Since ApoE's alteration of free intracellular calcium levels proved to be dose-dependent [52], differences in the amount of ApoE could play a role in the ApoE-isoform-dependent development of AD [56]. Indeed, standard Western blot analysis of hippocampal tissue blocks of 72 genotyped individuals has shown significantly lower levels of ApoE in APOE ε4 allele carriers as compared to APOE ε3 homozygotic individuals (W. Röckl, M.-A. Bassilikin and T.G. Ohm, unpublished work).

One potential mechanism for the pathology-associated decrease in ApoE protein was tested in a cell culture model. As known from previous studies, ApoE receptors (such as the LDL receptor-related protein) can bind βA4-amyloid and secreted APP [57–60]. The aim, therefore, was to test the hypothesis that, in binding to ApoE-producing astrocytes, βA4-amyloid might stop secretion or production of ApoE. Under control conditions, an ApoE-free medium was enriched over time with astrocyte-derived ApoE. This ApoE was secreted into the medium.

ApoE levels in the medium responded after increases in secretion were induced by stimulation with butyryl-cAMP, isoprenaline, arterenol and 5-hydroxytryptamine. Decreases were also induced, using phorbol esters, carbachol and clonidine (A. Cedazo-Minguez, U. Hamker, R.H. Vek, V. Meske, F. Albert, R.T. Cowburn and T.G. Ohm, unpublished work). The response was time- and dose-dependent, and suggests that the cultured cells were able to regulate ApoE secretion and perhaps ApoE production as well. With the addition of βA4-amyloid, the measurable level (ELISA detection threshold 250 pm ApoE/ml) of ApoE in the conditioned medium was drastically reduced and remained at detection thresholds even after 72 hours (U. Hamker, V. Meske, F. Albert and T.G. Ohm, unpublished work).

The use of various synthetic βA4-fragments (1–11, 1–16, 1–28, 1–38, 1–40, 1–42, 1–43, 10–20, 12–28, 25–35, 22–35 and 40–1) showed that 25–35 mer, 1–38 mer and longer fragments were most effective in triggering the reductions in secretion of ApoE. Interestingly, these fragments are those known to be neurotoxic *in vitro*. Life/death assays, however, showed that none of the tested fragments caused death of astrocytes within 72-hour observation intervals [61]. Control incubations of neurons, in marked contrast, confirmed the toxic potential at the concentrations used. These data argue in favour of the effect resulting from a regulatory mechanism rather than from the toxicity of the substances.

Confocal laser microscope analysis of βA4 and ApoE marked by indirect immunofluorescence showed most of the βA4-amyloid added to the astrocytes to be attached to the outside of the cells. ApoE was seen co-localized with βA4-amyloid particles (U. Hamker, V. Meske, F. Albert and T.G. Ohm, unpublished work). No free ApoE remained, suggesting that all of the pre-existing molecules had been bound to βA4-amyloid. Control cultures showed the normal picture of ApoE-producing cells with ApoE present in the Golgi apparatus and in vesicles. These images suggest that βA4-amyloid, even when not taken up by the cells, can bind all available ApoE secreted by the cell and stop its further synthesis. This interpretation was also supported by metabolic labelling studies. There was no difference observed in the total amount of marked proteins in astrocytes metabolically marked with ^{35}S-methionine when compared with astrocytes treated in the same fashion with the exception of an additional incubation with βA4-amyloid (100 vs 97%). In contrast, immunologically marked radioactive ApoE showed a statistically significant reduction after incubation with synthetic βA4-amyloid (1–40 mer) (100% vs 56%). Use of the reverse sequence of the 40–1 mer peptide of βA4-amyloid did not stop cellular ApoE production. Under these conditions, total labelled protein (100%) was even slightly increased (119%), an effect which was even more pronounced when looking specifically at ApoE (100 vs 147%) (U. Hamker, V. Meske, F. Albert and T.G. Ohm, unpublished work).

The results obtained further support the idea that the bioavailability of ApoE, which is associated with plasticity, is markedly reduced in the presence of βA4-amyloid. The development of AD is influenced by the affected individual's *APOE* genotype; carriers of the APOE ε4 allele begin to develop it much earlier, but progress with similar speed with respect to the formation of PHF-tau [12,16] and to the speed of their clinical deterioration. The mechanism outlined above presents two possibilities. The first is an isoform-specific difference in the production or secretion of ApoE. The second, noting that the basal production and secretion of ApoE is comparable among the various isoform carriers, attributes differences in the interaction of these isoforms with βA4-amyloid with differential influence of the kinetics by which the threshold for 'essential' ApoE levels is reached. Both ideas are supported by other findings. For example, ApoE4 and ApoE3 show different affinity to βA4 [62–65]. Even in hippocampal tissue free of βA4-amyloid, the protein levels of ApoE3 are roughly twice as high as in carriers of at least one APOE ε4 allele (W. Röckl, M.-A. Bassilikin and T.G. Ohm, unpublished work) and there has been a differential cellular accumulation/retention of ApoE with ApoE3>ApoE4 [66].

Until recently, ApoE had been thought to play a more direct role in plaque and tangle formation. The ApoE molecule, at least with respect to the non-neuronal systems studied before now, is known for its transport of lipids, particularly cholesterol. This opens the possibility that not ApoE itself, but rather its role in directing lipid transport, might be decisive for the development of AD. Indirect support for this view comes from observations of young individuals (aged 15–25 years) with a defect in intracellular cholesterol transport who develop severe mental dysfunction and show numerous PHF-tau tangles structurally and immunologically identical to those seen decades later in cases of AD [67–69].

These cases point to the possibility that changes in intracellular cholesterol levels or in the activity of cholesterol-controlled enzymes [70–72] could contribute to the development of the cellular pathology of AD. *In vitro* studies have already shown that a depletion of free cholesterol alters APP processing [73]. Interestingly, when rat primary neurons were cultured in a cholesterol-free medium under 3-hydroxy-3-methylglutaryl-coenzymeA reductase-mediated supression of endogenous cholesterol synthesis, an increase in tau phosphorylation and changes in the intraneuronal distribution of tau were evoked (V. Meske, F. Albert and T.G. Ohm, unpublished work). Under these conditions, the AT8-sensitive epitope was found to be phosphorylated. This epitope was suggested to be the one which is detected as being altered before tau becomes sensitive to silver stains specific for PHF-tau [74]. Since ApoE seems to be important in cell transport of excess cholesterol [75], the different ApoE isoforms could affect those processes to different degrees as well. However, it remains an open question whether cholesterol is the mediator in the AT8-epitope formation. Application of water-soluble cholesterol to neurons cultured in cholesterol-free media containing lovastatin did not prevent the formation of the AT8-sensitive epitope. The addition of mevalonate, by contrast, did so. This might indicate that the pathway is mevalonate rather than cholesterol dependent (V. Meske, F. Albert and T.G. Ohm, unpublished work). Given such a mechanism, the attempts of the neuron to maintain constant levels of cellular cholesterol may influence the activity of the enzymes responsible for its synthesis. As a consequence, differences in mevalonate concentrations might exist where no differences in cholesterol levels can be found. These differences with respect to mevalonate might, in turn, induce changes in geranylgeranyl- and/or farneysl-associated side reactions and lead, ultimately, to kinase activation or phosphatase inhibition.

We thank Christian Heath for critical reading of the manuscript and secretarial help. The studies were supported mainly by the Deutsche Forschungsgemeinschaft (Oh 48/4-2; Oh 48/1-3, SFB507 TPC2) and the EU Biomed-II program (project MICAT).

References

1. Alzheimer, A. (1907) *Allg. Z. Psychiatr. Psych. Gerichtl. Med.* **64**, 146–148
2. Ohm, T.G., Müller, H., Braak, H. and Bohl, J. (1995) *Neuroscience* **64**, 209–217
3. Haass, C., Lemere, C.A., Capell, A., Citron, M., Seubert, P., Schenk, D., Lannfelt, L. and Selkoe, D.J. (1995) *Nat. Med. (N.Y.)* **1**, 1291–1296
4. Hardy, J.A. and Higgins, G.A. (1992) *Science* **256**, 184–185
5. Walter, J., Grunberg, J., Schindzielorz, A. and Haass, C. (1998) *Biochemistry* **37**, 5961–5967
6. Hardy, J.A., Goate, A., Owen, M. and Rossor, M. (1989) *Lancet* **2**, 743
7. Hardy, J. (1997) *Trends Neurosci.* **20**, 154–159
8. Spillantini, M.G. and Goedert, M. (1998) *Trends Neurosci.* **21**, 428–433
9. Mandelkow, E.M. and Mandelkow, E. (1993) *Trends Biochem. Sci.* **18**, 480–483
10. Strittmatter, W.J. and Roses, A.D. (1996) *Ann. Rev. Neurosci.* **19**, 53–77
11. Houlden, H., Crook, R., Duff, K., Hutton, M., Collinge, J., Roques, P., Rossor, M. and Hardy, J. (1995) *Neurosci. Lett.* **188**, 202–204
12. Ohm, T.G., Kirca, M., Bohl, J., Scharnagl, H., Groß, W. and März, W. (1995) *Neuroscience*, **66**, 583–587
13. Corder, E.H., Saunders, A.M., Strittmatter, W.J., Schmechel, D.E., Gaskell, P.C., Rimmler, J.B., Locke, P.A., Conneally, P.M., Schmader, K.E., Tanzi, R.E., et al. (1995) *Neurology* 1323–1328
14. Nagy, Z., Esiri, M.M., Jobst, K.A., Johnston, C., Litchfield, S., Sim, E. and Smith, A.D. (1995) *Neuroscience* **69**, 757–761
15. Roses, A.D. (1994) *J. Neuropathol. Exp. Neurol.* **53**, 429–437
16. Ohm, T.G., Scharnagl, H., März, W. and Bohl, J. (1999) *Acta Neuropathol.* **98**, 273–280
17. Khatchaturian, Z.S. (1985) *Arch Neurol.* **31**, 545–548
18. Tierney, M.C., Fisher, R.H., Lewis, A.J., Zorzitto, M.L., Snow, W.G., Reid, D.W. and Nieuwstraten, P. (1988) *Neurology* **38**, 359–364
19. Hanger, D.P., Brion, J.P., Gallo, J.M., Cairns, N.J., Luthert, P.J. and Anderton, B.H. (1991) *Biochem. J.* **275**, 99–104
20. Lichtenberg, B., Mandelkow, E.M., Hagestedt, T. and Mandelkow, E. (1988) *Nature (London)* **334**, 359–362
21. Goedert, M., Jakes, R., Spillantini, M.G., Hasegawa, M., Smith, M.J. and Crowther, R.A. (1996) *Nature (London)* **383**, 550–553

22.   Goedert, M., Spillantini, M.G., Cairns, N.J. and Crowther, R.A. (1992) *Neuron* **8**, 159–168
23.   Goedert, M., Hasegawa, M., Jakes, R., Lawler, S., Cuenda, A. and Cohen, P. (1997) *FEBS Lett.* **409**, 57–62
24.   Gallyas, F. (1971) *Acta Morphol. Acad. Sci. Hung.* **19**, 1–8
25.   Braak, H., Braak, E., Ohm, T.G. and Bohl, J. (1989) *Neurosci. Lett.* **103**, 24–28
26.   Ohm, T.G., Braak, E. and Braak, H. (1989) *Neural Transm. (P-D Sect)* **1**, 111
27.   Lichtenberg Kraag, B., Mandelkow, E.M., Biernat, J., Steiner, B., Schroter, C., Gustke, N., Meyer, H.E. and Mandelkow, E. (1992) *Proc. Natl. Acad. Sci. U.S.A.* **89**, 5384–5388
28.   Biernat, J., Gustke, N., Drewes, G., Mandelkow, E.M. and Mandelkow, E. (1993) *Neuron* **11**, 153–163
29.   Anderton, B.H., Callahan, L., Coleman, P., Davies, P., Flood, D., Jicha, G.A., Ohm, T. and Weaver, C. (1998) *Progr. Neurobiol.* **55**, 595–610
30.   Praprotnik, D., Smith, M.A., Richey, P.L., Vinters, H.V. and Perry, G. (1996) *Acta Neuropathol.* 226–235
31.   Drewes, G., Trinczek, B., Illenberger, S., Biernat, J., Schmitt Ulms, G., Meyer, H.E., Mandelkow, E.M. and Mandelkow, E. (1995) *J. Biol. Chem.* **270**, 7679–7688
32.   Bancher, C., Braak, H., Fischer, P. and Jellinger, K.A. (1993) *Neurosci. Lett.* **162**, 179–182
33.   Terry, R.D., Masliah, E., Salmon, D.P., Butters, N., DeTeresa, R., Hill, R., Hansen, L.A. and Katzman, R. (1991) *Ann. Neurol.* **30**, 572–580
34.   Kang, J., Lemaire, H.G., Unterbeck,A., Salbaum, J.M., Masters, C.L., Grzeschik, K.H., Multhaup, G., Beyreuther, K. and Muller Hill, B. (1987) *Nature (London)* **325**, 733–736
35.   Beyreuther, K. and Masters, C.L. (1997) *Nature (London)* **389**, 677–678
36.   Campbell, S., Switzer, R.C. and Martin, T.L. (1987) *Soc. Neurosci. Abstr.* **13**, 678
37.   Abraham, C.R., Selkoe, D.J. and Potter, H. (1988) *Cell* **52**, 487–501
38.   Busciglio, J., Hartmann, H., Lorenzo, A., Wong, C., Baumann, K., Sommer, B., Staufenbiel, M. and Yankner, B.A. (1997) *J. Neurosci.* **17**, 5101–5107
39.   Weisgraber, K.H. (1994) *Adv. Protein Chem.* **45**, 249–302
40.   Mahley, R.W. (1988) *Science* **240**, 622–630
41.   Fleming, L.M., Weisgraber, K.H., Strittmatter, W.J., Troncoso, J.C. and Johnson, G. (1996) *Exp. Neurol.* **138**, 252–260
42.   Wang, X., Luebbe, P., Gruenstein, E. and Zemlan, F. (1998). *J. Neurosci. Res.* **51**, 658–665
43.   Strittmatter, W.J., Weisgraber, K.H., Goedert, M., Saunders, A.M., Huang, D., Corder, E.H., Dong, L.M., Jakes, R., Alberts, M.J., Gilbert, J.R., et al (1994) *Exp. Neurol.* **125**, 163–171
44.   Huang, D.Y., Weisgraber, K.H., Goedert, M., Saunders, A.M., Roses, A.D. and Strittmatter, W.J. (1995) *Neurosci. Lett.* **192**, 209–212
45.   Masliah, E., Cole, G.M., Hansen, L.A., Mallory, M., Albright, T., Terry, R.D. and Saitoh, T. (1991) *J. Neurosci.* **11**, 2759–2767
46.   Kurumatani, T., Fastbom, J., Bonkale, W.L., Bogdanovic, N., Winblad, B., Ohm, T.G. and Cowburn, R.F. (1998) *Brain Res.* **796**, 209–221
47.   Ohm, T.G., Schmitt, M., Bohl, J. and Lemmer, B. (1997) *Neurobiol. Aging* **18**, 275–279
48.   Ohm, T.G., Bohl, J. and Lemmer, B. (1991) *Brain Res.* **540**, 229–236
49.   Litersky, J.M., Johnson, G.V., Jakes, R., Goedert, M., Lee, M. and Seubert, P. (1996) *Biochem. J.*, **316**, 655–660
50.   Zheng Fischhofer, Q., Biernat, J., Mandelkow, E.M., Illenberger, S., Godemann, R. and Mandelkow, E. (1998) *Eur. J. Biochem.* **252**, 542–552
51.   Hartmann, H., Eckert, A. and Müller, W.E. (1994) *Biochem. Biophys. Res. Commun.* **200**, 1185–1192
52.   Müller, W., Meske, V., Berlin, K., Scharnagl, H., März, W. and Ohm, T.G. (1998) *Brain Pathol.* **8**, 641–653
53.   Dolmetsch, R.E., Xu, K. and Lewis, R.S. (1998) *Nature (London)* **392**, 933–936

54. Mattson, M.P., Cheng, B., Davis, D., Bryant, K., Lieberburg, I. and Rydel, R.E. (1992) *J. Neurosci.* **12**, 376–389

55. Cowburn, R.F., Wiehager, B. and Sundstrom, E. (1995) *Neurosci. Lett.* **191**, 31–34

56. Bertrand, P., Poirier, J., Oda, T., Finch, C.E. and Pasinetti, G.M. (1995) *Brain Res. Mol. Brain Res.* **33**, 174–178

57. Guillaume, D., Bertrand, P., Dea, D., Davignon, J. and Poirier, J. (1996) *J. Neurochem.* **66**, 2410–2418

58. Scharnagl, H., Winkler, K., Hüttinger, M., Wittmann, D., Nauck, M., Wieland, H., Gross,W., Ohm, T.G. and März, W. (1996) In *Apolipoprotein E and Alzheimer's Disease* (Roses, A.D., ed.) pp. 136–144, Springer Verlag, Berlin/Heidelberg,

59. Kounnas, M.Z., Moir, R.D., Rebeck, G.W., Bush, A.I., Argraves, W.S., Tanzi, R.E., Hyman, B.T. and Strickland, D.K. (1995) *Cell* **82**, 331–340

60. Scharnagl, H., Tisljar, U., Winkler, K., Hüttinger, M., Nauck, M.A., Groß, W., Wieland,H., Ohm, T.G., and März, W. (1999) *Lab. Invest.* **79**, 1271–1286

61. Meske, V., Hamker, U., Albert, F. and Ohm, T.G. (1998) *Neuroscience* **85**, 1151–1160

62. Strittmatter, W.J., Weisgraber, K.H., Huang, D.Y., Dong, L.M., Salvesen, G.S., Pericak Vance, M., Schmechel, D., Saunders, A.M., Goldgaber, D. and Roses, A.D. (1993) *Proc. Natl. Acad. Sci. U.S.A.* **90**, 8098–8102

63. Aleshkov, S., Abraham, C.R. and Zannis, V.I. (1997) *Biochemistry* **36**, 10571–10580

64. LaDu, M.J., Falduto, M.T., Manelli, A.M., Reardon, C.A., Getz, G.S. and Frail, D.E. (1994) *J. Biol. Chem.* **269**, 23403–23406

65. LaDu, M.J., Pederson, T.M., Frail, D.E., Reardon, C.A., Getz, G.S. and Falduto, M.T. (1996) *J. Biol Chem.* **270**, 9039–9042

66. Ji, Z.S., Pitas, R.E. and Mahley, R.W. (1998) *J. Biol. Chem.* **273**, 13452–13460

67. Auer, I.A., Schmidt, M.L., Lee, V.M., Curry, B., Suzuki, K., Shin, R.W., Pentchev, P.G., Carstea, E.D. and Trojanowski, J.Q. (1995) *Acta Neuropathol.* **90**, 547–551

68. Suzuki, K., Parker, C.C., Pentchev, P.G., Katz, D., Ghetti, B., D'Agostino, A. and Carstea, E.D. (1995) *Acta Neuropathol.* **89**, 227–238

69. Love, S., Bridges, L.R. and Case, C.P. (1995) *Brain* **118**, 119–129

70. Carstea, E.D., Morris, J.A., Coleman, K.G., Loftus, S.K., Zhang, D., Cummings, C., Gu, J., Rosenfeld, M.A., Pavan, W.J., Krizman, D.B., et al. (1997) *Science* **277**, 288–231

71. Liscum, L., Ruggiero, R.M. and Faust, J.R. (1989) *J. Cell Biol.* **108**, 1625–1636

72. Liscum, L. and Munn, N.J. (1999) *Biochim. Biophys. Acta* **1438**, 19–37

73. Simons, M., Keller, P., De Strooper, B., Beyreuther, K., Dotti, C.G. and Simons, K. (1998) *Proc. Natl. Acad. Sci. U.S.A.* **95**, 6460–6464

74. Braak, E., Braak, H. and Mandelkow, E.M. (1994) *Acta Neuropathol.* **87**, 554–567

75. Liscum, L. and Dahl, N.K. (1992) *J. Lipid Res.* **33**, 1239–1254

Biochem. Soc. Symp. **67**, 131–140
(Printed in Great Britain)

13

Regulation of gene expression by muscarinic acetylcholine receptors

Heinz von der Kammer[*][1],[2]**, Cüneyt Demiralay***,

Barbara Andresen*, **Claudia Albrecht***, **Manuel Mayhaus***

and Roger M. Nitsch[*][†]

*Center for Molecular Neurobiology, University of Hamburg, Martinistrasse 51, D-20246 Hamburg, Germany, and †Department of Psychiatry Research, University of Zürich, August-Forel-Strasse 1, CH-8008 Zürich, Switzerland

Abstract

In the brain, muscarinic acetylcholine receptors (mAChRs) are involved in higher cognitive functions including synaptic plasticity and memory. In Alzheimer's disease (AD) patients the cholinergic nervous system is severely damaged. In order to reinforce the cholinergic system, clinical tests were started to use cholinomimetic drugs to treat AD patients. To identify the genes involved in mAChR signalling, we used a differential display approach and found 11 genes that were readily activated by mAChR with 1 hour of activation. These included the transcription factors *Egr-1*, *Egr-2*, *Egr-3*, *c-Jun*, *Jun-D* and *Gos-3*; the growth regulator *hCyr61*; the signalling factors *NGFi-B* (nerve growth factor induced gene-B) and *Etr101*; the unknown gene *Gig-2* (for G-protein-coupled receptor induced gene 2); and the acetylcholinesterase gene (*ACHE*). Our data show that multiple immediate-early genes are under the control of mAChRs, and they suggest that these genes play important roles in coupling receptor stimulation to long-term neuronal responses. The results also suggest a feedback mechanism where up-regulated *ACHE* expression and accelerated breakdown of acetylcholine (ACh) at the cholinergic synapses limits increases in cholinergic transmission. Three hours after m1 mAChR activation a different pattern of gene expression was demonstrated. It included the novel genes *Gig-3* and *Gig-4*, as well as the LIM-only protein LM04. Like *ACHE*, these genes are target genes which may be under the control of the above immediate-early genes. Together, our data show that muscarinic

[1]To whom correspondence should be addressed, at the University of Hamburg.
[2]Present address: EVOTEC Neurosciences GmbH, Schnackenburgallee 114, 22525 Hamburg, Germany.

receptors induce a complex and sustained pattern of gene expression that may be involved in the regulation of cholinergic transmission as well as the control of cellular functions in post-synaptic cholinergic target cells. These results may contribute to a better understanding of the effects and side effects of cholino-mimetic treatment in AD patients.

Introduction

Muscarinic acetylcholine receptors (mAChRs) are members of a super-family of G-protein-coupled, cell-surface receptors [1,2]. Different subtypes of mAChRs include m1 and m3 mAChR, which are preferentially coupled to Gq/G11 proteins. They are present on somatodendritic plasma membranes of large pyramidal neurons throughout the cortex and the hippocampus, as well as on small cholinergic interneurons in the striatum. In contrast, m2 and m4 mAChRs are coupled to the G_i/G_0 proteins, and are predominantly localized to presynaptic terminals and the axons of the large basal forebrain projection neurons that innervate cortical and hippocampal cholinergic target cells. Postsynaptic mAChRs trigger a variety of distinct short-term and intermediate signalling cascades. These include phospholipase D, adenylate cyclase, phos-pholipase A_2, the generation of diacylglycerol, which activates protein kinase C and couples mAChRs to the ERK–MAP-kinase (extracellular signal-related protein kinase–mitogen-activated protein kinase) signalling cascade, activation of endoplasmic reticulum IP_3 receptors and stimulation of ligand-operated cell-surface Ca^{2+} channels, as well as voltage-gated potassium channels [3–10]. mAChRs are also involved in the activity-dependent regulation of the process-ing of the β-amyloid precursor protein (APP) by α-secretase [11–13]. This is associated with reduced generation of β-amyloid (Aβ) peptides [14–16], the principal component of amyloid plaques in Alzheimer's disease (AD) brains [17]. These experimental results together with the pathology of AD brains that show a progressive loss of cholinergic innervation from the basal forebrain to the cerebral cortex, hippocampus and amygdala [18–20], as well as the correla-tion of those changes to the cholinergic system with cognitive decline [21], led to the development of different therapeutic strategies that enhance cholinergic function [22,23]. One of these strategies is to use muscarinic agonists. Cellular responses of mAChRs include the activation of neurite outgrowth, the fine-tuning of membrane potentials and the regulation of mitogenic growth responses in cells that are not terminally differentiated [24]. In the brain, mAChRs are involved in long-term potentiation and synaptic plasticity [25]. Such plastic alterations in neuronal structure and function have been proposed to be associated with rapid and transient transcription of activity-dependent genes [26–29]. In order to identify genes that are regulated by mAChRs, we performed a differential mRNA display (DD) screen with HEK-293 cells stably transfected with m1 mAChR. We show here that several genes repre-senting three functional groups of proteins are readily induced by mAChRs.

Materials and methods

Cell culture experiments, DD, Northern blots, Western blots, mobility shift assays, co-transfections and promoter analysis were carried out as described previously [30,31].

Semiquantitative reverse transcriptase-PCR

HEK-293 cells stably transfected with m1 mAChR were treated with carbachol and 1 hour after stimulation total RNA was prepared using TRIZOL® reagent (Life Technologies, Karlsruhe, Germany) according to the manufacturer's instructions. Equal amounts of RNA (0.2 µg) were transcribed to cDNA in 20 µl reactions containing 20 µM dNTP, 10 µM DTT, 2 µl of Expand™ Reverse Transcriptase (Boehringer Mannheim, Mannheim, Germany), 1 µl of RNase OUT (Life Technologies, Karlsruhe, Germany) and 10 µM oligo-dT oligonucleotide. Reverse transcription was performed for 60 minutes at 42°C with a final denaturation step for 3 minutes at 95°C. Aliquots of 1 µl of the obtained cDNA were each subjected to PCR using primers corresponding to the hydrophilic form of human acetylcholinesterase {AChE; primer 1 = 1522(+), primer 2 = E6/2003(−) [32]} and corresponding to human glyceraldehyde-3-phosphate dehydrogenase (GAPDH; primer 1 = GTCATCAATGG AAATCCCATCACC, primer 2 = TGGCAGGTTTTCTAGACGGCAGG). PCRs were performed employing the corresponding primer (1 µM each), 2.5 mM $MgCl_2$, 100 µM dNTP (Amersham Pharmacia Biotech, Freiburg, Germany), and 0.5 units of Thermoprime Plus DNA polymerase (Advanced Biotechnologies, Hamburg, Germany) in a final volume of 25 µl. PCR cycle conditions were performed as follows: 94°C for 45 seconds, 62°C or 66°C (AChE or GAPDH respectively) for 1 minute and 72°C for 2 minutes. After each third cycle, starting with cycle number 24, one probe from each PCR was removed. DNA was separated by agarose gel electrophoresis and visualized by ethidium bromide staining and UV illumination.

Results and discussion

mAChRs regulate expression of several immediate-early genes

In order to identify genes that are regulated by mAChRs, we developed an mRNA differential display (DD) approach that yielded highly consistent results [30]. A set of 64 distinct random primers was specifically designed to approach a statistically comprehensive analysis of all mRNA species in a defined cell population. One-base anchor primers in combination with several random primers in the modified DD protocol were used in reactions employing total RNA obtained from HEK-293 cells stably expressing m1 mAChRs. By using 81 of 192 possible primer combinations to analyse mRNAs generated in response to 1 hour of m1 mAChR stimulation, we obtained 38 differential PCR products. Twenty-five of these were analysed and revealed 10 distinct immediate-early genes: *Egr-1*, *Egr-2*, *Egr-3*, *NGFi-B*, *Etr101*, *c-Jun*, *Jun-D*, *Gos-3*, and *hCyr61*, as well as the previously unknown gene *Gig-2* (Table 1).

All identified mAChR-inducible genes were immediate-early genes, consistent with the known mAChR-mediated induction of the transcription factor gene families Jun, Fos and Egr [33–41]. A more detailed study of the mAChR-coupled regulation of the Egr family showed that mAChRs can regulate Egr-1, Egr-2, Egr-3 and Egr-4 at the level of transcription, as well as functional protein synthesis [31]. Our data suggest that, among members of the Egr gene family, Egr-1 is the major target of the m1 receptor because competition experiments with Egr-1-specific antibodies almost completely blocked the binding of nuclear extracts to the Egr recognition sequence that is known to interact with all members of the Egr family. The ability of different mAChR subtypes to stimulate Egr-1 expression suggests that similar genes are controlled by ACh both in pre- and post-synaptic neuronal populations. Additional genes induced by m1 mAChR included *NGFi-B*, a transcription activator of the nuclear factor superfamily [42], and *Etr101*, an immediate-early gene with an unknown function [43]. Both genes were also found to be carbachol-inducible in independent studies [36,44,45].

Table 1 Differentially expressed genes induced by m1 mAChR activation.

Data represent numerical results from DD screens for m1 mAChR-inducible genes after 1 and 3 hours of receptor activation. DNA sequencing and data base analysis identified genes and novel gene tags. Verification of regulation of identified genes was done by Northern blot analyses.

Gene product	Protein function	Number of representing DD bands
After 1 hour of m1 mAChR activation		
Egr-1	Transcription factor	4
Egr-2	Transcription factor	1
Egr-3	Transcription factor	3
c-Jun	Transcription factor	3
Gos-3	Transcription factor	1
Jun-D	Transcription factor	1
NGFi-B	Transcription activator	1
Etr101	Unknown function	2
hCyr61	Growth promoter	2
Gig-2	Unknown	1
After 3 hours of m1 mAChR activation		
Egr-1	Transcription factor	2
Gig-3	Unknown	1
LM04	LIM-only protein	1
Gig-4	Unknown	1

mAChRs regulate expression of *hCyr61* and *Gig-2*

hCyr61, an immediate-early gene, is a member of the CCN gene family of *CTGF* (connective tissue growth factor), *Cyr61* and *Nov* that encode secretory signalling factors [46]. Cyr61 binds to integrin $a_v\beta_3$ at the cell surface [47], as well as to heparin-containing components of the extracellular matrix [48]. These interactions promote cell growth, adhesion, proliferation, chemotaxis and migration [49]. As a ligand of the integrin $a_v\beta_3$, Cyr61 induces angiogenesis, neovascularization and tumour growth [50]. By activation of m1 mAChRs, expression of hCyr61 was induced within 15 minutes with a maximum after 1 hour of stimulation [30].

Gig-2, a previously unknown gene, was found to be up-regulated by m1 mAChR within 40 minutes of stimulation, and it attained a maximum within 60–100 minutes of stimulation. Receptor stimulation also triggered Gig-2 expression in presence of cycloheximide, indicating that *Gig-2* is an immediate-early gene, and that receptor-coupled expression was independent of de-novo protein synthesis.

Both mAChR-overexpressing HEK-293 lines and primary cortical neurons responded to receptor stimulation with increased expression of both genes within 15 minutes, attained a maximum after 1 hour with sustained high expression for 4 hours. Increased expression of both hCyr61 and Gig-2 was coupled to mAChRs by protein kinase C, whereas cAMP failed to affect expression. In experiments *in vivo*, the muscarinic agonist pilocarpine strongly induced both hCyr61 and Gig-2 expression in neurons of several, but different, layers of the brain cortex, the hippocampal CA1 region and the putamen.

ACHE is an mAChR-regulated effector gene

Our studies show binding to, and activation of, Egr-promoter sequences followed by the synthesis of functional protein as a result of mAChR stimulation [31]. Egr-1 increases the promoter activity and gene expression of AChE, a serine hydrolase that catalyses the breakdown of ACh. Our data generated by using the AChE gene promoter fused to a luciferase reporter show that stimulation of m1 mAChR specifically increased AChE gene promoter activity [31]. Additional co-transfection experiments with the AChE gene promoter reporter construct together with a cytomegalovirus-driven expression plasmid for Egr-1 showed that overexpression of Egr-1 leads to an increase of transcription from the AChE gene promoter [31]. In order to analyse the transcription rate of AChE after mAChR activation, semiquantitative reverse transcriptase-PCR experiments were performed with m1 HEK-293 cells stimulated by carbachol (Figure 1). By comparison, kinetic PCR experiments with primer combinations for GAPDH as a control revealed that m1 mAChR activation leads to a significant induction of AChE mRNA expression. Moreover, *in vivo* experiments using adult rats that were treated with the cholinergic immuno-toxin 192 IgG-saporin revealed a dramatic decrease of AChE activity in cortex, hippocampus, and in the cholinergic cell bodies in the medial septum [51]. If confirmed for the subcortical cholinergic projection system in the brain, EGR-dependent regulation of AChE transcription may be involved in a receptor-coupled feedback control of cholinergic transmission also in the post-

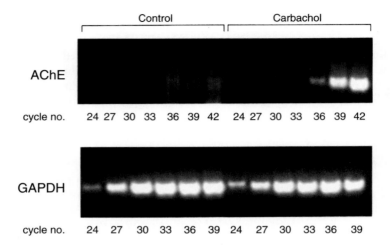

Figure 1 m1 mAChRs increase mRNA expression of AChE in m1 HEK-293 cells. Semiquantitative reverse transcriptase-PCR of total RNA from unstimulated (control) and carbachol-stimulated (1 hour of stimulation) m1 HEK-293 cells. PCR probes were analysed after different PCR cycle numbers. In comparison to the ubiquitously expressed GAPDH gene, AChE transcript was significantly increased after carbachol stimulation.

synaptic neurons. This would be an addition to the classical dogma that AChE is regulated in synaptic terminals of presynaptic neurons.

mAChRs regulate genes for late-response proteins

In order to identify additional mAChR-inducible target genes and late-response genes, we analysed, with DD, m1 HEK-293 cells 3 h after stimulation and identified 23 differential bands with 27 out of 192 possible primer combinations. Five of these revealed four distinct differentially expressed genes: *Egr-1*, *LM04*, and the two previously unknown genes *Gig-3* and *Gig-4* (Table 1). The differential band that corresponded to Egr-1 at this time was less intense than that after 1 hour of receptor activation. In contrast, Gig-4 expression was much stronger after 3 hours of receptor activation as compared to 1 hour (Figure 2). Similar results were revealed analysing time courses of gene expression of Gig-3 and LM04.

mAChRs induce multiple genes

Our studies show that the expression of many distinct genes is under the control of mAChRs. These results generate the hypothesis of mAChR regulation of gene expression (Figure 3). Activation of m1 AChRs induces the expression of two groups of immediate-early genes. These are: transcription factors including the Egr, Jun and Fos families, and early effector genes, including *Cyr61* and *Gig-2*, that are not directly related to transcriptional regulation. The biological functions of early effector genes may be directly involved in such cellular responses as growth, adhesion and plasticity. Transcription fac-

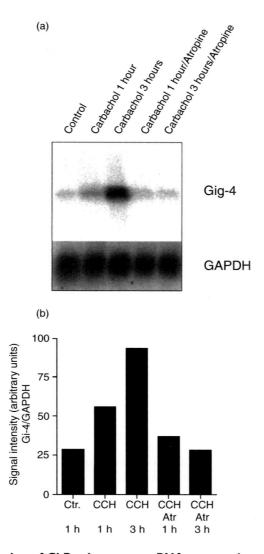

Figure 2 m1 mAChRs increase mRNA expression of Gig-4.
(a) Northern blot analysis of total RNA from unstimulated (control), carbachol-stimulated (hours of stimulation) m1 HEK-293 cells, and cells treated with atropine in parallel to carbachol. As compared to the GAPDH loading control, carbachol stimulation increased message levels of Gig-4 significantly after 3 hours of carbachol stimulation. Exposure time of the Gig-4 blot was 17 hours; exposure time of the GAPDH blot was 3 hours. (b) Quantification of Gig-4 mRNA level normalized with GAPDH mRNA level. Atr, Atropine; CCH, carbachol; Ctr., control.

tors induce a set of target genes that encode late effector proteins including AChE, LM04, Gig-3 and Gig-4. Both early and late effector proteins may act

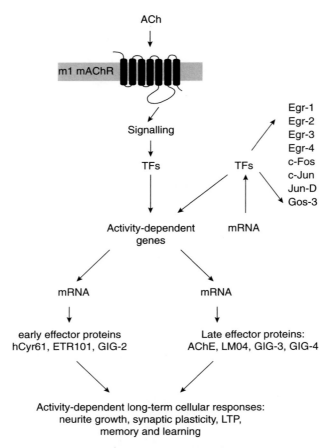

ACh

m1 mAChR

Signalling

TFs   TFs   Egr-1
                                                    Egr-2
                                                    Egr-3
                                                    Egr-4
                                                    c-Fos
                                                    c-Jun
                                                    Jun-D
                                                    Gos-3

Activity-dependent   mRNA
genes

mRNA   mRNA

early effector proteins   Late effector proteins:
hCyr61, ETR101, GIG-2   AChE, LM04, GIG-3, GIG-4

Activity-dependent long-term cellular responses:
neurite growth, synaptic plasticity, LTP,
memory and learning

Figure 3 Proposed regulation of gene expression stimulated by m1 mAChRs. We have shown that m1 mAChRs induce gene expression of transcription factors (TFs), early effector proteins and late effector proteins. The direct influence of these induced molecules to long-term cellular responses is hypothetical and needs to be proven in further studies. LTP, long-term potentiation.

together mediating such activity-dependent long-term cellular responses as neurite growth, synaptic plasticity, long-term potentiation, and memory and learning.

Cholinergic signalling in brains of Alzheimer's disease patients is heavily impaired as a result of the early and massive degeneration of the long basal forebrain projection neurons to brain hippocampus and cortex. In as much as EGR-dependent genes in post-synaptic cholinergic target cells are regulated by mAChR activity, expression of such genes may be decreased in AD. Post-mortem studies are required to test this hypothesis. Drugs designed to activate mAChRs, including AChE inhibitors and m1 agonists currently tested in clinical trials for the treatment of AD, may be expected to stimulate transcription of

Egr genes along with EGR-dependent target genes. *In vivo* studies are required to test whether pharmacological treatments designed to stimulate brain mAChRs increase AChE gene expression, along with AChE enzyme activity, and accelerated breakdown of ACh.

References

1. Bonner, T.I. (1989) *Trends Pharmacol. Sci.* (suppl.) 11–15
2. Wess, J. (1993) *Trends Pharmacol. Sci.* **14**, 308–314
3. Fukuda, K., Higashida, H., Kubo, T., Maeda, A., Akiba, I., Bujo, H., Mishina, M. and Numa, S. (1988) *Nature (London)* **335**, 355–358
4. Felder, C.C., Kanterman, R.Y., Ma, A.L. and Axelrod, J. (1989) *J. Biol. Chem.* **264**, 20356–20362
5. Sandmann, J., Peralta, E.G. and Wurtman, R.J. (1991) *J. Biol. Chem.* **266**, 6031–6034
6. Felder, C.C., Poulter, M.O. and Wess, J. (1992) *Proc. Natl. Acad. Sci. U.S.A.* **89**, 509–513
7. Felder, C.C., MacArthur, L., Ma, A.L., Gusovsky, F. and Kohn, E.C. (1993) *Proc. Natl. Acad. Sci. U.S.A.* **90**, 1706–1710
8. Crespo, P., Xu, N., Simonds, W.F. and Gutkind, J.S. (1994) *Nature (London)* **369**, 418–420
9. van Biesen, T., Hawes, B.E., Raymond, J.R., Luttrell, L.M., Koch, W.J. and Lefkowitz, R.J. (1996) *J. Biol. Chem.* **271**, 1266–1269
10. Lopez-Ilasaca, M., Crespo, P., Pellici, P.G., Gutkind, J.S., and Wetzker, R. (1997) *Science* **275**, 394–397
11. Nitsch, R.M., Slack, B.E., Wurtman, R.J. and Growdon, J.H. (1992) *Science* **258**, 304–307
12. Nitsch, R.M., Farber, S.A., Growdon, J.H. and Wurtman, R.J. (1993) *Proc. Natl. Acad. Sci. U.S.A.* **90**, 5191–5193
13. Farber, S.A., Nitsch, R.M., Schulz, J.G. and Wurtman, R.J. (1995) *J. Neurosci.* **15**, 7442–7451
14. Lee, R.K.K., Wurtman, R.J., Cox, A.J. and Nitsch, R.M. (1995) *Proc. Natl. Acad. Sci. U.S.A.* **92**, 8083–8087
15. Nitsch, R.M., Deng, M., Growdon, J.H. and Wurtman, R.J. (1996) *J. Biol. Chem.* **271**, 4188–4194
16. Nitsch, R.M., Deng, A., Wurtman, R.J. and Growdon, J.H. (1997) *J. Neurochem.* **69**, 704–712
17. Hung, A.Y., Haass, C., Nitsch, R.M., Qiu, W.Q., Citron, M., Wurtman, R.J., Growdon, J.H. and Selkoe, D.J. (1993) J. Biol. Chem. **268**, 22959–22962
18. Coyle, J.T., Price, D.L. and Delong, M.R. (1983) Science **219**, 1184–1190
19. Pearson, R.C.A., Esiri, M.M., Hiorns, R.W., Wilcock, G.K. and Powell, T.P.S. (1985) *Proc. Natl. Acad. Sci. U.S.A.* **82**, 4531–4533
20. Samuel, W., Terry, R.D., DeTeresa, R., Butters, N. and Masliah, E. (1994) *Arch. Neurol.* **51**, 772–778
21. Terry, R.D. and Katzman, R. (1983) *Ann. Neurol.* **14**, 497–506
22. Levey, A.I. (1996) *Proc. Natl. Acad. Sci. U.S.A.* **93**, 13541–13546
23. Ladner, C.J. and Lee, J.M. (1998) *J. Neuropathol. Exp. Neurol.* **57**, 719–731
24. Conklin, B.R., Brann, M.R., Buckley, N.J., Ma, A.L., Bonner, T.I. and Axelrod, J. (1988) *Proc. Natl. Acad. Sci. U.S.A.* **85**, 8698–8702
25. Di Chiara, G., Morelli, M. and Consolo, S. (1994) *Trends Neurosci.* **17**, 228–233
26. Morgan, J.I. and Curran, T. (1991) *Ann. Rev. Neurosci.* **14**, 421–451
27. Abraham, W.C., Mason, S.E., Demmer, J., Williams, J.M., Richardson, C.L., Tate, W.P., Lawlor, P.A. and Dragunow, M. (1993) *Neuroscience* **56**, 717–727
28. Huerta, P.T. and Lisman, J.E. (1993) *Nature (London)* **364**, 723–725
29. Miyashita, Y., Kameyama, M., Hasegawa, I. and Fukushima, T. (1998) *Neurobiol. Learn. Mem.* **70**, 197–211

30. von der Kammer, H., Albrecht, C., Mayhaus, M., Hoffmann, B., Stanke, G. and Nitsch, R.M. (1999) *Nucleic Acids Res.* **27**, 2211–2218
31. von der Kammer, H., Mayhaus, M., Albrecht, C., Enderich, J., Wegner, M. and Nitsch, R.M. (1998) *J. Biol. Chem.* **273**, 14538–14544
32. Karpel, R., Ben Aziz-Aloya, R., Sternfeld, M., Ehrlich, G., Ginzberg, D., Tarroni, P., Clementi, F., Zakut, H. and Soreq, H. (1994) *Exp. Cell Res.* **210**, 268–277
33. Blackshear, P.J., Stumpo, D.J., Huang, J.K., Nemenoff, R.A. and Spach, D.H. (1987) *J. Biol. Chem.* **262**, 7774–7781
34. Trejo, J. and Brown, J.H. (1991) *J. Biol. Chem.* **266**, 7876–7882
35. Ding, W.-Q., Larrson, C. and Alling, C. (1998) *J. Neurochem.* **70**, 1722–1729
36. Altin, J.G., Kujubu, D.A., Raffioni, S., Eveleth, D.D., Herschman, H.R. and Bradshaw, R.A. (1991) *J. Biol. Chem.* **266**, 5401–5406
37. Morita, K. and Wong, D.L. (1996) *J. Neurochem.* **67**, 1344–1351
38. Hughes, P. and Dragunow, M. (1994) *Mol. Brain Res.* **24**, 166–178
39. Ebihara, T. and Saffen, D. (1997) *J. Neurochem.* **68**, 1001–1010
40. Katayama, N., Iwata, E., Sakurai, H., Tsuchiya, T. and Tsuda, M. (1993) *J. Neurochem.* **60**, 902–907
41. Coso, O.A., Chiariello, M., Kalinec, G., Kyriakis, J.M., Woodgett, J. and Gutkind, S. (1995) *J. Biol. Chem.* **270**, 5620–5624
42. Maruyama, K., Tsukada, T., Ohkura, N., Bandoh, S., Hosono, T. and Yamagushi, K. (1998) *Int. J. Oncol.* **12**, 1237–1243
43. Shimizu, N., Ohta, M., Fujiwara, C., Sagara, J., Mochizuki, N., Oda, T. and Utiyama, H. (1991) *J. Biol. Chem.* **266**, 12157–12161
44. Arenander, A.T., de Vellis, J. and Herschman, H.R. (1989) *J. Neurosci. Res.* **24**, 107–114
45. Mittelstadt, P.R. and DeFranco, A.L. (1993) *J. Immunol.* **150**, 4822–4832
46. Bork, P. (1993) *FEBS Lett.* **327**, 125–130
47. Kireeva, M.L., Lam, S.C.T. and Lau, L.F. (1998) *J. Biol. Chem.* **273**, 3090–3096
48. Kireeva, M.L., Latinkic, B.V., Kolesnikova, T.V., Chen, C.-C., Yang, G.P., Abler, A.S. and Lau, L.F. (1997) *Exp. Cell Res.* **233**, 63–77
49. Kireeva, M.L., Mo, F., Yang, G.P. and Lau, L.F. (1996) *Mol. Cell. Biol.* **16**, 1326–1334
50. Babic, A.M., Kireeva, M.L., Kolesnikova, T.V. and Lau, L.F. (1998) *Proc. Natl. Acad. Sci. U.S.A.* **95**, 6355–6360
51. Nitsch, R.M., Rossner, S., Albrecht, C., Mayhaus, M., Enderich, J., Schliebs, R., Wegner, M., Arendt, T. and von der Kammer, H. (1998) *J. Physiol. (Paris)* **92**, 257–264

Biochem. Soc. Symp. **67**, 141–149
(Printed in Great Britain)

14

Oxidative signalling and inflammatory pathways in Alzheimer's disease

Ian Anderson*, Christy Adinolfi†, Susan Doctrow†,

Karl Huffman†, Ken A. Joy‡, Bernard Malfroy†, Peter Soden‡,

H. Tom Rupniak‡ and Julie C. Barnes‡[1]

*Cambridge Antibody Technology Ltd., The Science Park, Melbourn SG8 6JJ, U.K., †Eukarion, Inc., 6F Alfred Circle, Bedford, MA 01739, U.S.A., and ‡Department of Neuroscience, GlaxoWellcome Medicines Research Centre, Gunnel's Wood Road, Stevenage SG1 2NY, U.K.

Abstract

It is well established that inflammation and oxidative stress are key components of the pathology of Alzheimer's disease (AD), but how early in the pathological cascade these processes are involved or which specific molecular components are key, has not been fully elucidated. This paper describes the pharmacological approach to understand the molecular components of inflammation and oxidative stress on the activation of microglial cells and neuronal cell viability. We have shown that activation of microglia with the 42-amino-acid form of the β-amyloid peptide (Aβ42) activates the production of cyclo-oxygenase-2, the inducible form of nitric oxide synthase and tumour necrosis factor-α and there appears to be little interactive feedback between these three mediators. Moreover, we explore the effects of a series of salen-manganese complexes, EUK-8, -134 and -189, which are known to possess both superoxide and catalase activity. These compounds are able to protect cells from insults produced by hydrogen peroxide or peroxynitrite. Moreover, EUK-134 was also able to limit the output of prostaglandin E_2 from activated microglial cells. The mechanisms underlying these effects are discussed. Together, these data support a pivotal role for oxidative stress and inflammation as key mediators of the pathological cascade in AD and provide some ideas about possible therapeutic targets.

[1]To whom correspondence should be addressed.

Introduction

The role of oxidative stress and inflammation in Alzheimer's disease (AD) has been the subject of research in this field for many years and evidence has accumulated to support a critical involvement of both processes in this chronic neurodegenerative condition. Post-mortem studies in the AD brain have revealed consistent evidence of the damaging capabilities of some of the most potent free radical species, which include superoxide, peroxynitrite and the hydroxyl radical [1,2]. A role for inflammation in AD is even more compelling and is supported not only by post-mortem studies [3,4], but also by clinical epidemiology, which shows a reduced incidence of AD in patients prescribed anti-inflammatory drugs [5]. However, one of the major challenges to current research is to assess whether oxidative stress and brain inflammation contribute to the progressive nature of the pathology and clinical presentation of AD, or arise as secondary events, resulting from other more critical pathological processes. If either oxidative stress or brain inflammation prove to contribute substantially to the early pathology and subsequent clinical picture, then there will be a number of associated molecular targets that we can seriously consider as therapeutic strategies.

Considerable evidence exists to support the importance of microglial cells as the macrophages of the brain that mediate the inflammatory response [6,7].

Table 1 Effect of aggregated Aβ42 or LPS on the production of PGE$_2$, NO (measured as total nitrite) and TNF-α in primary rat and NTW8 microglial cells.

Primary rat microglial (PRM) cells were retrieved from mixed cell cultures prepared from cerebral cortex from neonatal (day 1) rats using the method described in [25]. Microglial cells were stimulated with aggregated Aβ42 (30 mM) or LPS (10 ng/ml) in the presence of interferon γ (100 or 10 units/ml, respectively) over 24 hours. Activation of microglial cells was quantified by release of the microglial products, NO (Griess assay), PGE$_2$ (ELISA) and TNF-α (ELISA) into the culture medium. The mean values from four separate experiments (performed in triplicate) and S.E.M. are shown. *$P < 0.05$, **$P < 0.01$ compared to control; Student's unpaired t test.

	PGE$_2$ (ng/ml)	NO$_x^-$ (μM)	TNF-α (ng/ml)
PRM cells			
Control	0.4±0.2	0.2±0.2	0.04±0.02
+ LPS	1.9±0.9*	29±4**	1.3±0.2**
Control	0.4±0.2	0.3±0.1	0.08±0.04
+ Aβ42	1.6±0.6*	29±8**	1±0.2**
NTW8 mouse microglial cell line			
Control	0.1±0.02	0±0.2	0.2±0.2
+ LPS	1.7±0.2**	34±1**	2.0±0.3**
Control	0.15±0.03	0.7±1	0.02±0.02
+ Aβ42	0.5±0.1*	23±3**	0.6±0.1*

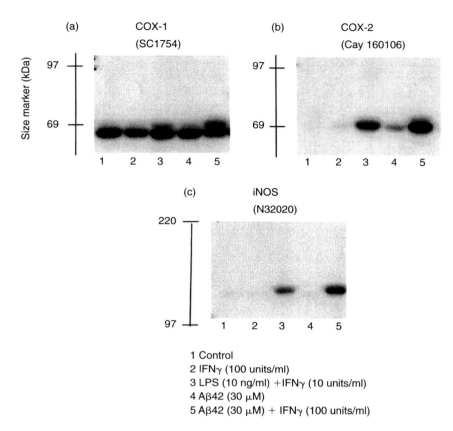

Figure 1 Effect of LPS or aggregated Aβ42 on COX-1, COX-2 and iNOS enzyme levels in NTW8 microglial cells (Western blot analysis). NTW8 cells were treated with Aβ42 (30 μM) or LPS (10 ng/ml) in the presence (100 or 10 units/ml, respectively) or absence of interferon γ (IFNγ). After 24 hour treatment, the cells were lysed in RIPA buffer. Cell lysates (50 μg of protein) were subjected to SDS-PAGE. The primary antibodies used were anti-COX-1 (Santa Cruz SC1754), anti-COX-2 (Cay160106) or anti-iNOS (Transduction Labs N32020).

Microglial cells are highly reactive cells that respond to a variety of stimuli by producing inflammatory mediators, such as tumour necrosis factor-α (TNF-α) and interleukin-1 [8,9]. Moreover, these cells can also produce free radical species, such as superoxide [10] and nitric oxide [11], which can combine to form the highly damaging radical peroxynitrite or, in the case of superoxide, can be converted to the hydroxyl radical by the action of superoxide dismutase (SOD) and the Fenton reaction. Such mediator release can have devastating consequences on neuronal integrity and pharmacological strategies to limit a reinforcing inflammatory cycle are likely to be highly beneficial.

Here, we have used a pharmacological approach to examine mediator release in activated microglia as well as to examine neuroprotective effects of

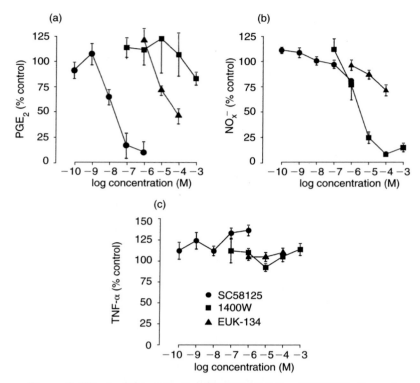

Figure 2 Effect of the selective COX-2 inhibitor SC58125, the selective iNOS inhibitor 1400W, and the SOD/catalase mimetic EUK-134, on the production of PGE$_2$, NO and TNF-α in primary rat microglial cells. Primary rat microglial cells were retrieved from mixed cell cultures prepared from the cerebral cortex of neonatal (day 1) rats using the method described in [25]. Cells were stimulated with LPS (10 ng/ml) and IFNγ (10 units/ml) in the presence of SC58125, 1400W or EUK-134. Activation of microglial cells was quantified by release of the microglial products, NO (Griess assay), PGE$_2$ (ELISA) and TNF-α (ELISA), into the culture medium. The data are expressed as the per cent product released compared to stimulated cells treated with vehicle (control). Values are means ± S.E.M. from 4–5 separate experiments (performed in triplicate).

specific agents. The clinical data with non-steroidal anti-inflammatory drugs (NSAIDs) [5] have triggered considerable interest in the cyclo-oxygenase (COX) enzymes, particularly the inducible form COX-2. Although NSAIDs are known to have actions other than COX inhibition [12,13], our data support a potential role for COX-2 in microglia-mediated brain inflammation. Activation of rat primary microglial cells or NTW8 cells, a microglial cell line [14], by the 42-amino-acid β-amyloid peptide (Aβ42) or lipopolysaccharide (LPS) increases prostaglandin E$_2$ (PGE$_2$), one of the pro-inflammatory products of the COX enzymes (Table 1). Western blot analysis in the NTW8 cells revealed that, whereas COX-1 was expressed constitutively (Figure 1a), activation of the microglia led to an associated increase in the expression of COX-2 (Figure

1b). In both primary microglia (Figure 2a) and NTW8 cells (data not shown, [14]), SC58125, a specific inhibitor of COX-2 [15], produced a concentration-dependent inhibition of PGE_2. These data suggest a critical role for COX-2 in producing pro-inflammatory COX products following microglial activation.

In addition to the production of PGE_2, there was a dramatic increase in the production of nitric oxide (NO) (measured as nitrite) and TNF-α (Table 1). The increase in NO was associated with a significant increase in the expression of the inducible form of the NO synthase (iNOS) enzyme (Figure 1c). Inhibitor studies in primary microglia showed that the increase in NO could be fully inhibited by the selective iNOS inhibitor, 1400W [16] (Figure 2b). Similar results were obtained in the NTW8 cells (data not shown, [14]). Interestingly, inhibition of the COX-2 enzyme failed to alter the production of NO or TNF-α (Figures 2b and 2c), nor did iNOS inhibition modify levels of PGE_2 and TNF-α (Figures 2a and 2c). These data suggest a lack of interactive feed-back between COX-2 and iNOS enzyme products.

To investigate the role of oxidative stress in the secretion of mediators from activated microglia cells as well as on neuronal integrity, we have employed a series of salen–manganese antioxidant complexes which, in cell-free systems, are known to act as SOD and catalase mimetics [17–19]. These compounds have also been shown to exhibit a broad neuroprotective profile both *in vivo* and *in vitro*. For example, in rat hippocampal slices, a prototype compound EUK-8 is protective against damage induced by anoxia/reoxygenation [20] or Aβ [21]. *In vivo*, the compounds prevent: paralysis induced by experimental autoimmune encephalitis [22]; dopaminergic neuronal damage induced by the 1-methyl-4-phenyl-1,2,3,6-tetrahydropyridine (MPTP) or 6-hydroxydopamine [19]; brain infarction in a rat stroke model [23]; and inhibit excitotoxic neuronal death, as well as earlier oxidative damage, in a rat model of temporal lobe epilepsy [24].

Here, we show the ability of these salen–manganese complexes to protect primary neurons, PC12 cells or human fibroblasts from insults mediated directly through specific oxidative insults. Three salen–manganese complexes, with struc-

Table 2 Effect of EUK-8, EUK-134 and EUK-189 on H_2O_2-mediated toxicity to rat primary neurons.

Primary neurons were prepared from embryonic (E18) rat cortex following papain dissociation. Cells were cultured for 24 hours in Neurobasal Medium (Gibco) prior to treatment with H_2O_2 in the presence of 100 μM salen–manganese compounds, at which concentration maximal protection was observed. After 24 hours cell viability was determined by MTT assay (Promega) and the data were expressed as the per cent protection relative to vehicle-treated controls.

Compound	% Neuroprotection
EUK-134	99±1
EUK-189	85±2
EUK-8	44±1

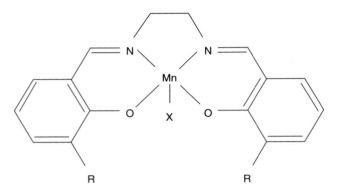

Figure 3 Basic structural template for three salen-manganese complexes. For EUK-8, R = H, X = Cl; EUK-134, R = OCH$_3$, X = Cl; and EUK-189, R = OCH$_2$CH$_3$, X = acetate.

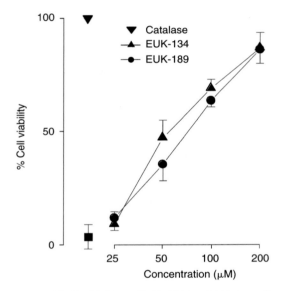

Figure 4 Effect of EUK-134 and EUK-189 on H$_2$O$_2$-mediated toxicity of human dermal fibroblasts. Human dermal fibroblasts were incubated for 18 hours with glucose and glucose oxidase, a H$_2$O$_2$-generating system (■), as well as the indicated concentrations of EUK-134 or EUK-189. Cytotoxicity was assessed using the XTT assay, as described previously [23]. In a standard assay monitoring the conversion of H$_2$O$_2$ to oxygen with a polarographic electrode [23], EUK-134 and EUK-189 had equivalent catalase activities, producing, respectively, 81±2 and 79±3 total nanomoles O$_2$ at an initial rate of 209±23 and 180±7 microM O$_2$/min. By comparison, EUK-8 was a weaker catalase, producing 22±1 total micromoles O$_2$ at an initial rate of 103±9 micromoles O$_2$/min and was inactive in this cytoprotective assay [23]. EUK-189, EUK-134 and EUK-8 showed equivalent SOD activities, assessed as described previously [23].

tures shown in Figure 3, were employed. We have previously reported ([23]; see also legend to Figure 4) that EUK-134 and EUK-8 have equivalent SOD activities, but EUK-134 is a more active catalase. Unlike EUK-8, EUK-134 was capable of protecting skin fibroblasts from enzymically generated H_2O_2-mediated toxicity (Figure 4). EUK-189 has SOD and catalase activities equivalent to those of EUK-134 (see legend to Figure 4) and is equally as effective at protecting cells from enzymically generated H_2O_2 (Figure 4). Similarly, in primary cortical neurons (Table 2), EUK-134 and EUK-189 were also fully protective against H_2O_2 toxicity, whereas EUK-8 was only partially active.

In contrast, when SIN-1 is the toxic agent, EUK-8 displayed a more robust protective effect, which was comparable to that of the other two analogues. SIN-1 is a compound that, by generating NO and superoxide, can lead to the production of peroxynitrite. In both primary cortical neurons (Figure 5a) and PC12 cells (Figure 5b), EUK-8, EUK-134 and EUK-189 were highly protective against SIN-1 toxicity. This observation is consistent with protection in this model being due to superoxide rather than H_2O_2 scavenging activity, although other potential mechanisms such as direct interactions with peroxynitrite may play a role.

In addition, when evaluated against mediator output from activated microglia, EUK-134 was able to partially inhibit PGE_2 produced following LPS stimulation (Figure 2A). Although we do not fully understand the mechanism by which EUK-134 inhibits PGE_2, the failure of EUK-134 to significantly suppress NO or TNF-α production suggests that a nuclear factor κB-mediated mechanism, affecting enzyme expression, is unlikely since nuclear factor-κB appears to be involved in the transcriptional regulation of COX-2, iNOS and TNF-α [26–28]. Moreover, we found no reduction in the amount of COX-2 enzyme expressed (data not shown). A more likely explanation is that the antioxidant is in some way interfering with the activity of this enzyme. COX-2 needs to generate radical species to function and the antioxidant compounds could effectively quench this process. This possibility is being explored.

Conclusions

These data confirm the sensitivity of microglia to respond to exogenous triggers such as Aβ42, by releasing a range of inflammatory mediators including COX products, cytokines and free radical species, for example NO. The data also confirm a role for COX-2 up-regulation in mediating the production of pro-inflammatory prostaglandins by these cells and support the possibility that the clinical data reported for NSAIDs in AD could be mediated through a COX-2-dependent mechanism.

The activity of the salen–manganese complexes to inhibit superoxide- and H_2O_2-mediated toxicity in culture systems concurs with their scavenging potencies in cell-free systems. The greater efficacy of EUK-134 over EUK-8 in an animal model of stroke [23] confirms the critical importance of both SOD and catalase activity *in vivo*. Moreover, the ability of EUK-134 to not only protect neurons, but also prevent protein nitration and reactive-oxygen-species-associated transcriptional activation prior to cell death [24], demon-

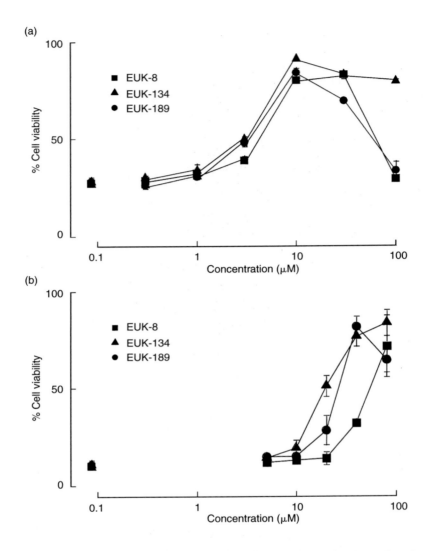

**Figure 5 Effect of EUK-8, EUK-134 and EUK-189 on SIN-1-mediated
toxicity of (a) rat primary neurons and (b) PC12 cells.** Primary neurons
were prepared from embryonic (E18) rat cortex following papain dissociation.
They were then cultured for 24 hours in Neurobasal Medium (Gibco) prior to
treatment with SIN-1 (800 μM) in the presence of EUK-8, 134 or 189. After
24 hours, cell viability was determined by MTT assay (Promega), and the data
were expressed as the per cent cell viability of vehicle-treated control cells.
PC12 cells (ATCC) were grown on collagen-coated multi-well plates in
medium (RPMI-1640; 10% inactivated horse serum, 5% fetal bovine serum, with
1% penicillin and streptomycin and 20 mM Hepes). Cytotoxicity was induced
by incubating cells with medium containing 2.5 mM SIN-1 for 18 hours, as well
as the indicated concentrations of EUK-8, EUK-134, or EUK-189. Cell viability
was assessed using the XTT reagent as described previously [23].

strates the link between an antioxidant effect in the brain and neuroprotection. Finally, the ability of EUK-134 to inhibit PGE_2 production from activated microglial cells suggests that antioxidant therapy may have an advantage over specific anti-inflammatory treatment such as COX-2 inhibitors, by virtue of being able to inhibit a number of processes that involve not only the generation of free radicals but also other potentially destructive inflammatory mediators.

References

1. Smith, M.A., Perry, G., Richey, P.L., Sayre, L.M., Anderson, V.E., Beal, M.F. and Kowall, N. (1996) *Nature (London)* **382**, 120–121
2. Good, P.F., Werner, P., Hsu, A., Olanow, C.W. and Perl, D.P. (1996) *Am. J. Pathol.* **149**, 21–28
3. McGeer, P.L. and McGeer, E.G. (1995) *Brain Res. Rev.* **21**, 195–218
4. Marx, F., Blasko, I., Pavelka, M. and Grubck-Luebenstein, B. (1998) *Exp. Gerontol.* **33**, 871–881
5. Breitner, J.C. (1996) *Neurobiol. Aging* **17**, 789–794
6. Gonzalez-Scarano, F. and Baltuch, G. (1999) *Ann. Rev. Neurosci.* **22**, 219–240
7. McGeer, P.L. and McGeer, E.G. (1999) *J. Leukocyte Biol.* **65**, 409–415
8. Griffin, W.S., Sheng, J.G., Royston, M.C., Gentleman, S.M., McKenzie, J.E., Graham, D.I., Roberts, G.W. and Mrak, R.E. (1998) *Brain Pathol.* **8**, 65–72
9. Benveniste, E.N. (1998) *Cytokine Growth Factor Rev.* **9**, 259–275
10. McDonald, D.R., Brunden, K.R and Landreth, G.E. (1997) *J. Neurosci.* **17**, 2284–2294
11. Meda, L., Cassatella, M.A., Szendrei, G.I., Otvos, Jr, L., Baron, P., Villalba, M., Ferrari, D. and Rossi, F. (1995) *Nature (London)* **374**, 647–650
12. Yin, M.-J., Yamamoto, Y. and Gaynor, R.B. (1998) *Nature (London)* **396**, 77–80
13. Lehmann, J.M., Lenhard, J.M., Oliver, B.B., Ringhold, G.M. and Kliewer, S.A. (1997) *J. Biol. Chem.* **272**, 3406–3410
14. Anderson, I.K., Choudry, S., Waslidge, N. and Rupniak, H.T.R. (1998) *Br. J. Pharmacol.* **120**, 272P
15. Seibert, K., Zhang, Y., Leahy, K., Hauser, S., Masferrer, J., Perkins, W., Lee, L. and Isakson, P. (1994) *Proc. Natl. Acad. Sci. U.S.A.* **91**, 12013–12017
16. Garvey, E.P., Oplinger, J.A., Furfine, E.S., Kiff, R.J., Laslo, F., Whittle, B.J.R. and Knowles, R.G. (1997) *J. Biol. Chem.* **272**, 4959–4963
17. Baudry, M., Etienne, S., Bruce, A., Palucki, M., Jacobsen, E. and Malfroy, B. (1993) *Biochem. Biophys. Res. Commun.* **192**, 964–968
18. Gonzalez, P.K., Zhuang, J., Doctrow, S.R., Malfroy, B., Benson, P.F., Menconi, M.J. and Fink, M.P. (1995) *J. Pharm. Exp. Ther.* **275**, 798–806
19. Doctrow, S.R., Huffman, K., Marcus, C.B., Musleh, W., Bruce, A., Baudry, M. and Malfroy, B. (1996) *Adv. Pharmacol.* **38**, 247–269
20. Musleh, W., Bruce, A., Malfroy, B. and Baudry, M. (1994) *Neuropharmacology* **33**, 929–934
21. Bruce, A.J., Malfroy, B. and Baudry, M. (1996) *Proc. Natl. Acad. Sci. U.S.A.* **93**, 2312–2316
22. Malfroy, B., Doctrow, S.R., Orr, P.L., Tocco, G., Fedoseyeva, E.V. and Benichou, G. (1997) *Cell. Immunol.* **177**, 62–68
23. Baker, K., Bucay Marcus, C., Huffman, K., Kruk, H., Malfroy, B and Doctrow, S.R. (1998) *J. Pharm. Exp. Ther.* **284**, 215–221
24. Rong, Y., Doctrow, S.R., Tocco, G. and Baudry, M. (1999) *Proc. Natl. Acad. Sci. U.S.A.* **96**, 9897–9902
25. Giulian, D. and Baker, T.J. (1986) *J. Neurosci.* **6**, 2163–2178
26. Swantek, J.L., Christerson, L. and Cobb, M.H. (1999) *J. Biol. Chem.* **274**, 11667–11671
27. Marks-Konczalik, J., Chu, S.C. and Moss, J. (1998) *J. Biol. Chem.* **273**, 22201–22208
28. Lukiw, W.J. and Bazan, N.G. (1998) *J. Neurosci. Res.* **53**, 583–592

Biochem. Soc. Symp. **67**, 151–162
(Printed in Great Britain)

15

Perturbed endoplasmic reticulum function, synaptic apoptosis and the pathogenesis of Alzheimer's disease

Mark P. Mattson[1], Devin S. Gary, Sic L. Chan and Wenzhen Duan

Laboratory of Neurosciences, National Institute on Aging, Gerontology Research Centre, 5600 Nathan Shock Drive, Baltimore, MD 21224, U.S.A.

Abstract

Endoplasmic reticulum (ER) appears to be a focal point for alterations that result in neuronal dysfunction and death in Alzheimer's disease (AD). Aberrant proteolytic processing and/or trafficking of the β-amyloid precursor protein (APP) in ER may promote neuronal degeneration by increasing the levels of the neurotoxic forms of β-amyloid (Aβ) and by decreasing the levels of the neuroprotective secreted form of APP (sAPPα).

Some cases of AD are caused by mutations in the genes encoding presenilin 1 (PS1). When expressed in cultured neuronal cells and transgenic mice, PS1 mutations cause abnormalities in ER calcium homoeostasis, enhancing the calcium responses to stimuli that activate IP_3- and ryanodine-sensitive ER calcium pools. Two major consequences of this disrupted ER calcium regulation are altered proteolytic processing of APP and increased vulnerability of neurons to apoptosis and excitotoxicity. The impact of PS1 mutations and aberrant APP processing is particularly great in synaptic terminals. Perturbed synaptic calcium homoeostasis promotes activation of apoptotic cascades involving production of Par-4 (prostate apoptosis response-4), mitochondrial dysfunction and caspase activation. Aβ42 (the 42-amino-acid form of Aβ) induces membrane lipid peroxidation in synapses and dendrites resulting in impairment of membrane ion-motive ATPases and glucose and glutamate transporters. This disrupts synaptic ion and energy homoeostasis thereby promoting synaptic degeneration. In contrast, sAPPα activates signalling pathways that protect

[1]To whom correspondence shold be addressed.

synapses against excitotoxicity and apoptosis. In the more common sporadic forms of AD, the initiating causes of the neurodegenerative cascade are less well defined, but probably involve increased levels of oxidative stress and impaired energy metabolism. Such alterations have been shown to disrupt neuronal calcium homoeostasis in experimental models, and may therefore feed into the same neurodegenerative cascade initiated by mutations in presenilins and APP. Perturbed synaptic ER calcium homoeostasis and consequent alterations in APP processing appear to be pivotal events in both sporadic and familial forms of AD.

Introduction

Alzheimer's disease (AD) is characterized by degeneration of synapses, neuronal death and associated deposition of β-amyloid (Aβ). Prior to the identification of AD-linked mutations in APP and presenilins, considerable evidence had accumulated that supported important roles for perturbed neuronal calcium homoeostasis and increased levels of oxidative stress in the pathogenesis of AD [1–5]. It also became evident that degeneration of synapses was strongly correlated with dementia in AD patients [6,7]. The identification of mutations in APP and the presenilins which cause early-onset inherited forms of AD has dramatically accelerated the process of determining the specific sequence of events that results in neuronal degeneration in AD. Studies of cultured cell lines and transgenic mice expressing APP and PS1 mutations have begun to delineate the molecular, biochemical and cell biological underpinnings of the neurodegenerative process in AD. This chapter describes recent findings originating from such studies, focusing on the alterations in endoplasmic reticulum (ER) function that appear to be the pivotal events that disrupt synaptic function and promote synapse degeneration and ultimately neuronal death in AD.

How do β-amyloid precursor protein (APP) mutations promote synaptic dysfunction and degeneration?

The gene encoding APP was the first to be identified as a locus for mutations that cause autosomal-dominant inherited AD [8]. Several different mutations have been identified. One mutation involves a single amino acid substitution located just N-terminal to the Aβ sequence, another mutation involves a two-residue change located just C-terminal to the Aβ sequence, and a third mutation involves a single amino acid change within the Aβ sequence. One consequence of these APP mutations is that they result in increased production of Aβ, particularly Aβ42 (the 42-amino-acid form of Aβ). Since Aβ has been shown to be neurotoxic, and to increase neuronal vulnerability to apoptosis and excitotoxicity, it has been proposed that the increase in Aβ production is the key alteration that leads to amyloid deposition and neuronal degeneration in patients with APP mutations [9]. The mechanism whereby Aβ damages neurons involves induction of membrane lipid peroxidation, which results in impairment of membrane ion-motive ATPases and glucose and gluta-mate transporters. This, in turn, promotes membrane depolarization and cellular energy depletion, and thereby renders neurons vulnerable to excitotox-icity and apoptosis [3,5,10–12].

APP is synthesized and glycosylated in the ER and is then 'sorted' to the plasma membrane, where it forms an integral membrane protein with one membrane-spanning domain [9]. An intriguing feature of APP is that it is enzymically cleaved in response to neuronal activity (depolarization and acti-vation of receptors is linked to phospholipase C activation) by a yet-to-be identified enzyme activity called α-secretase. The cleavage releases a large N-terminal domain, called sAPPα, from the cell surface. sAPPα plays important roles in modulating neuronal excitability, and in developmental and synaptic plasticity as indicated by the following findings. Exposure of cultured embry-onic hippocampal neurons to sAPPα results in activation of high-conductance, charybdotoxin-sensitive, potassium channels resulting in membrane hyperpo-larization and reduced calcium influx through voltage-dependent calcium channels and ionotropic glutamate receptor channels [13,14]. Dendrite out-growth in developing hippocampal neurons is increased following exposure to sAPPα [15]. Treatment of hippocampal slices from adult rats with sAPPα results in a shift in the frequency dependence of long-term depression of syn-aptic transmission, and an enhancement of long-term potentiation of synaptic transmission [16]. We have proposed that APP mutations promote neuronal degeneration by decreasing the levels of sAPPα [13,14,17] and, indeed, studies have documented that APP mutations do decrease production of sAPPα and that levels of sAPPα are decreased in the cerebrospinal fluid of AD patients [18,19].

Both Aβ and sAPPα exert direct effects on synaptic terminals. Such local effects of these APP derivatives are likely to play important roles in the early stages of AD (Figure 1). Studies of synaptosomes have shown that Aβ is able to induce membrane lipid peroxidation, and impair the function of ion, glucose and glutamate transporters in synaptic terminals [5,20]. These adverse effects of Aβ can be reduced by treating synaptosomes with antioxidants such as vitamin E and oestrogens [5,20,21]. Interestingly, Aβ and oxidative insults can induce local activation of apoptotic cascades involving prostate apoptosis response-4 (Par-4), caspases and mitochondrial dysfunction in dendrites and synaptic ter-minals [22–24]. The latter findings suggest that neuronal apoptosis in AD may be initiated by events occurring in synapses. Reduced levels of sAPPα may also promote synapse degeneration, since treatment of cultured hippocampal neu-rons with sAPPα decreases their vulnerability to synaptically driven excitotoxicity [13]. sAPPα can also protect synaptosomes against the damaging effects of exposure to Aβ and iron [25], as in intact neurons, the synaptoprotec-tive effects of sAPPα involve activation of a signalling pathway that employs cyclic GMP as a second messenger [14,25–27].

Finally, several observations suggest roles for alterations in ER function in the pathogenic actions of APP mutations. It has been proposed that APP mutations result in increased Aβ production because they alter trafficking of APP such that it is exposed to different enzymic environments [28–31]. Indeed,

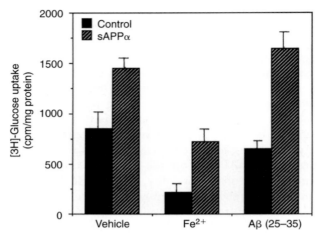

Figure 1 Direct actions of Aβ and sAPPα on synaptic terminals. Rat cortical synaptosomes were pretreated with sAPPα or saline (control). Synaptosomes were then exposed to either vehicle, Fe^{2+} or Aβ25–35 for 4 hours and the levels of radiolabelled glucose uptake were quantified. Values are means ± S.E.M. of determinations made in 4–6 synaptosome samples. Reproduced from Mattson, M.P., Cuo, Z.H. and Geiger, J.D. Secreted form of amyloid precursor protein enhances basal glucose and glutamate transport and protects against oxidative impairment of glucose and glutamate transport in synaptosomes by a cyclic GMP-mediated mechanism. (1999) J. Neurochem. **73 (2)**, 532–537, with permission. © (1999) Lippincott, Williams & Wilkins.

treatment of cells with agents that disrupt protein trafficking in the ER results in increased Aβ production. We recently provided evidence that perturbed ER calcium homoeostasis may contribute to the neurodegenerative effects of altered APP processing. Thus, agents such as dantrolene and xestospongin that block calcium release from ER can protect neurons against Aβ toxicity (Figure 2) [32,33]. In addition, treatment of cultured hippocampal neurons with sAPPα increases their resistance to apoptosis induced by thapsigargin, an agent that kills cells by inducing massive release of calcium from ER (Figure 2). On the other hand, metabolic stress and increased intracellular calcium levels alter APP processing such that levels of Aβ are increased and levels of sAPPα decreased [34,35]. Collectively, the data suggest that the neurodegenerative cascade in AD involves a feed-forward process in which metabolic compromise and perturbed calcium homoeostasis alter APP processing, inducing oxidative and metabolic stress and increasing levels of intracellular calcium (Figure 3).

How do presenilin mutations promote synaptic dysfunction and degeneration?

Several different laboratories have reported perturbed ER calcium regulation [32,33,36,37] and altered APP processing, resulting in increased production of Aβ42 and decreased production of sAPPα [38–40], as two consequences of expressing PS1 mutations in cultured cells. PC12

(a)   (b)

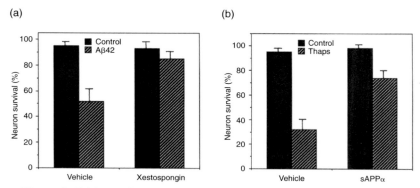

Figure 2 Evidence for the differential effects of Aβ and sAPPα on calcium release from ER and their roles in modifying neuronal death. Rat hippocampal cultures were pretreated for 2 hours with either 1 μM xestospongin (a) or 1 nM sAPPα (b). Cultures were then exposed to either 10 μM Aβ42 (a) or 1 μM thapsigargin (Thaps) (b) for 24 hours. Neuronal survival was quantified and values are means ± S.E.M. of determinations made in four separate cultures.

(pheochromocytoma) cells overexpressing PS1 mutations (Leu[286]→Val and Met[146]→Val) showed a significantly greater increase in levels of intracellular calcium, in response to activation of receptors linked to calcium release from

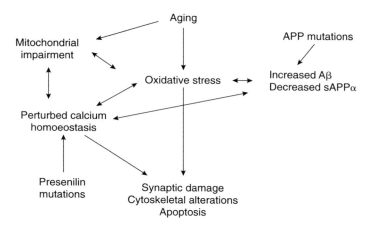

Figure 3 Inter-related mechanisms involved in the pathogenesis of sporadic and familial AD. In sporadic forms of AD, age-related increases in cellular oxidative stress and metabolic compromise result in altered proteolytic processing of APP, disruption of cellular calcium homoeostasis and mitochondrial dysfunction. In the case of presenilin mutations, the primary alteration appears to be perturbed ER calcium regulation which, in turn, results in altered APP processing and oxidative stress. Increased levels of oxidative stress and disruption of calcium homoeostasis result in neuronal apoptosis and excitotoxicity.

IP$_3$-sensitive stores, compared to untransfected PC12 cells and PC12 cells over-expressing wild-type PS1 ([32]; and M.P. Mattson, unpublished work]. PC12 cells overexpressing mutant PS1 exhibited increased vulnerability to apoptosis induced by trophic factor withdrawal and exposure to Aβ. This endangering action of the PS1 mutations could be counteracted by treating cells with agents that block calcium release from IP$_3$- and ryanodine-sensitive stores [32,33]. Thus, calcium release from ER is a necessary step in the pro-apoptotic actions of mutant PS1. Additional studies showed that overexpression of the calcium-binding protein calbindin [36] and treatment of cells with antioxidants [33] can counteract the pro-apoptotic action of mutant PS1, indicating that increased levels of cytoplasmic calcium and oxidative stress make important contribu-tions to the cell death process in such cell culture models.

Cells expressing mutant PS1 exhibit an abnormal pattern of activation of the anti-apoptotic transcription factor nuclear factor κB (NF-κB) following exposure to oxidative insults including Aβ [41]. Treatment with sAPPα pro-tected the cells against the pro-apoptotic actions of mutant PS1 and normalized the pattern of NF-κB activation. PC12 cells overexpressing mutant PS1 exhibit enhanced production of the pro-apoptotic protein Par-4 following trophic fac-tor withdrawal and exposure to Aβ [42]. The increased Par-4 production may contribute to reduced NF-κB activation [43].

More recently we showed that hippocampal neurons from PS1 mutant knockin mice are more vulnerable to excitotoxicity [44] and apoptosis [45] than are hippocampal neurons from wild-type mice. Calcium-imaging studies in hippocampal cultures from these mice showed that neurons expressing mutant PS1 exhibit enhanced calcium responses to glutamate when compared with wild-type neurons [44].

Presenilin mutations can cause local disruption of calcium homoeostasis and dysfunction in synapses. Synaptosomes prepared from the cerebral cortex of PS1 mutant transgenic mice exhibit enhanced elevations of intracellular cal-cium levels in response to membrane depolarization and exposure to Aβ, compared to synaptosomes from non-transgenic mice and mice overexpressing wild-type PS1 [46]. The magnitude of mitochondrial dysfunction and caspase activation induced by Aβ and a metabolic insult were also enhanced in synap-tosomes from PS1 mutant mice. Treatment of synaptosomes with the calcium chelator BAPTA-AM [(bis-(o-aminophenoxy)ethane-N,N,N',N'-tetra-acetic acid tetrakis (acetoxymethyl ester)] and dantrolene counteracted the adverse effects of the PS1 mutation on synaptic mitochondrial function, indicating that calcium release from ER was central to the adverse effects of PS1 mutations in synaptic terminals. More recently, Parent and colleagues [47] have demon-strated alterations in synaptic function in hippocampal slices from PS1 mutant transgenic mice. Collectively, the data support a key role for abnormal synaptic calcium homoeostasis and mitochondrial dysfunction in the pathogenic mecha-nism of PS1 mutations.

What is the specific mechanism whereby PS1 mutations disrupt ER cal-cium regulation? One possibility is that PS1 directly interacts with one or more calcium-regulating proteins and that PS1 mutations alter such interactions. Several candidates for such PS1-interacting proteins have recently been identified. Calsenilin is a cytoplasmic calcium-binding protein recently shown to interact with PS1 in the yeast two-hybrid assay [48]. Additional data in the latter study suggest that the calsenilin–PS1 interaction can alter enzymic cleavage of PS1. Also using the yeast two-hybrid approach, Kim and colleagues [49] reported that PS2 interacts with sorcin, a protein known to modulate the function of ryanodine receptors. However, PS1 did not interact with sorcin suggesting that this interaction may not play a role in the effects of presenilin mutations on ER calcium homoeostasis. Using a co-immunoprecipitation approach we have recently found that PS1 interacts with a ryanodine receptor complex in cultured neurons and mouse neocortical tissue [49a]. PS1 mutations might have indirect effects on ER calcium homoeostasis. For example, we recently found that levels of expression of the type 3 ryanodine receptor are greatly increased in PC12 cells overexpressing mutant PS1 [49a].

Role of the novel apoptotic protein Par-4 in synaptic apoptosis and AD

Par-4 is a 38 kDa protein identified by differential screening of prostate tumour cells for genes up-regulated during apoptosis [50]. Par-4 mRNA and protein levels were found to be increased in post-mortem brain tissue samples of hippocampus and inferior parietal cortex from AD patients compared to samples from age-matched control patients [42]. The latter study also showed that many neurofibrillary tangle-bearing neurons exhibit high levels of Par-4, suggesting that it increases specifically in neurons that degenerate. Experimental studies have shown that Par-4 protein levels increase rapidly in PC12 cells and primary hippocampal neurons in response to various apoptotic insults including trophic factor withdrawal and exposure to Aβ [42]. Suppression of the insult-induced increase in Par-4 levels, using antisense technology, prevents neuronal apoptosis, demonstrating a requirement for Par-4 in the cell death process [42]. Oxidative stress and calcium influx are triggers for Par-4 induction, and antioxidants and manipulations that reduce levels of intracellular calcium can suppress Par-4 expression [42,51]. Par-4 production occurs prior to, and is required for, mitochondrial dysfunction and caspase activation [42].

Par-4 contains both a leucine-zipper domain and a partially overlapping death domain near its C-terminus [50]. The leucine-zipper domain of Par-4 is required for its pro-apoptotic action since overexpression of Par-4 lacking the leucine-zipper domain does not promote apoptosis, and overexpression of the leucine-zipper domain alone acts in a dominant-negative manner to prevent apoptosis [42]. Several proteins have been identified that can interact with Par-4 and may mediate its pro-apoptotic action. Initial studies of tumour cells identified protein kinase Cζ (PKCζ) [52] as one protein that interacts with Par-4; the interaction inhibits the kinase activity of the enzyme. Data showing that activation of PKCζ can prevent apoptosis [53] suggest a role for the latter interaction in promoting apoptosis. We have found that Par-4 interacts with PKCζ in embryonic hippocampal neurons (S.L. Chan and M.P. Mattson, unpublished work). Interestingly, we also recently discovered that Par-4 suppresses activation of the anti-apoptotic transcription factor NF-κB [43]. Since PKCζ may mediate activation of NF-κB in cells exposed to potentially lethal insults, suppression of the PKCζ–NF-κB pathway may play an important role in the pro-apoptotic action of Par-4 (Figure 4). NF-κB exists in the cytoplasm of neurons in an inactive three-subunit complex that includes the transcription factor dimer (typically p50/p65 heterodimers) and an inhibitory subunit called I-κBα. NF-κB is activated when signals such as cytokines, calcium and oxidative stress induce phosphorylation of I-κB. This results in dissociation of the p50/p65 dimer which then translocates to the nucleus and binds to specific sequences in the enhancer region of target genes such as Mn-superoxide dismutase, calbindin and inhibitor of apoptosis (IAP) proteins [54].

Par-4 may play a particularly important role in post-synaptic terminals and dendrites. Exposure of synaptosomes and primary rat hippocampal cell cultures to apoptotic insults resulted in relatively rapid increases (1–2 hours) in Par-4 protein levels in dendrites and synaptic terminals [55]. Treatment of syn-

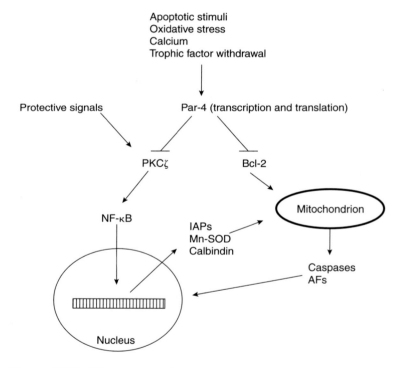

Figure 4 Working model of the mechanisms whereby Par-4 promotes neuronal apoptosis. Par-4 protein levels are rapidly increased in neurons following exposure to various apoptotic and excitotoxic insults. Available data suggest that Par-4 can suppress activation of the anti-apoptotic transcription factor NF-κB, apparently by suppressing activity of PKCζ, a kinase that can induce activation of NF-κB. In addition, Par-4 interacts with Bcl-2, and this interaction may lead to mitochondrial dysfunction and caspase activation. AF, apoptotic factor; IAP, inhibitor of apoptosis protein.

aptosomes with cycloheximide prevented the increases in Par-4 levels in synaptosomes following exposure to apoptotic insults, indicating that protein synthesis was required for Par-4 induction. These intriguing findings open a new avenue of investigation in the neuronal apoptosis field because they provide direct evidence that expression of a death-related protein can be induced locally in post-synaptic terminals. Moreover, Par-4 induction by apoptotic insults in synaptic terminals can be suppressed using antisense technology, and such suppression of Par-4 expression results in a marked attenuation of mitochondrial dysfunction and caspase activation [55]. Thus, Par-4 appears to play a central role in synaptic apoptotic cascades.

What about sporadic AD?

While studies of the pathogenic actions of APP and presenilin mutations have been invaluable in deciphering the molecular and cellular mechanisms underlying AD, the neurodegenerative process in the more common sporadic forms of AD remains unknown. The available data suggest the following scenario: subtle genetic factors, aging and the environment (e.g. diet, lifestyle, exposure to toxins or trauma) interact to increase levels of oxidative and metabolic stress in neurons. The latter statement is supported by compelling data demonstrating increased levels of oxyradical-mediated damage to proteins, lipids and DNA [56], and reduced glucose availability to cells [57] in the brain, during normal aging and more so in AD. Increased oxidative stress and reduced energy availability promote disruption of neuronal calcium homoeostasis. Perturbed calcium homoeostasis results in altered proteolytic processing of APP, which in turn leads to increased production of Aβ and decreased production of sAPPα. A vicious cycle is thus initiated that promotes neuronal apoptosis and excitotoxicity.

Genetic factors that may increase risk for sporadic AD are being identified. One such factor is *APOE* (apolipoprotein) genotype [58]; ApoE4 increases the risk, while ApoE2 decreases it. ApoEs appear to exert neurotrophic/neuroprotective actions, with ApoE2 and ApoE3 being more effective than ApoE4. We have recently found that ApoE2 protects neurons against oxidative injury by a mechanism that may involve binding of the toxic aldehyde product of lipid peroxidation, 4-hydroxynonenal [59]. The latter findings are intriguing because the differences between the three isoforms lie in cysteine residues at two positions (ApoE4 lacks cysteines at those residues, while ApoE3 and ApoE2 contain 1 and 2 cysteines respectively). 4-Hydroxynonenal covalently modifies proteins on cysteine residues. Thus, ApoE2 and ApoE3 isoforms may act to detoxify 4-hydroxynonenal under conditions of oxidative stress.

Environmental factors that may increase risk for AD include high calorie intake [60–62], history of head injury [63], low intake of antioxidants [64] and low level of mental challenges [65]. Reduced calorie intake may reduce the risk of developing AD by decreasing free radical production (a mechanism thought to underlie increased lifespan in animals maintained on a food restriction) and/or by enhancing cellular resistance to oxidative and metabolic insults

[66,67]. Living an intellectually enriched lifestyle may increase resistance of neurons to age-related degeneration by increasing production of neurotrophic factors and stress proteins [68]. What seems to be clear is that genetic and environmental factors converge on common neurodegenerative pathways involving oxidative stress, impaired energy metabolism and perturbed cellular calcium homoeostasis.

Implications for preventative and therapeutic approaches to AD

The following potentially beneficial preventative and therapeutic strategies are suggested by the kinds of data described above.

- Reduced calorie intake – this lifestyle approach may increase resistance of neurons to several age-related disorders including AD, Parkinson's disease, Huntington's disease and stroke [60,66,69]. This approach may be effective in both sporadic and familial forms of AD [61].
- Increased antioxidant intake – oxidative stress appears to make a major contribution to the neurodegenerative process in both sporadic and familial AD. Particularly valuable may be antioxidants that remove mitochondrial reactive oxygen species and suppress membrane lipid peroxidation.
- Drugs that stabilize neuronal calcium homoeostasis. Prototypical examples include dantrolene and xestospongin to suppress calcium release from ER, and calcium channel antagonists to suppress calcium influx through plasma membrane channels.
- Mental calisthenics – use of neuronal circuits increases their resistance to adversity. This may occur as a result of the up-regulation of neurotrophic factors and certain stress proteins [68].

This work was supported by the National Institute on Aging and the Alzheimer's Association.

References

1.   Mattson, M.P. (1990) *Neuron* 4, 105–117
2.   Nixon, R.A., Saito, K.I., Grynspan, F., Griffin, W.R., Katayama, S., Honda, T., Mohan, P.S., Shea, T.B. and Beerman, M. (1994) *Ann. N.Y. Acad. Sci.* 747, 77–91
3.   Mattson, M.P., Cheng, B., Davis, D., Bryant, K., Lieburg, I. and Rydel, R.E. (1992) *J. Neurosci.* 12, 376–389
4.   Goodman, Y. and Mattson, M.P. (1994) *Exp. Neurol.* 128, 1–12
5.   Mark, R.J., Hensley, K., Butterfield, D.A. and Mattson, M.P. (1995) *J. Neurosci.* 15, 6239–6249
6.   Terry, R.D., Masliah, E., Salmon, D.P., Butters, N., DeTeresa, R., Hill, R., Hansen, L.A. and Katzman, R. (1991) *Ann. Neurol.* 30, 572–580
7.   DeKosky, S.T., Scheff, S.W. and Styren, S.D. (1996) *Neurodegeneration* 5, 417–421
8.   Selkoe, D.J. (1993) *Trends Neurosci.* 16, 403–409
9.   Mattson, M.P. (1997) *Physiol. Rev.* 77, 1081–1132
10.   Mark, R.J., Lovell, M.A., Markesbery, W.R., Uchida, K. and Mattson, M.P. (1997) *J. Neurochem.* 68, 255–264

11.   Mark, R.J., Pang, Z., Geddes, J.W., Uchida, K. and Mattson, M.P. (1997) *J. Neurosci.* **17**, 1046–1054
12.   Blanc, E.M., Keller, J.N., Fernandez, S. and Mattson, M.P. (1998) *Glia* **22**, 149–160
13.   Mattson, M.P., Cheng, B., Culwell, A.R., Esch, F., Lieberburg, I. and Rydel, R.E. (1993) *Neuron* **10**, 243–254
14.   Furukawa, K., Barger, S.W., Blalock, E. and Mattson, M.P. (1996) *Nature (London)* **379**, 74–78
15.   Mattson, M.P. (1994) *J. Neurobiol.* **25**, 439–450
16.   Ishida, A., Furukawa, K., Keller, J.N. and Mattson, M.P. (1997) *NeuroReport* **8**, 2133–2137
17.   Smith-Swintosky, V., Pettigrew, L., Craddock, S., Culwell, A., Rydel, R. and Mattson, M.P. (1994) *J. Neurochem.* **63**, 781–784
18.   Palmert, M.R., Usiak, M., Mayeux, B., Raskind, M., Tourtellotte, W.W. and Younkin, S.G. (1990) *Neurology* **40**, 1028–1034
19.   Lannfelt, L., Basun, H., Wahlund, L.O., Rowe, B.A. and Wagner, S.L. (1995) *Nat. Med. (N.Y.)* **1**, 829–832
20.   Keller, J.N., Pang, Z., Geddes, J.W., Begley, J.G., Germeyer, A., Waeg, G. and Mattson, M.P. (1997) *J. Neurochem.* **69**, 273–284
21.   Keller, J.N. and Mattson, M.P. (1997) *J. Neurosci. Res.* **50**, 522–530
22.   Mattson, M.P., Keller, J.N. and Begley, J.G. (1998). *Exp. Neurol.* **153**, 35–48
23.   Mattson, M.P., Partin, J. and Begley, J.G. (1998) *Brain Res.* **807**, 167–176
24.   Duan, W., Rangnekar, V. and Mattson, M.P. (1999) *J. Neurochem.* **72**, 2312–2322
25.   Mattson, M.P., Guo, Z.H. and Geiger, J.D. (1999) *J. Neurochem.* **73**, 532–537
26.   Barger, S.W., Fiscus, R.R., Ruth, P., Hofmann, F. and Mattson, M.P. (1995) *J. Neurochem.* **64**, 2087–2096
27.   Furukawa, K., Sopher, B., Rydel, R.E., Begley, J.G., Martin, G.M. and Mattson, M.P. (1996) *J. Neurochem.* **67**, 1882–1896
28.   Cai, X., Golde, T. and Youkin, S. (1993) *Science* **259**, 514–516
29.   Citron, M., Vigo-Pelfrey, C., Teplow, D.B., Miller, C., Schenk, D., Johnston, J., Winblad, B., Venizelos, N., Lannfelt, L. and Selkoe, D.J. (1994) *Proc. Natl. Acad. Sci. U.S.A.* **91**, 11993–11997
30.   Haass, C., Hung, A., Selkoe, D. and Teplow, D. (1994) *J. Biol. Chem.* **269**, 17741–17748
31.   Haass, C., Lemere, C.A., Capell, A., Citron, M., Seubert, P., Schenk, D. and Selkoe, D. (1995) *Nat. Med. (N.Y.)* **1**, 1291–1296
32.   Guo, Q., Furukawa, K., Sopher, B.L., Pham, D.G., Robinson, N., Martin, G.M. and Mattson, M.P. (1996) *NeuroReport* **8**, 379–383
33.   Guo, Q., Sopher, B.L., Pham, D.G., Furukawa, K., Robinson, N., Martin, G.M. and Mattson, M.P. (1997) *J. Neurosci.* **17**, 4212–4222
34.   Gabuzda, D., Busciglio, J., Chen, L.B., Matsudaira, P. and Yankner, B.A. (1994) *J. Biol. Chem.* **269**, 13623–13628
35.   Querfurth, H.W. and Selkoe, D.J. (1994) *Biochemistry* **33**, 4550–4561
36.   Guo, Q., Christakos, S., Robinson, N. and Mattson, M.P. (1998) *Proc. Natl. Acad. Sci. U.S.A.* **95**, 3227–3232
37.   Leissring, M.A., Paul, B.A., Parker, I. and Cotman, C.W. and LaFerla, F.M. (1999) *J. Neurochem.* **72**, 1061–1068
38.   Scheuner, D. Eckman, C., Jensen, M., Song, X., Citron, M., Suzuki, N., Bird, T.D., Hardy, J., Hutton, M., Kukull, W., et al. (1996) *Nat. Med. (N.Y.)* **2**, 864–870
39.   Guo, Q., Sebastian, L., Sopher, B.L., Miller, M.W., Glazner, G.W., Ware, C.B., Martin, G.M. and Mattson, M.P. (1999) *Proc. Natl. Acad. Sci. U.S.A.* **96**, 4125–4130
40.   Ancolio, K., Marambaud, P., Dauch, P. and Checler, F. (1997) *J. Neurochem.* **69**, 2494–2499
41.   Guo, Q., Robinson, N. and Mattson, M. P. (1998) *J. Biol. Chem.* **273**, 12341–12351
42.   Guo, Q., Fu, W., Xie, J., Luo, H., Sells, S.F., Geddes, J.W., Bondada, V., Rangnekar, V.M. and Mattson, M.P. (1998) *Nat. Med. (N.Y.)* **4**, 957–962

43. Camandola, S. and Mattson, M.P. (2000) *J. Neurosci. Res.* **61**, 134–139

44. Guo, Q., Fu, W., Sopher, B.L., Miller, M.W., Ware, C.B., Martin, G.M. and Mattson, M.P. (1999) *Nat. Med. (N.Y.)* **5**, 101–107

45. Guo, Q., Sebastian, L., Sopher, B.L., Miller, M.W., Ware, C.B., Martin, G.M. and Mattson, M.P. (1999) *J. Neurochem.* **72**, 1019–1029

46. Begley, J.G., Duan, W., Duff, K. and Mattson, M.P. (1999) *J. Neurochem.* **72**, 1030–1039

47. Parent, A., Linden, D.J., Sisodia, S.S. and Borchelt, D.R. (1999) *Neurobiol. Dis.* **6**, 56–62

48. Buxbaum, J.D., Choi, E.K., Luo, Y., Lilliehook, C., Crowley, A.C., Merriam, D.E. and Wasco, W. (1998) *Nat. Med. (N.Y.)* **4**, 1177–1181

49. Kim, T.W., Pettingell, W.P. and Tanzi, R.E. (1998) *Soc. Neurosci. Abstr.* **34**, 757

49a. Chan, S.L., Mayne, M., Holden, C.P., Geiger, J.D. and Mattson, M.P. (2000) *J. Biol. Chem.* **275**, 18195–18200

50. Sells, S.F., Han, S.S., Muthukkumar, S., Maddiwar, N., Johnstone, R., Boghaert, E., Gillis, D., Liu, G., Nair, P., Monnig, S., et al. (1997) *Mol. Cell. Biol.* **17**, 3823–3832

51. Chan, S.L., Tammariello, S.P., Estus, S. and Mattson, M.P. (1999) *J. Neurochem.* **73**, 502–512

52. Diaz-Meco, M.T., Municio, M.M., Frutos, S., Sanchez, P., Lozano, J., Sanz, L. and Moscat, J. (1996) *Cell* **86**, 777–786

53. Berra, E., Municio, M.M., Sans, L., Frutos, S., Diaz-Meco, M.T. and Moscat, J. (1997) *Mol. Cell. Biol.* **17**, 4346–4354

54. Mattson, M.P., Culmsee, C., Yu, Z. and Camandola, S. (2000) *J. Neurochem.* **74**, 443–456

55. Duan, W., Rangnekar, V. and Mattson, M.P. (1999) *J. Neurochem.* **72**, 2312–2322

56. Markesbery, W.R. (1997) *Free Radic. Biol. Med.* **23**, 134–147

57. Mattson, M.P., Pedersen, W.A., Duan, W. and Camandola, S. (1999) *N.Y. Acad. Sci.* **893**, 154–175

58. Saunders, A.M., Strittmatter, W.J., Schmechel, D., George-Hyslop, P.H., Pericak-Vance, M.A., Joo, S.H., Rosi, B.L., Gusella, J.F., Crapper-MacLachlan, D.R., Alberts, M.J., et al. (1993) *Neurology* **43**, 1467–1472

59. Pedersen, W.A., Chan, S.L. and Mattson, M.P. (2000) *J. Neurochem.* **74**, 1426–1433

60. Bruce-Keller, A.J., Umberger, G., McFall, R. and Mattson, M.P. (1999) *Ann. Neurol.* **45**, 8–15

61. Zhu, H., Guo, Q. and Mattson, M.P. (1999) *Brain Res.* **842**, 224–229

62. Mayeux, R., Costa, R., Bell, K., Merchant, C., Tang, M.X. and Jacobs, D. (1999) *Neurology* **59**, S296–S297

63. Mayeux, R., Ottman, R., Maestre, G., Ngai, C., Tang, M.X., Ginsberg, H., Chun, M., Tycko, B. and Shelanski, M. (1995) *Neurology* **45**, 555–557

64. Morris, M.C., Beckett, L.A., Scherr, P.A., Hebert, L.E., Bennett, D.A., Field, T.S. and Evans, D.A. (1998) *Alzheimer Dis. Assoc. Disord.* **12**, 121–126

65. Stern, Y., Gurland, B., Tatemichi, T.K., Tang, M.X., Wilder, D. and Mayeux, R. (1994) *J. Am. Med. Assoc.* **271**, 1004–1010

66. Duan, W. and Mattson, M.P. (1999) *J. Neurosci. Res.* **57**, 195–206

67. Lee, J., Bruce-Keller, A.J., Kruman, Y., Chan, S.L. and Mattson, M.P. (1999) *J. Neurosci. Res.* **57**, 48–61

68. Mattson, M.P. and Lindvall, O. (1997) in *The Aging Brain* (Mattson, M.P. and Geddes, J.W., eds), pp. 299–345, JAI Press, Greenwich, CT

69. Yu, Z.F. and Mattson, M.P. (1999) *J. Neurosci. Res.* **57**, 830–839

Biochem. Soc. Symp. **67**, 163–175
(Printed in Great Britain)

16

Receptor–G-protein signalling in Alzheimer's disease

Richard F. Cowburn*[1], Cora O'Neill†,Willy L. Bonkale*,

Thomas G. Ohm‡ and Johan Fastbom*

*Karolinska Institute, NEUROTEC, Section for Geriatric Medicine, NOVUM, KFC,
S-141 86, Huddinge, Sweden, †Department of Biochemistry, University College,
Lee Maltings, Prospect Row, Cork, Ireland, and ‡Institute fur Anatomie, University
Klinikum Charité, D-10098 Berlin, Germany

Abstract

Based on radioligand binding studies, it has long been assumed that the
neurochemical pathology of Alzheimer's disease (AD) does not involve widespread changes in post-synaptic neurotransmitter function. However, more
recent studies suggest that receptor function in AD may be compromised due
to disrupted post-receptor signal transduction, in particular that mediated by
the G-protein regulated phosphoinositide hydrolysis and adenylate cyclase
(AC) pathways. The phosphoinositide hydrolysis pathway has been shown to
be altered at a number of levels in AD post-mortem brains, including impaired
agonist and G-protein regulation of phospholipase C, decreased protein kinase
C (PKC) levels and activity, and a reduced number of receptor sites for the second messenger, $Ins(1,4,5)P_3$. Of these, loss of $Ins(1,4,5)P_3$ receptors and PKC
in the entorhinal cortex and hippocampus correlates with AD-related neurofibrillary changes, as staged according to Braak's protocol. Disregulation of the
phosphoinositide hydrolysis pathway may therefore have consequences for the
progression of AD pathology. In contrast to the extensive pattern of disruption
seen with the phosphoinositide hydrolysis pathway, changes to AC signalling
in AD appear more circumscribed. Disruptions include a lesion at the level of
G_S-protein stimulation of AC and, at least in the hippocampus, reduced
enzyme activities in response to forskolin stimulation. Of these, the latter
change has been shown to precede neurofibrillary changes. Apart from a loss of
calcium/calmodulin sensitive AC isoforms, other components of this signalling pathway, including G-protein levels, G_i-protein mediated inhibition
and protein kinase A levels and activity, remain relatively preserved in the disorder.

[1]To whom correspondence should be addressed.

Introduction

The neuropathology of Alzheimer's disease (AD) is characterized by selective neuronal loss in association with two major lesions. Firstly, the extracellular deposition of the 39–43-residue β-amyloid (Aβ) peptide, in the cerebrovasculature [1] and cores of senile plaques [2], and secondly, the formation of paired helical filaments (PHFs) in intracellular neurofibrillary tangles (NFTs) [3], neuropil threads and senile plaque neurites. The principal component of PHFs is an abnormally hyperphosphorylated form of the microtubule-associated protein tau [4].

During the last 15–20 years there has been much debate as to which of the pathologies of amyloid deposition or PHF formation are most important for driving the process of AD. Proponents of amyloid deposition have drawn major support from the identification and understanding of the effects of disease-causing mutations in rare autosomal-dominant inherited forms of the disorder. Disease-causing mutations in the β-amyloid precursor protein (APP) gene, as well as in the unrelated presenilin 1 (PS1) and presenilin 2 (PS2) genes, have all been shown to affect APP metabolism to increase production of longer Aβ peptides (Aβ42/43) that have a greater propensity to form fibrils and thus deposit in the brain [5]. Such studies have provided the cornerstone of the 'amyloid cascade hypothesis' of AD, which in its simplest form states that altered APP metabolism generates excessive Aβ deposition in the form of senile plaques. This provides the driving force for a cascade of events including NFT formation, neuronal degeneration and inflammatory responses, finally resulting in the clinical symptomatology of dementia that brings the patient to the physician [6]. Other support for the amyloid cascade hypothesis has come from studies which demonstrated that Aβ is both directly neurotoxic and can also sensitize neurons to other injurious stimuli [7]. Alternatively, Mattson and colleagues have suggested that altered APP metabolism may contribute to the disease by decreasing the production of secreted APP (sAPP) derivatives that modulate neuronal excitability, neurite outgrowth, synaptogenesis and cell survival [8]. Alternatively, overproduction of the C-100–104 amino acids of APP may be responsible for neuronal death in AD [9].

Opponents of the amyloid cascade hypothesis argue that autosomal-dominant forms of AD are rare and that other primary cellular defects are necessary to explain the more common, late-onset, sporadic forms of AD. Furthermore, APP and PS gene mutations are now being shown to have multiple effects on vital cell signal transduction cascades. These effects may turn out to precede APP mis-metabolism and Aβ overproduction and/or to have separate neurodestructive roles. Notably, these include effects on signal transduction pathways known to be involved in apoptosis, heterotrimeric G-protein-coupled receptor signalling, cell survival and calcium signalling [9–12]. Evidence that Aβ deposition can occur in the normal aged brain without signs of either dementia or neuronal damage further suggests that amyloidosis may not be a phenomenon central to AD. Moreover, many studies have shown that the number and distribution of NFTs, rather than senile plaques, correlates better with clinical symptomatologies of dementia in AD [9]. The importance of NFT pathology to AD neurodegeneration is accentuated by the relative lack of neuronal loss or cognitive decline in transgenic animals with high *APP-* or *PS*-mutant-induced Aβ load.

The inability to establish a direct relationship (if one exists) between Aβ deposition and senile plaque development on the one hand, and tau hyperphosphorylation and development of PHFs and NFTs on the other, has led to the idea that these two pathologies may be coincidental to, as yet undiscovered, primary cellular events. One factor that has been suggested to underlie both the processes is that of altered signal transduction [13]. As summarized briefly below and reviewed extensively in chapters 4 and 7, a number of signal transduction pathways have been shown to contribute either directly or indirectly to APP metabolism and tau hyperphosphorylation. This is shown in schematic form in Figure 1.

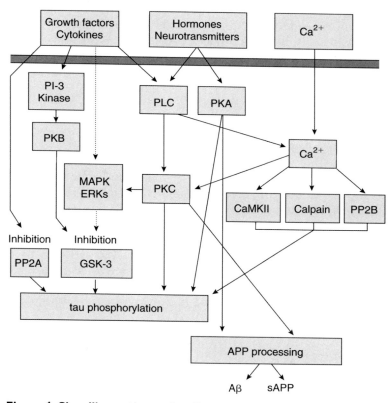

Figure 1 Signalling pathways implicated in APP metabolism and tau phosphorylation. Abbreviations used: CaMKII, calcium/calmodulin-dependent kinase II; ERK, extracellular signal-related protein kinase; MAPK, MAP kinase; PI-3 kinase, phosphoinositide 3-kinase; PKB, protein kinase B; PLC, phospholipase C. Re-drawn and modified from Neuroscience, **78**, Lovestone, S. and Reynolds, C.H., The phosphorylation of tau: a critical stage in neurodevelopment and neurodegenerative processes, 309–324, © (1997), with permission from Elsevier Science.

Signal transduction and APP metabolism

The Aβ peptide is derived from APP by the combined actions of a β-secretase, which cleaves just N-terminal of the Aβ sequence yielding a soluble secreted APP fragment (sAPPβ) and a C-100 fragment, which is cleaved by γ-secretase to yield Aβ. APP can also be processed by an alternative route that prevents generation of full-length Aβ and involves cleavage within the Aβ sequence by α-secretase to give a secreted N-terminal portion of APP (sAPPα) and a non-amyloidogenic C-terminal fragment of Aβ known as p3 [14,15].

The first suggestion that APP metabolism can be influenced by activation of signal transduction pathways came from studies showing that phorbol ester stimulation of protein kinase C (PKC) markedly increases the production of sAPP in a variety of transfected cell line systems [15–17]. Concomitant with an increased sAPPα secretion, PKC activation was shown to lower Aβ production [18], suggesting that PKC-stimulated α-secretase processing of APP can have direct consequences on Aβ production. However, it should be noted that the regulation of sAPP and Aβ production by PKC does not always occur in a mutually exclusive manner in neurons [15,19,20]. Nonetheless, the general consensus from these studies suggests that PKC-stimulated α-secretase processing of APP can have direct consequences for Aβ production.

Non-amyloidogenic, α-secretase APP processing has also been shown to be modulated upstream of PKC following activation of a number of neurotransmitter receptor types linked to the phosphoinositide hydrolysis pathway, including the acetylcholine muscarinic M_1 and M_3 [21–23] and glutamate metabotropic [24,25] receptor subtypes. Many of the heterotrimeric G-protein-coupled receptors, including acetylcholine muscarinic M_1, glutamate metabotropate as well as 5-hydroxytryptamine 2a and 2c receptor types, can also modulate sAPP production via phospholipase A_2 activation [26–28]. There is also evidence that processing of APP by α-secretase can be regulated by altered calcium homoeostasis [29,30].

The mechanisms underlying PKC-stimulated sAPP secretion have been suggested to involve the phosphorylation of proteins involved in the regulation of APP-containing secretory vesicle formation from the trans-Golgi network [31]. Xu and colleagues have also shown that cAMP-dependent protein kinase (PKA) can converge with PKC at the level of trans-Golgi network secretory vesicle formation to increase sAPP production [32]. However, in apparent contrast, Efthimiopoulos and colleagues showed that increased intracellular cAMP inhibits both constitutive and phorbol ester-stimulated sAPP secretion in C6 glioma cells [33]. Evidence that cAMP-mediated signalling has an adverse effect on APP metabolism is also provided by studies which show that cAMP regulates APP mRNA through transcriptional mechanisms [34,35], to give an accumulation of cell-associated APP holoprotein containing amyloidogenic Aβ peptides [36]. PKA and PKC may also exert their effects by phosphorylating other proteins which are involved in the regulation of APP secretase activity, including the presenilins [37].

Several early studies have also shown that sAPP release can be regulated by a wide variety of growth factor tyrosine kinase receptors [15]. However the interpretation of these results may have been confused by long-term effects of growth factors on APP expression. More recent studies have shown that short-term exposure to growth factors stimulates sAPP release in a mitogen-activated protein (MAP) kinase-dependent, PKC-independent fashion [15]. It has there-fore been suggested that G-protein-coupled receptors and growth factor recep-tors may converge to regulate sAPP and Aβ production at the level of MAP kinase signal transduction [15].

These data presented above, together with evidence that sAPP release is regulated by neuronal activity, have led to the suggestion that disturbances in neurotransmitter-receptor- and growth-factor-regulated signal transduction pathways could be the primary event causing altered α-secretase APP process-ing and a resulting increase in production of Aβ [38].

Signal transduction and tau hyperphosphorylation

The principle component of AD, PHFs, are an abnormally hyperphos-phorylated form of the microtubule-associated protein tau. The normal func-tion of tau is to bind to tubulin and promote microtubule assembly and stability. The tubulin-binding properties of tau are greatly diminished by its hyperphosphorylation to PHF-tau. Both proline-directed and non-proline-dependent protein kinases are likely to be important for PHF-tau hyperphos-phorylation [13,39].

The major proline-directed protein kinases that have been studied with respect to PHF-tau phosphorylation include MAP kinase, cdc2 (cell division control 2) kinase, cdk2 (cyclin-dependent kinase 2), cdk5 and glycogen syn-thase kinase-3 (GSK-3). Of these, GSK-3 induces AD-like tau phos-phorylation following transfection of cells with the enzyme, suggesting that this enzyme could be crucially involved in PHF-tau hyperphosphorylation [40]. GSK-3 has also been shown to be preferentially localized in NFT-bearing neurons [41] and the distribution of the active form of the enzyme parallels the spread of AD neurofibrillary changes [42].

Less attention has been given to the non-proline-dependent protein kinases such as PKA, PKC, casein kinases I and II and calcium/calmodulin-dependent kinase II (CaM kinase II), as it has been shown that tau is generally a poor substrate for these enzymes. However, although tau is a relatively poor substrate for PKA and PKC, these kinases may be important for unmasking sites otherwise inaccessible to the proline-dependent kinases. Thus it has been shown that prior phosphorylation of tau by PKA stimulates subsequent phos-phorylation by GSK-3 several fold [43,44]. Phosphorylation of tau by PKA also inhibits its proteolytic breakdown by the calcium-activated protease, cal-pain [45]. Also, as suggested by Lovestone and Reynolds, PKC may influence tau phosphorylation by activating MAP kinases leading in turn to an inhibition of GSK-3 activity [13]. Interestingly, GSK-3 signalling can be regulated by growth factors [46], G-proteins [47] and calcium signal transduction [48], once more suggesting that primary defects or down-regulation of these central brain survival pathways may converge to cause deregulation of both tau and APP metabolism in AD.

In addition to an overactive kinase input, the hyperphosphorylation of PHF-tau could occur as a result of decreased protein phosphatase activity in AD. Protein phosphatases PP2A and PP2B can revert tau that has been hyperphosphorylated *in vitro* by CaM kinase II, PKA, MAP kinase and cdc2 kinase to a normal-like state [49]. PP2A and PP2B can also catalyse AD PHF-tau dephosphorylation at select sites [50]. PP2B shows a selectively reduced expression in NFT-bearing neurons [41] and phosphatase enzyme activities may be reduced in AD brains [51].

Although hyperphosphorylation of tau prevents its binding to microtubules, it remains unclear as to whether tau hyperphosphorylation itself is necessary or sufficient for PHF formation [39]. Goedert and colleagues have shown that early interactions between tau and sulphated glycosaminoglycans can promote recombinant tau assembly into Alzheimer-like filaments, prevent tau binding to microtubules, and also stimulate tau protein phosphorylation [52,53].

Receptor–G-protein signalling in the AD brain

From the above it can be seen that there is a wealth of predominantly *in vitro* experimental data showing how various signalling pathways can contribute to APP metabolism and tau protein phosphorylation. In addition, it has been hypothesized that altered downstream signalling events may limit the successful outcome of neurotransmitter enhancement strategies for improving AD cognitive and behavioural deficits [54]. The following sections provide a summary of receptor–G-protein-mediated phospholipase C/PKC and adenylate cyclase/PKA signalling pathways in AD brains *post mortem*.

The phosphoinositide hydrolysis pathway in AD

The phosphoinositide hydrolysis pathway (as shown in its simplest form in Figure 2) has been shown to be disrupted at a number of levels in AD brains *post mortem*. The first evidence suggesting impaired phosphoinositide metabolism in AD was provided by Stokes and Hawthorne who reported 30–50% decreases in PtdIns, PtdIns4P and PtdIns(4,5)P_2 levels in AD anterior temporal cortex [55]. This may limit the available substrate pool for both G-protein-coupled receptors, through the phosphoinositide hydrolysis pathway, and growth factor signal transduction. Other workers subsequently showed that acetylcholine muscarinic M_1 receptor–G-protein coupling was disrupted in the parietal [56] and frontal [57] cortices and thalamus [58] in AD. In a more recent study Ladner and colleagues showed that M_1 receptor–G-protein uncoupling was disrupted in regions of the AD brain which showed abundant neuritic senile plaques, rather than NFT accumulation [59]. Data suggesting a muscarinic receptor–G-protein uncoupling in AD brain has also been provided by Cutler and colleagues in a study of carbachol-stimulated, low-K_m GTPase activity in the basal ganglia, superior frontal gyrus and hippocampus [60].

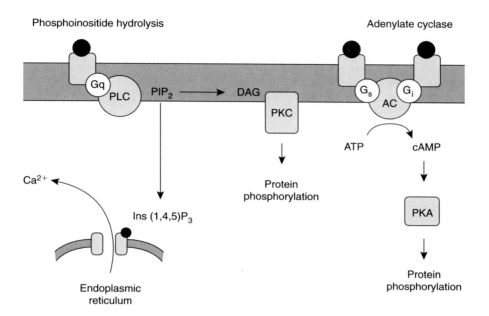

Figure 2 A simplified scheme of the prinicipal components of the phosphoinositide hydrolysis and adenylate cyclase (AC) signal transduction pathways. The key components of the phosphoinositide hydrolysis pathway include the effector enzyme phospholipase C (PLC), the receptor activation of which is regulated by an intermediate heterotrimeric G-protein, termed Gq. Receptor and G-protein activation of PLC results in the hydrolysis of PtdIns(4,5)P_2 (PIP$_2$) to give the second messengers diacylglycerol (DAG) and Ins(1,4,5)P_3. DAG in turn activates PKC, whereas Ins(1,4,5)P_3 mediates intracellular calcium homoeostasis. AC activity can be either stimulated or inhibited, depending upon the receptor type occupied. Receptor stimulation and inhibition of AC occurs via G_s- and G_i-proteins, respectively, and results in altered production of cAMP, an important intracellular second messenger for ion channel gating and protein phosphorylation via PKA.

More direct evidence for an impaired regulation of the phosphoinositide hydrolysis pathway in AD has come from studies on the regulation of phospholipase C activity following either neurotransmitter-receptor or G-protein activations. Jope and colleagues reported that the hydrolysis of exogenous [³H]phosphatidylinositol was significantly reduced in the AD prefrontal cortex in response to muscarinic [61–64], glutamate metabotropic, histamine and 5-hydroxytryptamine receptor agonists [64]. Decreased [³H]phosphatidylinositol hydrolysis was also seen following direct G-protein activation with GTPγS and aluminium fluoride [64]. This, together with data showing that Gq protein α-subunit levels are relatively preserved in a number of AD brain regions [61,64–66], implies that the disrupted regulation of phosphoinositide hydrolysis in the AD brain is likely to result from an altered Gq protein function.

Dysregulated phosphoinositide hydrolysis in AD brain has also been demonstrated using physiological mixtures of exogenous phosphoinositides [67] and [³H]PtdIns(4,5)P_2 [68] as enzyme substrates, although it should be noted that others have failed to show this deficit [69,70].

The most consistent deficit found in phosphoinositide hydrolysis signalling in AD brains is that of an altered PKC regulation. The PKC deficit was first shown by Cole and colleagues who reported reduced [³H]phorbol-dibutyrate binding to PKC and reduced PKC enzyme activities in particulate fractions of AD frontal cortex [71]. The reduction in PKC activity in AD has been suggested to involve a defective sensitivity of the enzyme to the cofactors phosphatidylserine, calcium and diacylglycerol [72]. However, data from other studies indicate that altered PKC activities in AD brains are likely to reflect a loss of the protein. Thus, Masliah and colleagues showed decreased concentrations of PKCβII and PKCα in particulate fractions of AD hippocampus and mid-frontal cortex [73]. Similarly, Shimohama and colleagues reported significantly reduced levels of PKCβ in membranous fractions from AD temporal cortex [74]. Matsushima and colleagues also reported a reduced level of PKCε in AD temporal cortex, which occurred in the absence of altered levels of two other calcium-independent isoforms, namely PKCδ and PKCζ [75].

Masliah and colleagues have suggested that PKC alterations may occur early in AD and have consequences for the development of disease pathology. These workers showed that early or diffuse Aβ-containing plaques without PHF-containing neuritic components showed strong immunostaining for PKCβII, which was associated with the membranes of cellular processes extending into these structures [76]. Further data showing that PKCβII levels and PKC-dependent P86 phosphorylation were reduced in the neocortex of clinically non-demented individuals with cortical plaques, led to the idea that there is a PKCβII aberration in AD that precedes clinical deficits and correlates with neuritic plaque rather than with NFT formation [76].

In apparent contrast to the above, we have provided evidence that reduced PKC levels correlate well with the progression of AD-related neurofibrillary changes. By performing [³H]phorbol 12,13-dibutyrate autoradiography, according to a protocol devised by Braak and Braak, on sections of entorhinal cortex and anterior hippocampus staged for disease pathology [77], we showed that PKC levels in the entorhinal cortex, subiculum, CA1, CA2, CA3 and CA4 pyramidal layers, as well as dentate gyrus, decline with the progressive accumulation of neurofibrillary changes, but not amyloid deposition [78].

The phosphoinositide hydrolysis pathway has also been shown to be disrupted in AD brains at the level of the intracellular actions of the second messenger Ins(1,4,5)P_3. Both Young and colleagues [79] and Garlind and colleagues [80] have demonstrated significant reductions in the binding of [³H]Ins (1,4,5)P_3 to receptor sites in homogenates of AD parietal cortex, hippocampus, superior frontal and superior temporal cortices, as well as cerebellum. Haug and colleagues also reported that reduced Ins(1,4,5)P_3 receptor protein levels in AD temporal cortex, as determined by immunoblotting, correlated with a semi-quantitative score for neuritic plaque and NFT accumulation [81]. More recently, we showed that $Ins(1,4,5)P_3$ receptor loss in the entorhinal cortex, subiculum and CA1 pyramidal layer of the anterior hippocampus correlated with staging for both neurofibrillary changes and amyloid deposition [78].

Adenylate cyclase in AD

In contrast to the multiple deficits seen in the phosphoinositide hydrolysis pathway, disrupted adenylate cyclase (AC) signalling (see Figure 2 for scheme) in AD brains appears more restricted because it occurs primarily at the level of neurotransmitter receptor–G_s-protein–enzyme coupling. Analogous to the deficit in muscarinic M_1 receptor–Gq protein coupling described above, it has been shown that β-adrenoceptor–G-protein coupling is impaired in AD temporal [82] and frontal [83] cortices. Other evidence for an impaired G_s-protein function in AD has come from studies of AC enzyme activities in the disorder. Using assay conditions favouring G_s-protein stimulation of calcium/calmodulin-insensitive AC isoforms, we reported that the G-protein activators, GTPγS and aluminium fluoride, gave markedly reduced stimulations of enzyme activity in membranes prepared from AD hippocampus; frontal, temporal and occipital cortices; angular gyrus; and cerebellum, as compared to controls. In the same studies it was observed that forskolin stimulations of enzyme catalytic activity were not significantly different between AD and control groups [84–86]. These studies have been interpreted as indicating a specific lesion at the level of G_s-protein–AC interactions and are in general agreement with those published in independent studies of AC regulation in AD hippocampus [87,88]. In contrast, however, Ross and colleagues did not see an impaired G_s-protein–AC interaction in AD neocortex. This discrepancy may reflect differences in assay conditions for an enzyme with many different isoforms and regulators [89].

Of the above studies it should be noted that Ohm and colleagues, in addition to finding an impaired G_s-protein regulation of AC, also saw reduced forskolin-stimulated enzyme activities in AD hippocampus [87]. This suggested a loss of AC enzyme units in AD and has been corroborated by more recent immunoblotting studies using isoform-specific antibodies. Yamamoto and colleagues showed a significant loss of the AC type I and II, but not IV or V/VI, isoforms in AD parietal cortex [90,91]. The loss of the calcium/calmodulin-sensitive type I isoform was further shown to correlate with reduced basal and forskolin-stimulated enzyme activities measured in the presence, but not absence, of calcium and calmodulin [91]. This raised the possibility that loss of AC enzyme units in the AD brain is restricted to the calcium/calmodulin-sensitive isoforms of this enzyme. The G_s-protein–AC dysregulation in the AD brain is unlikely to result from gross changes in total G_s protein α-subunit ($G_{s\alpha}$) levels [85,89,92], although in some brain regions subtle changes in different isoforms of $G_{s\alpha}$ may be important [85]. The suggestion that alterations in AC activity may be related to the progression of AD pathology came from a study showing that reduced forskolin-stimulated enzyme activities in the hippocampus occur prior to the development of severe neurofibrillary changes [93].

The idea that disrupted receptor–G-protein regulation of AC occurs selectively at the level of the stimulatory G_s-protein input to the enzyme has received support from a number of studies that have shown that inhibitory coupling of receptors, including the noradrenaline α_2 [94], 5-hydroxy-tryptamine 1A [95], somatostatin [96], adenosine A_1 [88] and k1 opiate [97] types, to presumed G_i and G_o proteins is relatively intact in AD neocortex. In AD superior temporal cortex, the number of high-affinity, G-protein-coupled muscarinic M_2 receptor sites even appears to be increased [98,99]. However, muscarinic M_2 receptor G-protein coupling may be compromised in brain regions that show severe senile plaque and NFT pathology, such as the hippocampus [99]. Inhibition of AC enzyme activity following either direct G_i-protein activation [100] or stimulation via somatostatin or adenosine A_1 receptor types [88] is also preserved in a number of AD brain regions.

AC signalling deficits in the AD brain do not appear to be accompanied by widespread changes in PKA levels and activity [94,101]. In a recent autoradiographic study of the dentate gyrus and CA1–CA4 hippocampal subfields we showed that [^{3}H]cAMP binding to PKA did not show marked changes with respect to staging for AD neurofibrillary pathology or amyloid deposition. In contrast, apparent levels of soluble PKA in the entorhinal cortex were found to be decreased with the progression of both of these pathologies [102]. Licameli and colleagues reported that immunoreactivities for the regulatory (RIIβ) subunits of type II PKA were similar in AD and control hippocampal pyramidal neurons, but substantially decreased in the superior temporal and occipital cortices [103].

Summary

This chapter has provided an overview of current knowledge of the integrity of receptor–G-protein-mediated signalling in the AD brain *post mortem*. Given the involvement of these pathways in APP metabolism and tau phosphorylation, it is feasible that disrupted signalling may play a pivotal role in initiating and/or exacerbating the progressive neurodegeneration seen in AD [13,62,104]. This scenario is supported by recent data showing that the loss of different signalling components, such as PKC and $Ins(1,4,5)P_3$ receptor levels, correlates with the staged progression of neurofibrillary changes and amyloid deposition.

References

1.   Glenner, G.G. and Wong, C.W. (1984) *Biochem. Biophys. Res. Commun.* **120**, 885–890
2.   Masters, C.L., Simms, G., Weinman, N.A., Multhaup, G., McDonald, B.L. and Beyreuther, K. (1985) *Proc. Natl. Acad. Sci. U.S.A.* **82**, 4245–4249
3.   Kidd, M. (1963) *Nature (London)* **197**, 192–193
4.   Grundke-Iqbal, I., Iqbal, K., Tung, Y.C., Quinlan, M., Wisniewski, H.M. and Binder, L.I. (1986) *Proc. Natl. Acad. Sci. U.S.A.* **83**, 4913–4917
5.   Hardy, J. (1997) *Trends Neurosci.* **20**, 154–159
6.   Hardy, J.A. and Higgins, G.A. (1992) *Science* **256**, 184–185
7.   Iversen, L.L., Mortishire-Smith, R.J., Pollack, S.J. and Shearman, M.S. (1995) *Biochem. J.* **311**, 1–16

8.   Mattson, M.P. (1997) *Physiol. Rev.* **77**, 1081–1132
9.   Neve, R.L. and Robakis, N.K. (1998) *Trends Neurosci.* **21**, 15–19
10. Gervais, F.G., Xu, D., Robertson, G.S., Vaillancourt, J.P., Zhu, Y., Huang, J., LeBlanc, A., Smith, D., Rigby, M., Shearman, M.S., et al. (1999) *Cell* **97**, 395–406
11. Yamatsuji, T., Matsui, T., Okamoto, T., Komatsuzaki, K., Takeda, S., Fukumoto, H., Iwatsubo, T., Suzuki, N., Asami-Odaka, A., Ireland, S., et al. (1996) *Science* **272**, 1349–1352
12. Zhang, Z., Hartmann, H., Do, V.M., Abramowski, D., Sturchler-Pierrat, C., Staufenbiel, M., Sommer, B., van de Wetering, M., Clevers, H., Saftig, P., et al. (1998) *Nature (London)* **395**, 698–702
13. Lovestone, S. and Reynolds, C.H. (1997) *Neuroscience* **78**, 309–324
14. Selkoe, D.J. (1996) *Cold Spring Harbor Symp. Quant. Biol.* **61**, 587–596
15. Mills, J. and Reiner, P.B. (1999) *J. Neurochem.* **72**, 443–460
16. Caporaso, G.L., Gandy, S.E., Buxbaum, J.D., Ramabhadran, T.V. and Greengard, P. (1992) *Proc. Natl. Acad. Sci. U.S.A.* **89**, 3055–3059
17. Checler, F.J. (1995) *J. Neurochem.* **65**, 1431–1444
18. Hung, A.Y., Haass, C., Nitsch, R.M., Qiu, W.Q., Citron, M., Wurtman, R.J., Growdon, J.H. and Selkoe, D.J. (1993) *J. Biol. Chem.* **268**, 22959–22962
19. LeBlanc, A.C., Koutroumanis, M. and Goodyer, C.G. (1998) *J. Neurosci.* **18**, 2907–2913
20. Dyrks, T., Mönning, U., Beyreuther, K. and Turner, J. (1994) *FEBS Lett.* **349**, 210–214
21. Buxbaum, J.D., Oishi, M., Chen, H.I., Pinkas-Kramarski, R., Jaffe, E.A., Gandy, S.E. and Greengard, P. (1992) *Proc. Natl. Acad. Sci. U.S.A.* **89**, 10075–10078
22. Nitsch, R.M., Slack, B.E., Wurtman, R.J. and Growdon, J.H. (1992) *Science* **258**, 304–307
23. Wolf, B.A., Wertkin, A.M., Jolly, Y.C., Yasuda, R.P., Wolfe, B.B., Konrad, R.J., Manning, D., Ravi, S., Williamson, J.R. and Lee, V.M. (1995) *J. Biol. Chem.* **270**, 4916–4922
24. Lee, R.K., Wurtman, R.J., Cox, A.J. and Nitsch, R.M. (1995) *Proc. Natl. Acad. Sci. U.S.A.* **92**, 8083–8087
25. Jolly-Tornetta, C., Gao, Z.Y., Lee, V.M. and Wolf, B.A. (1998) *J. Biol. Chem.* **273**, 14015–14021
26. Emmerling, M.R., Moore, C.J., Doyle, P.D., Carroll, R.T. and Davis, R.E. (1993) *Biochem. Biophys. Res. Commun.* **197**, 292–297
27. Nitsch, R.M., Deng, M., Growdon, J.H. and Wurtman, R.J. (1996) *J. Biol. Chem.* **271**, 4188–4194
28. Nitsch, R.M., Deng, M., Wurtman, R.J. and Growdon, J.H. (1997) *J. Neurochem.* **69**, 704–712
29. Buxbaum, J.D., Ruefli, A.A., Parker, C.A., Cypess, A.M. and Greengard, P. (1994) *Proc. Natl. Acad. Sci. U.S.A.* **91**, 4489–4493
30. Querfurth, H.W. and Selkoe, D.J. (1994) *Biochemistry* **33**, 4550–4561
31. Xu, H., Greengard, P. and Gandy, S. (1995) *J. Biol. Chem.* **270**, 23243–23245
32. Xu, H., Sweeney, D., Greengard, P. and Gandy, S. (1996) *Proc. Natl. Acad. Sci. U.S.A.* **93**, 4081–4084
33. Efthimiopoulos, S., Punj, S., Manolopoulos, V., Pangalos, M., Wang, G.P., Refolo, L.M. and Robakis, N.K. (1996) *J. Neurochem.* **67**, 872–875
34. Shekarabi, M., Bourbonnière, M., Dagenais, A. and Nalbantoglu, J. (1997) *J. Neurochem.* **68**, 970–978
35. Bourbonnière, M., Shekarabi, M. and Nalbantoglu, J. (1997) *J. Neurochem.* **68**, 909–916
36. Lee, R.K., Araki, W. and Wurtman, R.J. (1997) *Proc. Natl. Acad. Sci. U.S.A.* **94**, 5422–5426
37. Shin, J.-E., Koh, J.-Y. and Mook-Jung, I. (1999) *Neurosci. Lett.* **269**, 99–102
38. Nitsch, R.M. and Growdon, J.H. (1994) *Biochem. Pharmacol.* **47**, 1275–1284
39. Goedert, M. (1996) *Ann. N.Y. Acad. Sci.* **777**, 121–131
40. Lovestone, S., Hartley, C.L., Pearce, J. and Anderton, B.H. (1996) *Neuroscience* **73**, 1145–1157
41. Pei, J.J., Sersen, E., Iqbal, K. and Grundke-Iqbal, I. (1994) *Brain Res.* **655**, 70–76

42. Pei, J.J., Braak, E., Braak, H., Grundke-Iqbal, I., Iqbal, K., Winblad, B. and Cowburn, R.F. (1999) *J. Neuropathol. Exp. Neurol.* **58**, 1010–1019

43. Blanchard, B.J., Raghunandan, R. and Roder, H.M. (1994) *Biochem. Biophys. Res. Commun.* **200**, 187–194

44. Singh, T.J., Zaidi, T., Grundke-Iqbal, I. and Iqbal, K. (1995) *FEBS Lett.* **358**, 4–8

45. Litersky, J.M. and Johnson, G.V.W. (1992) *J. Biol. Chem.* **267**, 1563–1568

46. Cross, D.A., Alessi, D.R., Cohen, P., Andjelkovich, M. and Hemmings, B.A. (1995) *Nature (London)* **378**, 785–789

47. Dale, T.C. (1998) *Biochem. J.* **329**, 209–223

48. Hartigan, J.A. and Johnson, G.V. (1999) *J. Biol. Chem.* **274**, 21395–21401

49. Goedert, M., Jakes, R., Qi, Z., Wang, J.H. and Cohen, P. (1995) *J. Neurochem.* **65**, 2804–2807

50. Gong, C.X., Grundke-Iqbal, I. and Iqbal, K. (1994) *Neuroscience* **61**, 765–772

51. Gong, C.–X., Shaikh, S., Wang, J.–Z., Zaidi, T., Grundke-Iqbal, I. and Iqbal, K. (1995) *J. Neurochem.* **65**, 732–738

52. Goedert, M., Jakes, R., Spillantini, M.G., Hasegawa, M., Smith, M.J. and Crowther, R.A. (1996) *Nature (London)* **383**, 550–553

53. Hasegawa, M., Crowther, R.A., Jakes, R. and Goedert, M. (1997) *J. Biol. Chem.* **272**, 33118–33124

54. Fowler, C.J., O'Neill, C., Garlind, A. and Cowburn, R.F. (1990) *Trends Pharmacol. Sci.* **11**, 183–184

55. Stokes, C.E. and Hawthorne, J.N. (1987) *J. Neurochem.* **48**, 1018–1021

56. Smith, C.J., Perry, E.K., Perry, R.H., Fairbairn, A.F. and Birdsall, N.J.M. (1987) *Neurosci. Lett.* **82**, 227–232

57. Flynn, D.D., Weinstein, D.A. and Mash, D.C. (1991) *Ann. Neurol.* **29**, 256–262

58. Warpman, U., Alafuzoff, I. and Nordberg, A. (1993) *Neurosci. Lett.* **150**, 39–43

59. Ladner, C.J., Celesia, C.G., Magnuson, D.J. and Lee, J.M. (1995) *J. Neuropathol. Exp. Neurol.* **54**, 783–789

60. Cutler, R., Joseph, J.A., Yamagami, K., Villalobos-Molina, R. and Roth, G.S. (1995) *Brain Res.* **664**, 54–60

61. Jope, R.S., Song, L., Li, X. and Powers, R. (1994) *Neurobiol. Aging* **15**, 221–226

62. Jope, R.S. (1996) *Alzheimer's Dis. Rev.* **1**, 2–14

63. Jope, R.S., Song, L. and Powers, R.E. (1997) *Neurobiol. Aging* **18**, 111–120

64. Greenwood, A.F., Powers, R.T.E. and Jope, R.S. (1995) *Neuroscience* **69**, 125–138

65. Shanahan, C., Deasy, M., Ravid, R. and O'Neill, C. (1995) *Biochem. Soc. Trans.* **23**, 363S

66. Li, X., Greenwood, A.F., Powers, R. and Jope, R.S. (1996) *Neurobiol. Aging* **17**, 115–122

67. Crews, F.T., Kurian, P. and Freund, G. (1994) *Life Sci.* **55**, 1992–2002

68. Ferraro-DiLeo, G. and Flynn, D.D. (1993) *Life Sci.* **53**, 439–444

69. Wallace, M.A. and Claro, E. (1993) *Neurochem. Res.* **18**, 139–145

70. Alder, J.T., Chessell, I.P. and Bowen, D.M. (1995) *Neurochem. Res.* **20**, 769–771

71. Cole, G., Dobkins, K., Hansen, L.A., Terry, R.D. and Saitoh, T. (1988) *Brain Res.* **452**, 165–174

72. Wang, H.–Y., Pisano, M.R. and Friedman, E. (1994) *Neurobiol. Aging* **15**, 293–298

73. Masliah, E., Cole, G.M., Shimohama, S., Hansen, L.A., DeTeresa, R., Terry, R.D. and Saitoh, T. (1990) *J. Neurosci.* **10**, 2113–2124

74. Shimohama, S., Narita, M., Matsushima, H., Kimura, J., Kameyama, M., Hagiwara, M., Hidaka, H. and Taniguchi, T. (1993) *Neurology* **43**, 1407–1413

75. Matsushima, H., Shimohama, S., Chachin, M., Taniguchi, T. and Kimura, J. (1996) *J. Neurochem.* **67**, 317–323

76. Masliah, E., Cole, G.M., Hansen, L.A., Mallory, M., Allbright, T., Terry, R.D. and Saitoh, T. (1991) *J. Neurosci.* **11**, 2759–2767

77. Braak, H. and Braak, E. (1991) *Acta Neuropathol.* **82**, 239–259

78.   Kurumatani, T., Fastbom, J., Bonkale, W.L., Bogdanovic, N., Winblad, B., Ohm, T.G. and
      Cowburn, R.F. (1998) *Brain Res.* **796**, 209–221
79.   Young, L.T., Kish, S.J., Li, P.P. and Warsh, J.J. (1988) *Neurosci. Lett.* **94**, 198–202
80.   Garlind, A., Cowburn, R.F., Forsell, C., Ravid, R., Winblad, B. and Fowler, C.J. (1995)
      Brain Res. **681**, 160–166
81.   Haug, L.-S., Østvold, A.C., Cowburn, R.F., Garlind, A., Winblad, B. and Walaas, S.I.
      (1996) *Neurodegeneration* **5**, 169–176
82.   Cowburn, R.F., Vestling, M., Fowler, C.J., Ravid, R., Winblad, B. and O'Neill, C. (1993)
      Neurosci. Lett. **155**, 163–166
83.   Wang, H.-Y. and Friedmann, E. (1993) *Neurosci. Lett.* **173**, 37–39
84.   Cowburn, R.F., O'Neill, C., Ravid, R., Alafuzoff, I., Winblad, B. and Fowler, C.J. (1992)
      J. Neurochem. **58**, 1409–1419
85.   O'Neill, C., Fowler, C.J., Wiehager, B., Ravid, R., Winblad, B. and Cowburn, R.F. (1994)
      Brain Res. **636**, 193–201
86.   Bonkale, W.L., Fastbom, J., Wiehager, B., Ravid, R., Winblad, B. and Cowburn, R.F. (1996)
      Brain Res. **737**, 155–161
87.   Ohm, T.G., Bohl, J. and Lemmer, B. (1991) *Brain Res.* **540**, 229–236
88.   Schnecko, A., Witte, K., Bolh, J., Ohm, T. and Lemmer, B. (1994) *Neurosci. Lett.* **644**,
      291–296
89.   Ross, B.M., McLaughlin, M., Roberts, M., Milligan, G., McCulloch, J. and Knowler, J.T.
      (1993) *Brain Res.* **622**, 35–42
90.   Yamamoto, M., Ozawa, H., Saito, T., Frolich, L., Riederer, P. and Takahata, N. (1996)
      NeuroReport **7**, 2965–2970
91.   Yamamoto, M., Ozawa, H., Saito, T., Hatta, S., Riederer, P. and Takahata, N. (1997)
      J. Neural. Transm. **104**, 721–732
92.   McLaughlin, M., Ross, B.M., Milligan, G., McCulloch, J. and Knowler, J.T. (1991)
      J. Neurochem. **57**, 9–14
93.   Ohm, T.G., Schmitt, M., Bohl, J. and Lemmer, B. (1997) *Neurobiol. Aging* **18**, 275–279
94.   O'Neill, C., Fowler, C.J., Wiehager, B., Cowburn, R.F., Alafuzoff, I. and Winblad, B.
      (1991) *Brain Res.* **563**, 39–43
95.   O'Neill, C., Cowburn, R.F., Wiehager, B., Alafuzoff, I., Winblad, B. and Fowler, C.J.
      (1991) *Neurosci. Lett.* **133**, 15–19
96.   Bergström, L., Garlind, A., Nilsson, L., Alafuzoff, I., Fowler, C.J., Winblad, B. and
      Cowburn, R.F. (1991) *J. Neurol. Sci.* **105**, 225–233
97.   Garlind, A., Cowburn, R.F., Wiehager, B., Ravid, R., Winblad, B. and Fowler, C.J. (1995)
      Neurosci. Lett. **185**, 131–134
98.   Hérnandez-Hérnandez, A., Adem, A., Ravid, R. and Cowburn, R.F. (1995) *Neurosci. Lett.*
      186, 57–60
99.   Cowburn, R.F., Wiehager, B., Ravid, R. and Winblad, B. (1996) *Neurodegeneration* **5**,
      19–26
100. Cowburn, R.F., O'Neill, C., Ravid, R., Winblad, B. and Fowler, C.J. (1992) *Neurosci. Lett.*
      141, 16–20
101. Meier-Ruge, W., Iwangoff, P. and Reichlmeier, K. (1984) *Arch. Gerontol. Geriatr.* **3**,
      161–165
102. Bonkale, W.L., Cowburn, R.F., Ohm, T.G., Bogdanovic, N. and Fastbom, J. (1999) *Brain
      Res.* **818**, 383–396
103. Licameli, V., Mattiace, L.A., Erlichman, J., Davies, P., Dickson, D. and Shafit-Zagardo, B.
      (1992) *Brain Res.* **578**, 61–68
104. Fowler, C.J. (1997) *Brain Res. Rev.* **25**, 373–380

Biochem. Soc. Symp. **67**, 177–194
(Printed in Great Britain)

17

Dysfunctional intracellular calcium homoeostasis: a central cause of neurodegeneration in Alzheimer's disease

Cora O'Neill*[1], Richard F. Cowburn†, Willy L. Bonkale†, Thomas G. Ohm‡, Johan Fastbom†, Mark Carmody* and Mary Kelliher*

*Department of Biochemistry, University College, Lee Maltings, Prospect Row, Cork, Ireland, †Karolinska Institute, NEUROTEC, Section for Geriatric Medicine, NOVUM, KFC, S-141 86, Huddinge, Sweden, and ‡Institute fur Anatomie, University Klinikum Charité, D-10098 Berlin, Germany

Abstract

The clinical symptoms of all forms of Alzheimer's disease (AD) result from a slowly progressive neurodegeneration that is associated with the excessive deposition of β-amyloid (Aβ) in plaques and in the cerebrovasculature, and the formation of intraneuronal neurofibrillary tangles, which are composed primarily of abnormally hyperphosphorylated tau protein. The sequence of cellular events that cause this pathology and neurodegeneration is unknown. It is, however, most probably linked to neuronal signal transduction systems that become misregulated in the brains of certain individuals, causing excessive Aβ to be formed and/or deposited, tau to become aggregated and hyperphosphorylated and neurons to degenerate. We hypothesize that a progressive alteration in the ability of neurons to regulate intracellular calcium, particularly at the level of the endoplasmic reticulum, is a crucial signal transduction event that is linked strongly to the initiation and development of AD pathology. In this chapter we will discuss the key findings that lend support to this hypothesis.

[1]To whom correspondence should be addressed.

Cellular mechanisms proposed to underlie the neurodegeneration of AD: where does calcium fit in?

Calcium (Ca^{2+}) has long been implicated as a key life and death signal for neurons [1] and many studies support a key role for deregulated Ca^{2+} homoeostasis in the neurodegenerative processes of AD [2–4]. Although it is indisputable that Ca^{2+} is involved in the neurodegeneration of AD, it has been difficult to evaluate whether dysfunctions in neuronal Ca^{2+} metabolism are a proximal cause or an associated consequence of the disease pathology. For dysfunctional Ca^{2+} homoeostasis to be a primary cause of the neurodegeneration of AD, it should occur early on in the disease and have the potential to cause progressive β-amyloid deposition, abnormal tau hyperphosphorylation and selective neuronal cell death. Evidence outlined in this chapter indicates that this could be the case. Findings discussed below also support the possibility that dysfunctional Ca^{2+} homoeostasis is a driving force for AD pathology, secondary to increased Aβ, increased C-100 [the 100 C-terminal amino acids of the β-amyloid precursor protein (APP)] and/or reciprocal decreased sAPPα (a secreted product of APP processing) in the disease. Recent findings have also shown that mutations in presenilin 1 and presenilin 2, which cause familial forms of AD, deregulate intracellular Ca^{2+} homoeostasis [5]. Together, this data suggests that altered Ca^{2+} homoeostasis may be a common cellular instigator for neurodegeneration in both sporadic and familial forms of AD

Neuronal Ca^{2+} homoeostasis

Intracellular Ca^{2+} ([Ca^{2+}]i) is a critical neuronal second messenger playing a vital role in synaptic transmission and the maintenance of neuronal function and survival [1,5]. Neurons possess elaborately controlled systems for regulating and responding to changes in [Ca^{2+}]i because of its crucial and powerful signalling role. (Figure 1 shows a simplified scheme of the mechanisms which control [Ca^{2+}]i homoeostasis.) Briefly, intraneuronal Ca^{2+} is derived from sources both outside and inside the cell. Ca^{2+} enters the cell through voltage- and ligand-operated ion channels and is also released within the cell from endoplasmic reticulum (ER) stores by activation of Ins(1,4,5)P_3 (IP$_3$) receptors (IP$_3$Rs) and ryanodine receptors (RyRs). In general IP$_3$Rs respond to IP$_3$ which is produced through agonist activation of the phosphatidylinositol signalling pathway, whereas RyRs are directly responsive to [Ca^{2+}]i, so-called Ca^{2+}-induced Ca^{2+} release.

A variety of other proteins play a crucial role in maintaining [Ca^{2+}]i homoeostasis. These include: the SERCA (sarcoplasmic/endoplasmic-reticulum Ca^{2+}-ATPase) pump, which accumulates Ca^{2+} into the ER; Ca^{2+}-ATPase and Na^+/Ca^{2+} membrane exchangers in the plasma membrane, which move Ca^{2+} out of the cell; and Ca^{2+}-binding proteins which sequester free Ca^{2+}. The mitochondria also sequester some of the Ca^{2+} signal and Ca^{2+} shuttles between the ER and mitochondria. The maintenance of [Ca^{2+}]i homoeostasis in neu-

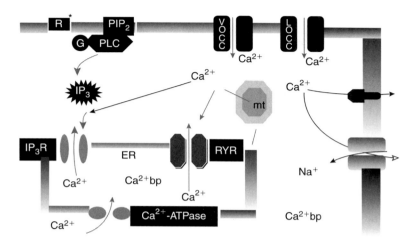

Figure 1 Scheme of the primary components operating to control neuronal Ca^{2+} concentrations. Ca^{2+} enters neurons through either voltage- or ligand-operated Ca^{2+} channels (VOCC and LOCC), and is removed from the neuron by Ca^{2+} pumps or Na$^+$/Ca^{2+} exchange. Release of intracellular Ca^{2+} from ER stores occurs either by activation of Ins(1,4,5)P_3 (IP$_3$) receptors in response to IP$_3$ produced by agonist activation of receptors (R*) linked to the phosphatidylinositol cycle, or by activation of ryanodine receptors (RyR) which are activated primarily by Ca^{2+}. Ca^{2+} is pumped into the ER by Ca^{2+}-ATPase proteins and sequestered by a variety of binding proteins (bp) both within the ER and in the cytosol. Ca^{2+} also accumulates in the mitochondria (mt) and can shuttle between the mitochondria and ER. Abbreviations used: PIP$_2$, PtdIns(4,5)P_2.

rons relies heavily upon the ER and the interplay between and responses of the IP$_3$R, the RyR and the SERCA pump and their respective control proteins [1].

APP metabolism and neuronal calcium homoeostasis

The influence of Ca^{2+} on APP processing

Altered APP processing to overproduce Aβ42/43 is believed to be a primary event in the pathological cascade that is AD [6]. Proteolytic degradation of APP, by the combined action of two proteases dubbed β-secretase and γ-secretase, produces the Aβ peptide [6]. β-secretase cleaves APP immediately N-terminal to the Aβ sequence yielding a large, soluble, secreted APP fragment, sAPPβ, and a C-100 fragment. C-100 is subsequently processed by γ-secretase to yield Aβ which is predominantly 42/43 and 40 amino acids long. These Aβ peptides are secreted but can also be found inside neurons. Aβ42 accounts for only 10% of the secreted Aβ but is the major fibrillogenic species found accumulated in senile plaques of AD. APP can also be endoproteolytically cleaved at the cell surface within the Aβ sequence by α-secretase generating sAPPα and the non-amyloidogenic 3 kDa (p3) Aβ peptide.

It has been widely shown that APP processing can be modulated by cell signal transduction pathways including Ca^{2+} ([7]; see also chapter 16). Of interest, firstly with respect to intracellular Ca^{2+} signalling, is the finding that Aβ42 localizes to the ER in neurons but does not appear to do so in other cell types [8,9]. This suggests that the ER may be an important site for generating Aβ42. In agreement with this studies have shown that activation of ER Ca^{2+} release from RyRs in HEK-293 cells increased total Aβ and p3 secretion fourfold [10]. This effect was potentiated by thapsigargin and cyclopiazonic acid agents which raise $[Ca^{2+}]i$ by preventing its reuptake into the ER [10]. Other studies have reported that thapsigargin could either increase or decrease Aβ release, depending on the concentration used, and that it could increase formation of soluble APP (sAPP) from CHO cells overexpressing APP_{751} following down-regulation of protein kinase C (PKC) [11]. In contrast to these findings, Nitsch and colleagues did not observe any changes in the levels of sAPP release in 3T3 cells following treatment with thapsigargin [12]. Treatment of cells with the Ca^{2+} ionophore A23187 has also been shown to up-regulate total Aβ production, this effect appeared to be dependent on extracellular Ca^{2+} [13]. The exact relationship between the release and uptake of Ca^{2+} and the processing of APP in the ER remains to be defined, particularly in neurons where APP processing differs from that detected in cell lines of peripheral origin [14]. The mechanism(s) underlying the effect of disrupted ER Ca^{2+} signalling on APP processing may involve alteration of the exit or export of APP or C-100 from the ER, and/or alteration in the regulation of Ca^{2+}-dependent cofactors/proteins controlling the secretase enzymes, or indeed direct effects of Ca^{2+} on the secretase enzymes that cleave APP. In this respect, the regulation of ER Ca^{2+} release exerted by the presenilin proteins may influence their role in γ-secretase processing of APP (see section on presenilins).

The influence of Aβ, C-100 and sAPP on Ca^{2+} homoeostasis

A greater quantity of work has focused upon the effects of APP and its metabolites on Ca^{2+} homoeostasis than on the effect of Ca^{2+} homoeostasis on APP processing. The overall outcome of this work suggests that overproduction of Aβ and its precursor C-100 or diminished production of sAPPα has a primary effect on neuronal Ca^{2+} homoeostasis. This is proposed to initiate a pathological neuronal cell death cascade that could potentially be inhibited by blocking these detrimental Ca^{2+} responses. Work examining the effect of Aβ on Ca^{2+} homoeostasis has been performed in a variety of cell culture systems using a broad array of Aβ types, Aβ preparation methods and Aβ concentrations. Primarily, studies have used micromolar concentrations of Aβ40 and Aβ25–35 peptides with fewer studies using Aβ42. It is still unclear which species of Aβ is neurotoxic, e.g. protofibrils, oligomers or higher-molecular-mass species (see chapter 1), and whether the Aβ is only neurotoxic outside the neuron or can be toxic upon intracellular production. Results have shown that Aβ peptides can induce neurotoxicity by increasing $[Ca^{2+}]i$ [15] which can involve enhanced excitatory-amino-acid- and Ca^{2+}-ionophore-induced Ca^{2+}

fluxes [16–18]. In agreement with this, Aβ peptides have been shown to affect Ca^{2+} uptake into PC12 cells [19] and cortical and hippocampal neurons [20]. They have also been shown to increase the activity of Ca^{2+}-channel proteins, including the L-type voltage-operated Ca^{2+} channels [21,22], possibly through mitogen-activated protein (MAP) kinase phosphorylation of the channel [23], and N-type voltage-gated Ca^{2+} channels [24]. The IP_3 Ca^{2+}-release channel has been shown to exhibit enhanced $[^3H]IP_3$ binding in the presence of Aβ peptides [25] and also to mobilize Ca^{2+} in response to Aβ peptides [26]. The involvement of voltage-operated Ca^{2+} channels in Aβ-induced neurodegeneration is further confirmed by findings that Aβ-induced neurodegeneration can be blocked by nimodipine and Co^{2+} [21,22]. Aβ peptides have also been found to impair K^+-dependent Ca^{2+} flux [27,28] and to block Na^+/K^+-ATPase activity, thus indirectly impairing the removal of excess $[Ca^{2+}]i$ by ion-exchange pumps [29,30].

The mechanism(s) by which Aβ affects such a range of the cellular Ca^{2+} signalling machinery and the relevance of the *in vitro* work to the situation that occurs *in vivo* is unknown. The observation that Aβ40 [31,32] and Aβ42 [33] can insert into synthetic lipid bilayers and reconstituted lipid vesicles as a Ca^{2+}-carrying ionophore may be important. In this respect the localization of Aβ42 to the ER in neurons and the identification of specific binding sites for Aβ in the ER [34] suggest the possibility that Aβ42 may disrupt ER Ca^{2+} homoeostasis by inserting into ER membranes. The exact sequence of signalling events by which Aβ-induced increases in $[Ca^{2+}]i$ cause neuronal cell death is not entirely clear but it has been proposed to trigger intracellular events that eventually cause cell dysfunction and death, including oxidative stress and activation of apoptotic cell death pathways.

C-100, cleaved from APP by β-secretase, which includes the Aβ sequence has also been shown to affect Ca^{2+} homoeostasis. Studies have shown that PC12 cells expressing C-100 show altered Ca^{2+} handling [35] and exhibit enhanced sensitivity to the Ca^{2+} ionophore A23187 [36], with this peptide also showing the ability to propagate intercellular Ca^{2+} waves [37]. Further studies have shown that this APP fragment inhibits the Na^+/Ca^{2+}-exchanger activity in SK-N-SH cells [38] and decreases the activity of the Mg^{2+}/Ca^{2+}-ATPase of the ER, suggesting that this peptide, which is only found inside neurons, can inhibit the ability of the ER to sequester Ca^{2+} in AD [39].

sAPPα has also been found to modulate $[Ca^{2+}]i$, where it normalizes $[Ca^{2+}]i$ increases induced by cellular insults including Aβ. Increases in the second messenger cGMP and its responsive cGMP-dependent kinase [40], and activation of the transcription factor nuclear factor κB (NF-κB) [41], have been shown to be involved in the Ca^{2+}-normalizing effect of sAPPα. sAPPα has also been found to activate K^+ channels [42], an effect that was mimicked by cGMP and that reduced Ca^{2+} influx [42,43], suggesting that activation of K^+ channels and membrane hyperpolarization may be the primary neuroprotective target of sAPPα. In summary it is believed that increased production of Aβ in association with decreased production of sAPPα will have detrimental effects on the neuronal Ca^{2+} signalling machinery activating cell death pathways in the AD brain.

Presenilin modulation of Ca^{2+} homoeostasis

Disrupted Ca^{2+} homoeostasis may be a common cellular pathway for neurodegeneration both in sporadic and familial forms of AD. This evolves from findings showing that presenilin 1 (PS1) and presenilin 2 (PS2) mutations which cause familial forms of AD, cause disruptions in intracellular Ca^{2+} homoeostasis which can cause neurodegeneration. The effect of presenilin mutations on Ca^{2+} homoeostasis primarily targets the ER, affecting both IP_3R- and RyR-induced Ca^{2+} release (see chapter 15). This fits in with the cellular localization of the presenilins, which are detected predominantly in the ER [44–46]. Results have shown that familial AD-causing PS1 mutations enhance Ca^{2+}release in a variety of systems including: cells transfected with PS1 mutants [47,48]; mutant PS1 knockin mice [49]; synaptosomes prepared from transgenic mice expressing mutant PS1 [50]; and fibroblasts from patients with familial AD [51,52]. Increased $[Ca^{2+}]i$ levels and resultant neurotoxic responses to Aβ and other stressors induced by PS-1 mutations could be blocked by dantrolene, an inhibitor of RyR-induced Ca^{2+} release [47,48,50], suggesting that the neurodegenerative effect induced by PS1 mutations involves disruption of RyR-induced Ca^{2+} release from the ER. Recent results confirm this and have shown that PS2 interacts with the Ca^{2+}-binding protein sorcin [53], a known modulator of RyR activity [54], which influences the interaction of RyRs with L-type Ca^{2+} channels [55], and that RyR expression levels are enhanced by PS1 mutations (see chapter 15). PS1 mutations have also been found to affect the IP_3 receptor, where IP_3-evoked Ca^{2+} signals were found to be potentiated significantly by PS1 mutants, in *Xenopus* oocytes [56]. Furthermore, fibroblasts from patients with PS1 mutations, and PC12 cells transfected with PS1 mutants, exhibit increased Ca^{2+} release from intracellular stores in response to agonists that activate the phosphatidylinositol signal transduction system [47,51,52].

The importance of ER Ca^{2+} release in the neurodegeneration of AD is shown by findings which demonstrate that blocking enhanced ER Ca^{2+} release, particularly with dantrolene which targets the RyR can protect against the neurodegeneration initiated by PS mutations and Aβ. The relationship between PS mutant-induced increases in Aβ42 production and ER Ca^{2+} homoeostasis remains to be determined. In this respect it is of importance to investigate whether increased Aβ42 production is a cause or consequence of ER Ca^{2+}-release dysfunction.

Calcium signalling and tau hyperphosphorylation

Tau proteins are the predominant component of the paired helical filaments (PHFs) in intracellular neurofibrillary tangles (NFTs), neuropil threads and neuritic plaques of the AD brain. PHF-tau differs from normal tau by several post-translational modifications, including hyperphosphorylation, altered glycosylation and altered proteolysis. Tau hyperphosphorylation is regarded as the major driving force for PHF formation and severely affects tau function, reducing its ability to bind to and stabilize microtubules, thus leading to disturbances in neuronal microtubular function in the AD brain [57,58].

Tau hyperphosphorylation must ensue through deregulation of one or several signal transduction cascades regulating kinases and/or phosphatases targeting tau [57]. However, the cellular mechanisms contributing to phosphorylation of tau to form PHFs in AD are still unclear and appear to be complex. Presently the consensus is that the proline-directed kinases, including: glycogen synthase kinase-3 (GSK-3); cyclin-dependent kinases, cdc(2) (cell division control) and CDK5 (p35): and MAP kinases, extracellular signal-related protein kinase, c-jun N-terminal kinase and p38 MAP kinase, are prominently involved in tau phosphorylation [57]. Of these, GSK-3β is believed to be a crucial physiological kinase for tau, and studies have shown that GSK-3 preferentially localizes to NFT-bearing neurons [59] and that the distribution of the active form of the enzyme parallels the spread of AD neurofibrillary changes [60]. Phosphorylation of tau by non-proline-directed kinases also occurs. These include protein kinase A (PKA), myristoylated alanine-rich C-kinase, calcium/calmodulin-dependent kinase II (CaM kinase II), casein kinase I and II and protein kinase C (PKC), some of which have been shown to act synergistically with the proline-directed kinases in the phosphorylation of tau [57]. The protein phosphatases PP2A, PP2B and PP1 also have important roles in the regulation of the phosphorylation state of tau and can dephosphorylate tau that has been phosphorylated by many of the above kinases, converting it to a normal form [61]. It has also been shown that PP2A and PP2B can catalyse tau dephosphorylation in PHFs prepared from AD brains [62].

Intracellular Ca^{2+} signals of varying amplitude and frequency are vital regulators of cellular kinase and phosphatases [63,64]. It is therefore possible that hyperphosphorylation of tau is an event downstream of a primary defect of $[Ca^{2+}]i$ homoeostasis. In this respect it has been shown that Ca^{2+} can control many of the kinases and phosphatases implicated in tau phosphorylation including GSK-3β, the MAP kinase family, the cyclin-dependent kinases and many of the non-proline-directed protein kinases, particularly PKA, PKC and CaM kinase II, plus the Ca^{2+}-dependent phosphatase PP2B or calcineurin. Transient increases in $[Ca^{2+}]i$ have been shown to cause persistent tyrosine phosphorylation and activation of GSK-3β resulting in prolonged site-selective increases in tau phosphorylation [65]. It has also been shown that Ca^{2+} influx through the N-methyl-D-aspartate (NMDA) receptors dephosphorylates tau [67]. Impaired Ca^{2+} influx through the NMDA receptor may thus cause tau hyperphosphorylation possibly through down-regulation of the CaM kinase II–Akt-pathway [68] which would cause activation of GSK-3β.

Results have shown that calcineurin can dephosphorylate tau at select sites [62] and can revert tau that has been phosphorylated *in vitro* by CaM kinase II, PKA, MAP kinase and cdc(2) kinase to a normal-like state [61] that can bind to microtubules and promote tubulin polymerization. These results suggest that impaired calcineurin activity in the AD brain can lead to neurofibrillary pathology. Ca^{2+} has been shown to regulate other aspects of tau function other than the kinases and phosphatases that phosphorylate tau. These include the ability to induce aggregates of PHF-tau but not normal human tau [69], and the proteolysis of tau by calpains [70].

Studies of the direct effect of altering $[Ca^{2+}]i$ on the state of tau phosphorylation within cells have for the most part not investigated the response to changes in the amplitude and frequency of the Ca^{2+} signal, which plays an important role in mediating phosphorylation-dependent cell function. Rather, these studies have simply totally up-regulated intracellular Ca^{2+} using agents such as Ca^{2+} ionophores. These studies have found that the treatment of primary neuronal cultures with Ca^{2+} ionophores both increases [17,71] and decreases [72] tau phosphorylation. Ca^{2+} ionophore treatment of human neuroblastoma cells was also shown to result in both increases [73] and decreases [74] in tau phosphorylation. Further studies have shown that increasing intracellular Ca^{2+} by activation of NMDA receptors results in the dephosphorylation of tau in rat brain slices [75] and cortical neuronal cultures [72]. More in-depth studies are needed to define which aspects of $[Ca^{2+}]i$ signalling control tau phosphorylation, and how this relates to the effects of Ca^{2+} on APP metabolism.

Ca^{2+} signal transduction dysfunction in the AD brain

Regulation of $[Ca^{2+}]i$ homoeostasis is impaired in the post-mortem AD brain when compared to control brains, which correlates with the *in vitro* work outlined above. This occurs at a number of levels including alterations in Ca^{2+}-channel proteins and the status of many Ca^{2+}-activated enzymes, such as key neuronal proteases, kinases and phosphatases. Prominent among the Ca^{2+}-channel defects are critical alterations in the IP_3R and RyR Ca^{2+}-release channels of the ER, which are affected at very early stages of AD pathology and in the specific brain areas which are damaged in the disease. Work by our groups suggests that a primary, but slowly progressive impairment in the control of Ca^{2+} release from the ER in AD brain, would have a downstream effect on an array of vital Ca^{2+}-regulatable systems and on ER function in neurons, thus causing progressive neuronal damage and AD pathology and neuronal loss. Figure 2 shows the proposed model.

IP_3Rs and RyRs in AD

The activation of IP_3R and RyR ER Ca^{2+}-release channels plays a crucial role in regulating diverse Ca^{2+} signals and an array of neuronal functions such as excitability, release of transmitters, synaptic plasticity, gene expression and neuronal survival, being central to efficient receptor communication and co-ordination in brain [1]. Disruption of efficient ER Ca^{2+} release would be expected to have a negative effect on all of the above neuronal functions, many of which are known to be impaired in the AD brain.

The first evidence suggesting that Ca^{2+} release from the ER was impaired in the AD brain *post mortem* was provided by Young and colleagues [76] who reported significant reductions in the number of $[^3H]IP_3$ binding sites in

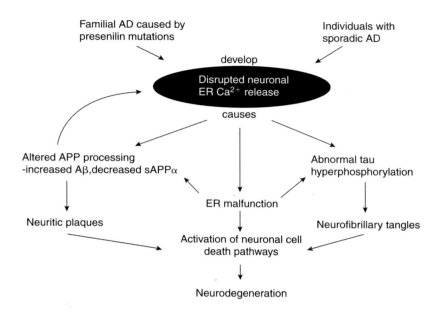

Figure 2 Simplified model outlining mechanisms by which disrupted neuronal Ca²⁺ release from the ER may cause the neurodegeneration and pathology of AD.

homogenates of AD parietal cortex and hippocampus, but not in the frontal, occipital or temporal cortices, when compared to control brains. This study was confirmed by Garlind and colleagues [77], who detected reduced [³H]IP₃ binding in the same brain regions and also in AD temporal cortex, frontal cortex and cerebellum when compared to matched control brains. Subsequently it was reported that reduced IP₃R levels in the AD temporal cortex, as determined by immunoblotting (using an antisera that did not discriminate between IP₃R isoforms), correlated with a semi-quantitative score for neuritic plaque and NFT accumulation [78]. In agreement with this it has been shown that IP₃R loss in the entorhinal cortex, subiculum and CA1 pyramidal layer of the anterior hippocampus correlated with the staging for both neurofibrillary changes and amyloid deposition [79]. These latter results strongly suggest that progressive loss of IP₃R and [³H]IP₃ binding sites in AD is linked mechanistically to the development of disease pathology.

Historically RyRs have been little examined in human brain and not at all in neurodegenerative disorders. This has been an oversight as RyRs may be as or more important than IP₃Rs when considering human brain Ca²⁺ homoeostasis in AD. This is owing to the presence of RyR, particularly RyR-2, in areas that are susceptible to degeneration in AD [80,81] and to the fact that the unit conductance for RyR is about 10 times that of IP₃R. Our group was the first to examine the integrity of the RyR in the AD brain [82]. These studies found that the B_{max} (maximum number of binding sites) for [³H]ryanodine binding was reduced significantly in areas of the brain affected by AD pathology (temporal cortex) but not in areas which are relatively unaffected pathologically (putamen, occipital cortex). This reduction in B_{max} was due in part to loss of the RyR-2 isoform, which was the only RyR isoform detected in the human brain temporal cortex. Deficiencies in the ability of magnesium and Ruthenium Red to inhibit [³H]ryanodine binding were also found, suggesting that the RyRs are impaired functionally in AD brain. Autoradiographical analysis of [³H]ryanodine binding in sections of entorhinal cortex and anterior hippocampus staged for disease pathology, according to a protocol devised by Braak and Braak [83], found that [³H]ryanodine binding was significantly and selectively increased in areas of the hippocampus (CA1, subiculum) which succumb to early (Stage I–II) neurofibrillary pathology, compared to brain sections from matched neurologically normal control cases. This up-regulation effect was selective for RyRs, as [³H]IP₃ or [³H]phorbol 12,13-dibutyrate binding was not increased in these same sections [79]. Following on from this, [³H]ryanodine binding decreased progressively in a fashion that correlated with the advancement of neurofibrillary pathology in the hippocampus and also with Aβ build-up in some hippocampal regions. At the end-stage of the disease, loss of [³H]ryanodine binding was extremely severe in the hippocampal sections (74–84%), suggesting that RyR Ca^{2+}-release function is radically impaired once neurofibrillary pathology becomes severe (Stage V–VI) [82]. This would have severe repercussions for efficient neuronal function. We believe that the initial up-regulation of [³H]ryanodine binding and increased RyR Ca^{2+} release may precede initial neuronal pathology in vulnerable brain regions.

Further studies in our group have shown that levels of cytosolic FKBP12 (FK506-binding protein MW 12 kDa), a key modulatory protein for both RyRs and IP₃Rs [84], is significantly and selectively reduced in brain regions affected by the pathology of AD [85]. This loss of FKBP12 correlates positively with the loss of RyR-2 and [³H]ryanodine binding in the disease ([85] and M. Carmody, M. Kelliher and C. O'Neill, unpublished work) suggesting that loss of FKBP12 may be linked mechanistically to RyR-2 dysfunction in the disease. Loss of FKBP12 is known to have severe repercussions on RyR function, rendering these calcium channels 'leaky' and unable to exhibit full conductance states [84,86], a situation that may thus occur in the AD brain.

Such an alteration in both RyRs and IP₃Rs as detected in AD would be expected to put the ER under progressive and eventually substantial stress, a phenomenon that has been hypothesized to underlie neuronal degeneration [5] and which will influence vital ER functions including protein folding, secretion, aggregation and export [87]. This impairment of RyR and IP₃R responses would also severely compromise key neuronal signal transduction pathways that underlie cognitive and higher mental function. Inherent in this is impaired function of the vast array of enzymes and binding proteins that are controlled by temporal and spatial increases in $[Ca^{2+}]i$ brought about by RyR and IP₃R which is discussed in the sections below.

Ca^{2+}-dependent enzymes in the AD brain

Many key Ca^{2+}-regulated enzymes have been found to be impaired in AD brain. These include: proteases, including the calpains; kinases, including PKC; CaM kinase II; the phosphatase calcineurin; and oxidative stress-linked enzymes including nitric oxide synthase (NOS) and phospholipase A$_2$ (PLA$_2$) Other key Ca^{2+}-regulated signalling molecules such as adenylate cyclase and phospholipase C are also dysfunctional in AD brain and are discussed in chapter 16.

Ca^{2+}-dependent proteases in the AD brain

One of the most thoroughly studied groups of Ca^{2+}-dependent proteases are the calpains, which are Ca^{2+}-activated cysteine proteases. There are two isoenzymes, calpain I and calpain II, which require micromolar and millimolar levels of Ca^{2+} respectively for full activity *in vitro*. These proteases regulate protein function by limited proteolysis. Both isoforms have been found to be consistently up-regulated in the brains of patients with AD [88–90]. Grynspan and colleagues [88] have shown that active calpain II accumulates in NFTs and is an early-appearing pervasive component of the neurofibrillary pathology in the disease. Studies by Tsuji and colleagues [91] have detected significantly increased levels of calpain II in cytosolic fractions from AD brains *post mortem* when compared to control tissue. It is possible that increased Ca^{2+} release from RyRs is responsible for calpain II activation in the hippocampus at early stages of AD although this has not been investigated. Calpain II has been shown to be activated at very early stages of neurofibrillary pathology in the entorhinal cortex and hippocampus. This would be consistent with the up-regulation of [^{3}H]ryanodine binding sites observed by us in these regions at early stages in the development of neurofibrillary pathology. Calpain mobilization and its long-term and abnormal activation are believed to be a major contributor to proteolysis and removal of cytoskeletal fragments during NFT formation. It is also believed to play an important role in aggregation events, particularly of the cytoskeleton, while also cleaving and modulating kinases and phosphatases that modulate cytoskeletal proteins including tau.

Calpain activity is thought also to be necessary for apoptotic cell death in certain systems [92,93] and to proteolytically cleave enzymes and proteins involved in apoptosis. Amongst these are the caspase protease family which are believed to play a key role in apoptotic cell death pathways in the nervous system [92] and have been shown to be regulated by [Ca^{2+}]i and calpains [92,94,95]. Work is presently emerging to support a role for the caspase protease family in the neurodegeneration of AD [96,97]. An extensive study of the integrity of these cysteine proteases in the AD brain has not been performed. However, studies have detected a 50–100% elevation in caspase I or interleukin-1β-converting enzyme (ICE) in the hippocampus of AD brains compared to controls [98], with overexpression of ICE-α cDNA also reported in the AD brain [99]. Furthermore, transcription factors activated by caspase-1, such as NF-κB, can be induced by elevated [Ca^{2+}]i and drive important responses to neuronal stress. Activated NF-κB p65 has been shown to be up-regulated in the AD brain [100] where it has been found to associate with the plaque pathology of the disease [101,102].

Ca^{2+}-activated kinases in the AD brain

Central and critical alterations in the PKC family of enzymes have been described in the brains of AD patients. PKC dysfunction has been the most consistent and reported alteration in the phosphoinositide signalling pathway in AD brain and is discussed in detail in chapter 16. Disrupted intracellular Ca^{2+} homoeostasis may be a driving force for PKC dysfunction in AD as the conventional PKC isoforms (α, βI, βII and γ) are regulated by Ca^{2+} and show reduced activity in AD brain compared to control tissue.

CaM kinase II is one of the most abundant kinases in the brain and has a key role in memory function and synaptic plasticity [103,104]. This Ca^{2+}-dependent kinase is widely expressed in neurons vulnerable to AD pathology and has been shown to be differentially modulated in AD, where it is shown to be associated with PHF [105,106]. The finding that GSK-3β is overactive in the brains of AD patients compared to controls, and that the active form of the enzyme co-localizes with NFTs in the disease, suggests that the enzyme is mis-regulated in AD. This altered regulation may include loss of the normal inhibitory input to GSK-β induced by growth factors, wingless (wnt)/β-catenin signalling and also by CaM kinase II activation, all of which can increase the kinase activity of Akt to phosphorylate and inactivate GSK-3β.

Ca^{2+}-dependent phosphatases in the AD brain

PP2B or calcineurin is expressed at very high levels in the brain and can dephosphorylate PHF-tau *in vitro* as mentioned above. Calcineurin has a variety of roles in the nervous system including: the regulation of Ca^{2+} release from IP_3R and RyR, neurotransmitter release, synaptic plasticity and neuronal survival/apoptosis. Studies examining calcineurin in the brain *post mortem* detected a co-localization of calcineurin with NFT and a selective reduction of calcineurin expression in neurons containing NFTs [59]. Furthermore, knock-out mice lacking the gene for the calcineurin catalytic subunit show accumulation of phosphorylated tau in the hippocampus [107]. Initial immunoblot analysis did not detect any difference in total levels of calcineurin when co-mapping homogenates prepared from AD and matched control brains [108,109]. However, more detailed studies by Ladner and colleagues [110] detected reduced calcineurin activity in the AD brain, which correlated inversely with NFT and neuritic plaque density and which was selective to areas pathologically affected by the disorder.

Ca^{2+}-activated NOS and PLA_2 in the AD brain

The integrity of Ca^{2+}-activated enzymes involved in Ca^{2+}-induced oxidative stress pathways in the brain, including the neuronal and endothelial isoforms of NOS (nNOS and eNOS) and PLA_2, has been examined in AD brains. NOS has received the most attention, owing to the key role that NO is believed to play in neurodegenerative pathways. Results from investigations examining the integrity of NOS in AD brain have been somewhat contradictory. Thus some investigations have shown nNOS-containing neurons to be susceptible to neurodegeneration, with decreased levels of nNOS detected in the entorhinal cortex and hippocampus of AD brains [111,112] compared to controls. Whereas other investigations have reported nNOS-containing neurons to be resistant to the neurodegeneration of AD [113]. The eNOS enzyme has been reported to be aberrantly expressed in the AD brain compared to control brain tissue [114]. Studies performed in our group have detected a selective impairment of the nNOS isoform in areas pathologically affected by AD with highly significant reductions in nNOS levels in the presence of unaltered nNOS activity, suggesting a loss of control of this enzyme in AD ([115] and M. Kenny, R. Ravid and C. O'Neill, unpublished work).

PLA_2 activates the arachidonic acid cascade leading to the generation of multiple eicosanoids, many of which are believed to play a role in the inflammatory process. PLA_2 is activated by very low levels of Ca^{2+} and thought to control receptor-mediated eicosanoid production. Ross and colleagues have detected significant reductions in PLA_2 activity, both in the presence and absence of Ca^{2+} in the parietal and temporal cortex of AD brains compared to control brains [116]. On the other hand, Stephenson and colleagues, showed elevations in cytosolic PLA_2 immunoreactivity in AD brains suggestive of the presence of an increased inflammatory response mechanism through this pathway in the disease [117].

Ca^{2+}-binding proteins in AD

Ca^{2+}-binding proteins buffer intracellular Ca^{2+} levels and regulate many Ca^{2+}-dependent processes playing a vital role in maintaining efficient Ca^{2+} homoeostasis in the brain. In general, many of the Ca^{2+}-binding proteins investigated so far in the AD brain are expressed to much higher levels in interneurons than in pyramidal neurons, the latter being the major neuronal type to degenerate in AD. These Ca^{2+}-binding proteins include: parvalbumin, calretilin, and calbindin 28K. The general consensus from work performed is that neurons containing these binding proteins are resistant to the neurodegeneration of AD [118–121]. Some investigations have detected a selective loss of calbindin 28K in specific cortical layers of the AD brain, when compared to control brains [122,123], with more recent results also detecting subfield- and layer-specific changes in parvalbumin and calretilin in the entorhinal cortex in AD [124]. A more specific study of the functional integrity and profile of the Ca^{2+}-binding proteins of pyramidal neurons would be beneficial in elucidating whether changes in the function or expression of these proteins are linked to the Ca^{2+}-induced neurodegenerative pathways of AD.

Summary and future directions

Disrupted Ca^{2+} release from the ER, particularly from the RyR, is one of the earliest changes described in neuronal Ca^{2+} homoeostasis in the AD brain. We believe that slowly progressive impairments in both the RyR and IP_3R cause the progressive deregulation of a number of critical Ca^{2+}-dependent enzymes to induce cellular stress leading to the neurodegeneration and pathology of AD. This raises the exciting possibility that targeting these ER Ca^{2+} channels to negate their malfunction may protect against the neurodegeneration of AD. In the future, experiments examining the role of the RyR, IP_3R and ER functions in neurodegeneration will be important. In this respect, development of neuronal expression systems, both cell lines and transgenic animals, for normal and genetically modified RyRs and IP_3Rs will provide valuable information about the role of these receptors in brain function and neurodegeneration.

We are grateful to the Health Research Board of Ireland, the Alzheimer Society of Ireland and Enterprise Ireland for the financial support of our research work.

References

1.   Berridge, M.J., Bootman, M.D. and Lipp, P. (1998) *Nature (London)* **395**, 645–648
2.   Mattson, M.P. (1990) *Neuron* **4**, 105–117
3.   Mark, R.J., Hensley, K., Butterfield, D.A. and Mattson, M.P. (1995) *J. Neurosci.* **15**, 6239–6249
4.   Mattson, M.P., Furukawa, K., Bruce, A.J., Mark, R.J. and Blanc, E.M. (1996) in *Molecular Mechanisms of Dementia* (Wasco, W. and Tanzi, R.E., eds.), pp. 103–143, Human Press, Totowa, New Jersey
5.   Mattson, M.P., Guo, Q., Furukawa, K. and Pedersen, W.A. (1998) *J. Neurochem.* **70**, 1–14
6.   Selkoe, D.J. (1999) *Nature (London)* **399**, A23–A31
7.   Mills, J. and Reiner, R.B. (1999) *J. Neurochem.* **72**, 443–460
8.   Cook, D.G., Forman, M.S., Sung, J.C., Leight, S., Kolson, D.L., Iwatsubo, T., Lee, V.M.-Y. and Doms, R.W. (1997) *Nat. Med. (N.Y.)* **3**, 1021–1023
9.   Hartman, T., Bieger, S.C., Bruhl, B., Tienari, P.J., Ida, N., Allsop, D., Roberts, G.W., Masters, C.L., Dotti, C.G., Unsicker, K. and Beyreuther, K. (1997) *Nat. Med. (N.Y.)* **3** 1016–1020
10. Querfurth, H.W., Jiang, J.M., Geiger, J.D. and Selkoe, D.J. (1997) *J. Neurochem.* **69**, 1580–1591
11. Buxbaum, J.D., Ruefli, A.A., Parker, C.A., Cypess, A.M. and Greengard, P. (1994) *Proc. Natl. Acad. Sci. U.S.A.* **91**, 4489–4493
12. Nitsch, R.M., Deng, M., Growdon, J.H. and Wurtman, R.J. (1996) *J. Biol. Chem.* **271**, 4188–4194
13. Querfurth, H.W. and Selkoe, D.J. (1994) *Biochemistry* **33**, 4550–4561
14. LeBlanc, A.C., Xue, R. and Gambetti, P (1996) *J. Neurochem.* **66**, 2300–2310
15. Mattson, M.P. (1997) *Physiol. Rev.* **77**, 1081–1132
16. Yankner, B.A., Duffy, L.K. and Kirschener, D.A. (1990) *Science* **250**, 279–282

17. Mattson, M.P., Cheng, B., Davis, D., Bryan, K., Lieberberg, I. and Rydel, R.E. (1992) *J. Neurosci.* **12**, 376–389
18. Scorziello, A., Meucci, O., Florio, T., Fattore, M., Forloni, G., Salmon, M. and Schettini, G. (1996) *J. Neurochem.* **66**, 1995–2003
19. Fukuyama, R., Wadhwani, K.C., Galdzicki, Z., Rapoport, S.I. and Ehrenstein, G. (1994) *Brain Res.* **667**, 269–272
20. Ueda, K., Shinohara, S., Yagami, T., Asakura, K. and Kawasaki, K. (1997) *J. Neurochem.* **68**, 265–271
21. Weiss, J.H., Pike, C.J. and Cotman, C.W. (1994) *J. Neurochem.* **62**, 372–375
22. Copani, A., Bruno. V., Battaglia, G., Leanza, G., Pelliteri, R., Russo, A., Stanzani, S. and Nicoletti, F. (1995) *Mol. Pharmacol.* **47(5)**, 890–897
23. Ekinci, F.J., Malik, K.U. and Shea, T.B. (1999) *J. Biol. Chem.* **274**, 30322–30327
24. Price, S.A., Held, B. and Pearson, H.A. (1998) *NeuroReport* **9**, 539–545
25. Cowburn, R.F., Wiehager, B. and Sundstrom, E. (1995) *Neurosci. Lett.* **191**, 31–34
26. Ishigawa, H., Ozawa, H., Saito, T., Takahara, N. and Takemura, H. (1998) *Life Sci.* **62**, 705–713
27. Mattson, M.P. (1994) *Ann. N.Y. Acad. Sci.* **747**, 50–76
28. Good, T.A. and Murphy, R.M. (1996) *Proc. Natl. Acad. Sci. U.S.A.* **93**, 15130–15135
29. Mark, R.J., Blanc, E.M. and Mattson, M.P. (1997) *Mol. Neurobiol.* **12**, 211–224
30. Bores, G.M., Smith, C.P., Wirtz-Brugger, F. and Giovanni, A. (1998) *Brain Res. Bull.* **46**, 423–427
31. Arispe, N., Pollard, H.P. and Rojas, E. (1994) *Ann. N.Y. Acad. Sci.* **747**, 256–266
32. Lin, H., Zhu, Y.J. and Lal, R. (1999) *Biochemistry* **58**, 11189–11196
33. Rhee, S.K., Quist, A.P and Lal, R. (1998) *J. Biol. Chem.* **273**, 13379–13382
34. Yan, S.D., Fu, J., Sorto, C., Chen, X., Zhu, H., Al-Mohanna, F., Collison, K., Zhu, A., Stern, E., Saido, T., et al., (1997) *Nature (London)* **389**, 689–695
35. Pascale, A., Bhagavan A., Nelson, T.J., Neve, R.L., McPhie, D.L. and Etcheberrigaray, R. (1999) *Brain Res. Mol. Brain Res.* **72**, 205–213
36. McKeon-O'Malley, C., Wells, J., Fine, R., Ullman, M.D. and Volicer, L. (1999) *Brain Res. Mol. Brain Res.* **72**, 103–107
37. Lynn, B.D., Marrotta, C.A. and Nagu, J.I. (1995) *Neurosci. Lett.* **199**, 21–24
38. Kim, H.S., Lee, J.H. and Suh, Y.H. (1999) *NeuroReport* **10**, 113–116
39. Kim, H.S., Park, C.H. and Suh, Y.H. (1998) *NeuroReport* **9**, 3875–3879
40. Barger, S.W. and Mattson, M.P. (1996) *Brain Res. Mol. Brain Res.* **40**, 116–126
41. Barger, S.W., Horster, D., Furukawa, K., Goodman, Y., Krieglstein, J. and Mattson, M.P. (1995) *Proc. Natl. Acad. Sci. U.S.A.* **92**, 9328–9332
42. Furukawa, K., Sopher, B.L., Rydel, R.E., Begley, J.G., Pham, D.G., Martin, G.M., Fox, M. and Mattson, M.P. (1996) *J. Neurochem.* **67**, 1882–1896
43. Furukawa, K., Barger, S.W., Blalock, E.M. and Mattson, M.P. (1996) *Nature (London)* **379**, 74–78
44. Walter, J., Capell, A., Grunberg, J., Pesold, B., Schindzielorz, A., Prior, R., Podlinsky, M.B., Fraser, P., St George-Hyslop, P., Selkoe, D.J. and Haass, C. (1996) *Mol. Med.* **2**, 673–691
45. Cook, D.G., Sung, J.C., Golde, T.E., Felsenstein, K.M., Wojczyk, B.S., Tanzi, R.E., Trojanowski, J.O., Lee, V.M.-Y. and Doms, R.W. (1996) *Proc. Natl. Acad. Sci. U.S.A.* **93**, 9223–9228
46. Kovacs, D.M., Faussset, H.J., Page, K.J., Kim, T.W., Moir, R.D., Merriam, D.E., Hollister R.D., Hallmark, O.G., Mancini, R., Felsenstein, D.H., et al. (1996) *Nat. Med. (N.Y.)* **2**, 224–229
47. Guo, Q., Furukawa, K., Sopher, B.L., Pham, D.G., Xie, J., Robinson, N., Martin, G.M. and Mattson, M.P. (1996) *NeuroReport* **6**, 379–383
48. Guo, Q., Sopher, B.L., Pham, D.G., Furukawa, K., Robinson, N., Martin, G.M. and Mattson, M.P. (1997) *J. Neurosci.* **17**, 4212–4222

49. Guo, Q., Fu, W., Sopher, B.L., Miller, M.W., Ware, C.B., Martin, G.M. and Mattson, M.P. (1999) *Nat. Med. (N.Y.)* **5**, 101–107

50. Begley, J.G., Duan, W., Chan, S., Duff, K. and Mattson, M.P. (1999) *J. Neurochem.* **72**, 1030–1039

51. Ito, H., Oka, K., Etcheberrigaray, R., Nelson, T.J., McPhie, D.L., Tofel-Grehl, B., Gibson, G.E. and Alkon, D.L. (1994) *Proc. Natl. Acad. Sci. U.S.A.* **91**, 534–538

52. McCoy, K.R., Mullins, R.D., Newcomb, T.G., Ng, G.M., Paulinkova, G., Polinsky, R.J., Nee, L.E. and Sisken, J.E. (1993) *Neurobiol. Aging* **14**, 447–455

53. Kim, T.W., Pettingell, W.P. and Tanzi, R.E. (1998) *Soc. Neurosci. Abstr.* **24**, 757

54. Meyers, M.B., Pickel, V.M., Sheu, S.S., Sharma, V.K., Scotto, K.W. and Fishman, G.I. (1995) *J. Biol. Chem.* **270**, 26411–26418

55. Meyers, M.B., Puri, T.S., Chien, A.J., Gao, T., Hsu, P.H., Hosey, M.M. and Fishman, G.I. (1998) *J. Biol. Chem.* **273**, 18930–18935

56. Leissring, M.A., Paul, B.A., Parker, I., Cotman, C.W. and La Ferla, F.M. (1999) *J. Neurochem.* **72**, 1061–1068

57. Lovestone, S. and Reynolds, C.H. (1997) *Neuroscience* **78**, 309–324

58. Goedert, M. (1996) *Ann. N.Y. Acad. Sci.* **777**, 121–131

59. Pei, J.J., Sersen, E., Iqbal, K. and Grundke-Iqbal, I. (1994) *Brain Res.* **655**, 70–76

60. Pei, J.J., Braak, E., Braak, H., Grundke-Iqbal, I., Iqbal, I., Winblad, B. and Cowburn, R.F. (1999) *J. Neuropathol. Exp. Neurol.* **58**, 1010–1019

61. Goedert, M., Jakes, R., Qi, Z., Wang, J.H. and Cohen, P. (1995) *J. Neurochem.* **65**, 2804–2807

62. Gong, C.Q., Grundke-Iqbal, I. and Iqbal, K. (1994) *Neuroscience* **61**, 765–772

63. Berridge, M.J. (1997) *J. Exp. Biol.* **200**, 315–319

64. Berridge, M.J. (1998) *Neuron* **21**, 13–26

65. Hartigan, J.A. and Johnson, G.V.W. (1999) *J. Biol. Chem.* **274**, 21395–21401

66. Reference deleted

67. Fleming, L.M. and Johnson, G.V. (1995) *Biochem. J.* **309**, 41–47

68. Yano, S., Tokumitsu, H. and Soderling, T.R. (1998) *Nature (London)* **396**, 584–587

69. Yang, L.S. and Ksiezak-Reding, H. (1999) *J. Neurosci. Res.* **55**, 36–43

70. Litersky, J.M. and Johnson, G.V.H. (1992) *J. Biol. Chem.* **267**, 1563–1568

71. Mattson, M.P., Engle, M.G. and Rychlik, B. (1991) *Mol. Chem. Neuropathol.* **15**, 117–142

72. Adamec, E., Mercken, M., Beerman, M.L., Didier, M. and Nixon, R.A. (1997) *Brain Res.* **757**, 93–101

73. Shea, T.B., Prabhakar, S. and Ekinci, F.J. (1997) *J. Neurosci. Res.* **49**, 759–768

74. Xie, H.Q. and Johnson, G.V.W. (1998) *J. Neurosci. Res.* **53**, 153–164

75. Fleming, L.M. and Johnson, G.V. (1995) *Biochem. J.* **309**, 41–47

76. Young, L.T., Kish, S.J., Li, P.P. and Warsh, J.J. (1988) *Neurosci. Lett.* **94**, 198–202

77. Garlind, A., Cowburn, R.F., Forsell, C., Ravid, R., Winblad, B. and Fowler, C.J. (1995) *Brain Res.* **681**, 160–166

78. Haug, L.-S., Ostwald, A.C., Cowburn, R.F., Garlind, A., Winblad, B. and Walaas, S.I. (1996) *Neurodegeneration* **5**, 169–176

79. Kuramatani, T., Fastbom, J., Bonkale, W.L., Bogdamovic, N., Winblad, B., Ohm, T.G. and Cowburn, R.F. (1998) *Brain Res.* **796**, 209–221

80. Giannini, G., Conti, A., Mammarella, S., Scrobogna, M. and Sorrentino, V. (1995) *J. Cell Biol.* **128**, 893–904

81. Furuichi, T., Furutama, D., Hakamatama, Y., Nakai, J., Takeshima, H. and Mikoshiba, K. (1994) *J. Neurosci.* **14**, 4794–4805

82. Kelliher, M., Fastbom, J., Cowburn, R.F., Bonkale, W., Ohm, T.G., Ravid, R., Sorrentino, V. and O'Neill, C. (1999) *Neuroscience* **92**, 499–513

83. Braak, H. and Braak, E. (1991) *Acta Neuropathol. (Berlin)* **82**, 239–259

84. Marks, A.R. (1996) *Phys. Rev.* **3**, 631–649

85.   Carmody, M., Kelliher, M., Ravid, R. and O'Neill, C. (1998) *Neurobiology of Aging* 19, 551, 210
86.   Brilliantes, A.M.B., Ondrias, K., Scott, A., Kobrinsky, E., Ondriasova, M.C., Moschell, T., Jayaraman, M., Landers, B.E., Ehrlich, B.E. and Marks, A.R. (1994) *Cell* 77, 513–524
87.   Aridor, M. and Balch, W.E. (1999) *Nat. Med. (N.Y.)* 5, 745–751
88.   Grynspan, F., Griffin, W.R., Cataldo, A., Katayama, A. and Nixon, R.A. (1997) *Brain Res.* 763, 145–158
89.   Nixon, R.A., Saito, K.I., Grynspan, F., Griffin, W.R., Katayama, S., Honda, T., Mohan, P.S., Shea, T.B. and Beerman, M. (1994) *Ann. N.Y. Acad. Sci.* 747, 77–91
90.   Saito, K.I., Elce, J.S., Hamon, J.E. and Nixon, R.A. (1993) *Proc. Natl. Acad. Sci. U.S.A.* 90, 2628–2632
91.   Tsuji, T., Shimohama, S., Kimura, J. and Shimuzu, K. (1998) *Neurosci. Lett.* 248, 109–112
92.   Chan, S.L. and Mattson, M.P. (1999) *J. Neurosci. Res.* 58, 167–190
93.   Porn-Ares, M.I., Samali, A. and Orrenius, S. (1998) *Cell Death Differ.* 5, 1028–1033
94.   Moran, J., Itoh, T., Reddy, U.R., Chen, M., Alnemri, E.S. and Pleasure, D. (1999) *J. Neurochem.* 73, 568–577
95.   Takedera, T., Matsuda, I. and Ohyashiki, T. (1999) *J. Neurochem.* 73, 548–556
96.   Le Blanc, A., Liu, H., Goodyer, C., Bergeron, C. and Hammond, J. (1999) *J. Biol. Chem.* 274, 23426–23436
97.   Uetsuki, T., Takemoto, K., Nishimura, I., Okamoto, M., Ninobe, M., Momoi, T., Miura, M. and Yoshikawa, K. (1999) *J. Neurosci.* 19, 6955–6964
98.   Zhu, S.G., Sheng, J.G., Jones, R.A., Brewer, M.M., Zhou, X.Q., Mrak, R.E. and Griffin, W.S. (1999) *J. Neuropathol. Exp. Neurol.* 58, 582–587
99.   Desjardins P. and Ledoux, S. (1998) *Neurosci. Lett.* 244, 69–72
100. Ferrer, I., Marti, E., Lopez, E. and Tortosa, A. (1998) *Neuropathol. Appl. Neurobiol.* 24, 271–277
101. Kitamura, Y., Shimohama, S., Ota, T., Matsuoka, Y., Nomura, Y. and Taniguchi, T. (1997) *Neurosci. Lett.* 237, 17–20
102. Kaltschmidt, B., Uherek, M., Volk, B., Baeuerle, P.A. and Kaltschmidt, C. (1997) *Proc. Natl. Acad. Sci. U.S.A.* 94, 2642–2647
103. Micheau, J. and Riedel, G. (1999) *Cell Mol. Life Sci.* 55, 534–548
104. Nicholl, R.A. and Malenka, R.C. (1999) *Ann N.Y. Acad. Sci.* 868, 515–525
105. Xiao, J., Perry, G., Troncoso, J. and Monteiro, M.J. (1996) *J. Neuropathol. Exp. Neurol.* 55, 954–963
106. Simonian, N.A., Elvhage, T., Czernik, A.J., Greengard, P. and Hyman, B.T. (1994) *Brain Res.* 657, 294–299
107. Kayyali, U.S., Zhang, W., Yee, A.G., Seidman, J. and Potter, H. (1997) *J. Neurochem.* 68, 1668–1678
108. Gong, C.-X., Singh, T.J., Grunke-Iqbal, I. and Iqbal, K. (1994) *J. Neurochem.* 62, 803–806
109. Billingsley, M.L., Ellis, C., Kincaid, R.L., Martin, J., Schmidt, M.L., Lee, V.M. and Trojanowski, J.Q. (1994) *Exp. Neurol.* 126, 178–184
110. Ladner, C.J., Czech, J., Maurice, J., Lorens, S.A. and Lee, J.M. (1996) *J. Neuropathol. Exp. Neurol.* 55, 924–931
111. Thorns, V., Hansen, L. and Masljah, E. (1998) *Exp. Neurol.* 150, 14–20
112. Norris, P.J., Faull, R.L. and Emson, P.C. (1996) *Brain Res. Mol. Brain Res.* 41, 36–49
113. Hyman, B.T., Marzloff, K., Wenniger, J.J., Dawson, T.M., Bredt, D.S. and Snyder, S.H. (1992) *Ann. Neurol.* 32, 818–820
114. de La Monte, S.M. and Bloch, K.D. (1997) *Mol. Chem. Neuropathol.* 30, 135–159
115. Kenny, M., Walsh, R., Ravid, R. and O'Neill, C. (1998) *Neurobiology of Aging* 19, 551, 218
116. Ross, B.M., Moszczynska, A., Erlich, J. and Kish, S.J. (1998) *J. Neurochem.* 70, 786–793
117. Stephenson, D.T., Lemere, C.A., Selkoe, D.J. and Clemens, J.A. (1996) *Neurobiol. Dis.* 3, 51–63

118.   Solodkin, A., Veldhuizen, S. and Van Hoesen, G.W. (1996) *J. Neurosci.* **16**, 3311–3321
119.   Sampson, V.L., Morrison, J.H. and Vickers, J.C. (1998) *Exp. Neurol.* **145**, 295–302
120.   Maguire-Zeiss, K.A., Li, Z.W., Shimoda, L.M. and Hamill, R.W. (1995) *Brain Res. Mol. Brain Res.* **30**, 362–366
121.   Hof, P.R., Nimchinsky, E.A., Celio, M.R., Bouras, C. and Morrison, J.H. (1993) *Neurosci. Lett.* **152**, 145–148
122.   Nishiyama, E., Ohwada, J., Iwamoto, N. and Arai, H. (1993) *Neurosci. Lett.* **163**, 223–226
123.   Ferrer, I., Tunon, T., Soriano, E., del Rio, A., Iraizoz, I., Fonseca, M. and Guionnet, N. (1993) *Clin. Neuropathol.* **12**, 53–58
124.   Mikkonen, M., Alafuzoff, I., Tapiola, T., Soininen, H. and Miettinen, R. (1999) *Neuroscience* **92**, 515–532

Biochem. Soc. Symp. **67**, 195–202
(Printed in Great Britain)

18

Transgenic mouse models of Alzheimer's disease: phenotype and mechanisms of pathogenesis

Karen Duff

Nathan Kline Institute, 140 Old Orangeburg Rd, Orangeburg, NY 10962, U.S.A.

Abstract

A range of transgenic mice have been created to model Alzheimer's disease. These include mice expressing human forms of the amyloid precursor protein, the presenilins and, more recently, tau. Several of the models develop features of the disease including amyloid pathology, cholinergic deficits, neurodegeneration and cognitive impairment. Progress in the characterization and use of these model animals is discussed.

Introduction

Alzheimer's disease (AD) is a progressive neurodegenerative disease. Most cases of AD occur sporadically, but familial forms of the disease have been most widely studied because of the insight they give into disease aetiology. Genetic causes of the disease are heterogeneous and include mutations or variants in several genes including those for amyloid precursor protein (APP), the presenilins (PS) and apolipoprotein E [1]. The disease phenotype is remarkably consistent and includes the accumulation of β-amyloid (Aβ) and its deposition into senile plaques, the formation of tau-containing tangles, reactive gliosis, neurodegeneration, cholinergic deficit and cognitive impairment.

The first transgenic mouse to develop a robust AD-related phenotype was described in 1995 by the Exemplar/Athena Neuroscience group [2]. This line known as PDAPP, overexpresses mutant APP at levels high enough to generate sufficient Aβ for extracellular deposits (plaques) to form in relevant regions of the brain. In 1996, a second line (Tg2576) was created by Karen Hsiao and colleagues, which also made sufficient amyloid for deposits to form. In addition, this mouse showed age-related cognitive impairment [3]. Subsequently, other cDNA mice [4,5] and mice overexpressing genomic constructs [6] have also been shown to form amyloid in old age. Several groups have created transgenic mice that overexpress mutant PS [7–9] but these mice do not show amyloid deposition, most likely because they have insufficient levels of the Aβ peptide.

Most of the current work on transgenic mice focuses on the cellular response to amyloid accumulation and its relevance to AD. Very recently, the PDAPP line of mice has been used to test the feasibility of modulating amyloid levels by immunization with Aβ [10]. The results of this experiment suggest that amyloid modulation is indeed possible, and that some of the secondary effects of amyloidosis (gliosis and neuritic changes) can be prevented. This work opens up a new direction in amyloid research and may well have a significant impact on the development of human therapies.

Recent advances in phenotype assessment in transgenic models of AD

Amyloidosis

Several studies aimed to modulate the amyloid phenotype by crossing in other transgenes such as PS1 or transforming growth factor-β. The studies showed that when a PS1 mutant mouse was crossed with a mouse overexpressing APP, the levels of Aβ42/43 (the 42/43-amino-acid Aβ peptide) were increased in the double transgenic. This elevation had a profound influence on the age at which amyloid deposition could first be detected [6,11,12]. In one cross, the age at which amyloid deposits were first identified was reduced from 9–12 months to 10–12 weeks [12a], which is the earliest age at which amyloid has been reported. When transforming growth factor-β cDNA mice are crossed with a line overexpressing APP, amyloid deposition was again accelerated and was far more prominent in the vasculature [13]. Apart from demonstrating that these pathways interact, one outcome of the crossed-mouse studies is to enhance, and in some cases modify, the phenotype, providing us with better models.

Presenilin transgenics

In terms of the amyloid phenotype seen in AD, the most significant phenotype in the mutant PS transgenics continues to be the specific elevation of Aβ42/43 [7–9]. Mutant PS2 transgenics that show elevation in Aβ42/43 have also recently been created [14], which strengthens the argument that APP and the presenilins interact, either directly as suggested by Wolfe et al. [15] or indirectly, and that PS mutations cause AD through APP/Aβ modulation.

Studies of knockout PS1 animals have shown that PS1 plays an important role in development. Lack of the protein leads to a deficiency in somitogenesis during early embryogenesis, which results in severe skeletal abnormalities and prenatal death [16,17]. These abnormalities strongly resemble those seen in Notch knockout mice [18] and this observation, coupled with several studies *in vivo* and *in vitro*, suggests that Notch and PS1 interact in some way to affect normal cellular function, which downstream may affect signalling, differentiation and development [19].

PS1 has been strongly implicated in other signalling pathways as several potential components of signal transduction pathways have been identified as PS-interacting proteins. These include several proteins containing an armadillo repeat region, a 42-amino-acid motif that has been identified in proteins involved in cell-to-cell adhesion, protein–protein interaction and signal transduction. The best known of these is β-catenin. Both β-catenin, and its homologue δ-catenin, have been shown to interact with PS1 [20]. The effect of PS1 mutations on β-catenin stability, and hence its downstream effects, are controversial. In transgenic mice and human familial AD brain homogenates, for example, mutations in PS1 are linked to increased degradation of β-catenin [21], whereas other studies have suggested no effect or increased activity for the wild-type and mutant PS1 protein [22–24]. It remains unclear quite how PS1 mutations might lead to AD through a β-catenin pathway, although in addition to the effect on Aβ42 they are thought to affect the action of glycogen synthase kinase-β and hence tau phosphorylation (for a review, see Alzheimer forum panel discussion at www.alzforum.org/members/forums/journals/catenin/index.html).

Neurodegeneration

The human AD brain shows extensive neurodegeneration, both in cholinergic neurons of the nucleus basalis [25], and in non-cholinergic neurons throughout the cortex and hippocampus. Studies have shown that fibrillar Aβ peptides are toxic to neurons in culture [26] and the overproduction of human Aβ in the brains of transgenic mice was therefore expected to cause extensive neurodegeneration. Several of the best characterized mouse models have been examined for overt cell loss [27–29] but neither PDAPP, Tg2576 nor the Tg2576/PS1 cross-mouse show significant cell loss, even though amyloid burden exceeds 30%. One model has been reported to show significant cell loss, but only in the hippocampus [29]. Although overt cell loss is not seen in mice such as Tg2576/PS1, neurites in close proximity to amyloid deposits are severely dystrophic [29a]. In addition, magnetic resonance imaging (MRI) has revealed differences in the volume of structures such as the lateral ventricles and the corpus callosum between mice with and without amyloid, which may reflect loss of neuropil or shrinkage of cells rather than cell death itself (J. Helpern, K. Duff, R. Nixon, T. Wisneiwski and M. De Leon, unpublished work). Although the field is in its infancy, the application of functional and structural MRI to the analysis of models is predicted to have a significant impact, especially as longitudinal analyses, including the effects of drug treatments, can be performed on the same mouse.

Cholinergic deficits

Although modulation of the cholinergic system has been a therapeutic treatment for AD dementia for many years, investigations into the response of cholinergic neurons to amyloid insult have only recently been performed in transgenic mice. Immunohistochemical analysis has shown that cholinergic markers accumulate in swollen abnormal neurites around amyloid deposits in the cortex [4]. Our own studies have shown that in the early stages of deposition, neurons in the nucleus basalis of depositing mice appear normal, but their projection areas in certain regions of the cortex show a significant reduction in synapse density and size [30]. Further work to assess how cholinergic neurons in all areas of the brain respond to increasing amyloid burden and age is underway as cholinesterase inhibitors are currently considered to be valid therapeutic agents for AD.

Cognitive impairments and neurodegeneration

Recreating human cognitive impairment is perhaps the greatest challenge facing genetic engineers working on transgenic models of human dementia. Mice are genetically less suitable for behavioural testing than rats as performance data on normal mice from different strains are often contradictory. Despite these reservations, most of the transgenic mice that form amyloid deposits have been tested for cognitive impairment. The PDAPP mouse [31,32], Tg2576 [3] and the Tg2576/PS1 cross-mouse [12] have all shown a deficit in tests of hippocampal dysfunction before amyloid deposits form, which strongly suggests that overt amyloid accumulation/deposition is not responsible for this early cognitive impairment. Deficits in water maze performance that correlate with increasing age and amyloid burden and with decreasing long-term potentiation have been reported for Tg2576 [3,33]. Recent studies with Tg2576 and the Tg2576/PS1 cross suggest that amyloid/age-related deficits in tests such as the radial arm maze (and especially the radial arm water maze) may be more informative than the regular Morris water maze and that appreciable cognitive impairment may be a feature of mice with extensive amyloid deposits (D. Quartermain, T. Wisneiwski and K. Duff, unpublished work).

Tau pathology

One of the major deficits in the current AD mice is the lack of tau pathology. In humans, tau pathology takes the form of intracellular tangles of an abnormally phosphorylated form of the tau protein, which associates into paired helical filaments. Amyloid plaques and tau tangles are both pathognomic features of human AD, and their relative contribution to the disease has long been disputed. The identification of AD-causing mutations in APP and the presenilins, however, adds weight to the amyloid based hypothesis of pathogenesis, which assumes that tau abnormalities are a secondary lesion that form in response to amyloid accumulation. To investigate this link, transgenic mice with extensive amyloid burden have been examined for abnormal tau pathology by immunohistochemical analysis. This work has shown that amyloid deposits in transgenic mice are ringed by dystrophic neurites that are immunoreactive for markers of phospho-tau epitopes such as phosphoserine[202] [4,34]. These epitopes are phosphorylated to some degree in the normal brain, but are hyperphosphorylated in the AD brain. In the mice, it is not yet clear whether the immunoreactivity around deposits reflects local hyperphosphorylation of tau, or simple elevation of tau protein levels in response to neuritic damage. In the human AD brain, subsets of neurons are also immunolabelled with antibodies to both tyrosine phospho-tau and the signalling protein fyn which is an src, non-receptor tyrosine kinase [35]. Co-immunoprecipitation has shown that the N-terminus of tau and the SH3 (src homology) domain of fyn interact directly, suggesting that tau may be involved in signal transduction pathways [36]. Interestingly, fyn binds another signalling protein, FAK [37], which is itself up-regulated by Aβ [38]. Ongoing work includes a study of how FAK, fyn, tau and Aβ interact in transgenic animals with and without elevated amyloid.

It is clear, however, that tau pathology does not develop further in the transgenic animals. This suggests that either Aβ/amyloid accumulation is not detrimental to tau or differences between the mouse and human brain preclude the formation of pathogenic tau as suggested by Yankner and colleagues [39]. We have recently created a line of transgenic mice that overexpress all isoforms of human tau under the control of the human tau promoter [40]. These mice not only provide a humanized tau environment in which amyloid deposition can be elicited through crossbreeding, but they also generate animal models in which both normal and abnormal tau biology can be studied. The latter is perhaps particularly significant in light of the recent identification of mutations in tau that cause frontotemporal dementia with Parkinsonism linked to chromosome 17 [41–43], as some of the mutations result in an imbalance of the normal tau isoform ratios; a situation that is reproduced in the transgenic mice.

Summary

Transgenic models of AD continue to gain credibility as more features of the human disease are shown to be represented in the mice. They are, however, still incomplete models as neither tau pathology nor extensive cell loss has been generated in the models created so far. Despite these shortcomings, they are excellent models of amyloidosis and have been highly informative in advancing our understanding of *in vivo* responses to amyloid insult, and the mechanism by which other AD-related genes cause the disease.

References

1.   Cruts, M. and Van Broeckhoven, C. (1998) Molecular genetics of Alzheimer's disease. *Ann. Med.* **30**, 560–565

2.   Games, D., Adams, D., Alessandrini, R., Barbour, R., Berthelette, P., Blackwell, C., Carr, T., Clemena, J., Donaldson, T., Gillespie, F., et al. (1995) Alzheimer-type neuropathology in transgenic mice overexpressing V717F β-amyloid precursor protein. *Nature (London)* **373**, 523–527

3.   Hsiao, K., Chapman, P., Nilsen, S., Eckman, C., Harigaya, Y., Younkin, S., Yang, F. and Cole, G. (1996) Correlative memory deficits, Aβ elevation and amyloid plaques in transgenic mice. *Science* **274**, 99–102

4.   Sturchler-Pierrat, C., Abramowski, D., Duke, M., Wiederhold, K.H., Mistl, C., Rothacher, S., Ledermann, B., Burki, K., Frey, P., Paganetti, P.A., et al. (1997) Two amyloid precursor protein transgenic mouse models with Alzheimer disease-like pathology. *Proc. Natl. Acad. Sci. U.S.A.* **94**, 13287–13292

5.   Nalbantoglu, J., Tirado-Santiago, G., Lahsaini, A., Poirier, J., Goncalves, O., Verge, G., Momoli, F., Welner, S.A., Massicotte, G., Julien, J.P. and Shapiro, M.L. (1997) Impaired learning and LTP in mice expressing the carboxy terminus of the Alzheimer amyloid precursor protein. *Nature (London)* **387**, 500–505

6.   Lamb, B.A., Bardel, K.A., Kulnane, L.S., Anderson, J.J., Holtz, G., Wagner, S.L., Sisodia, S.S. and Hoeger, E.J. (1999) Amyloid production and deposition in mutant amyloid precursor protein and presenilin-1 yeast artificial chromosome transgenic mice. *Nat. Neurosci.* **8**, 695–697

7.   Duff, K., Eckman, C., Zehr, C., Yu, X., Prada, C.M., Perez-tur, J., Hutton, M., Buee, L., Harigaya, Y., Yager, D., et al. (1996) Increased amyloid-Aβ42(43) in brains of mice expressing mutant presenilin 1. *Nature (London)* **383**, 710–713

8.   Borchelt, D.R., Thinakaran, G., Eckman, C.B., Lee, M.K., Davenport, F., Ratovitsky, T., Prada, C.M., Kim, G., Seekins, S., Yager, D., et al. (1996) Familial Alzheimer's disease-linked presenilin 1 variants elevate Abeta1-42/1-40 ratio in vitro and in vivo. *Neuron* **17**, 1005–1013

9.   Citron, M., Westaway, D., Xia, W., Carlson, G., Diehl, T., Levesque, G., Johnson-Wood, K., Lee, M., Seubert, P., Davis, A., et al. (1997) Mutant presenilins of Alzheimer's disease increase production of 42-residue amyloid β-protein in both transfected cells and transgenic mice. *Nat. Med. (N.Y.)* **3**, 67–68

10. Schenk, D., Barbour, R., Dunn, W., Gordon, G., Grajeda, H., Guido, T., Hu, K., Huang, J., Johnson-Wood, K., Khan, K., et al. (1999) Immunization with amyloid-beta attenuates Alzheimer-disease-like pathology in the PDAPP mouse. *Nature (London)* **400**, 173–177

11. Borchelt, D.R., Ratovitski, T., van Lare, J., Lee, M.K., Gonzales, V., Jenkins, N.A., Copeland, N.G., Price, D.L. and Sisodia, S.S. (1997) Accelerated amyloid deposition in the brains of transgenic mice co-expressing mutant presenilin 1 and amyloid precursor proteins. *Neuron* **19**, 939–945

12. Holcomb, L., Gordon, M.N., McGowan, E., Yu, X., Benkovic, S., Jantzen, P., Wright, K., Saad, I., Mueller, R., Morgan, D., et al. (1998) Accelerated Alzheimer-type phenotype in transgenic mice carrying both mutant amyloid precursor protein and presenilin 1 transgenes. *Nat. Med. (N.Y.)* **4**, 97–100

12a McGowan, E., Sanders, S., Iwatsubo, T., Takeuchi, A., Saido, T., Zehr, C., Yu, X., Uljon, S.E., Wang, R., Mann, D., et al. (1999) Amyloid phenotype characterization of transgenic mice over-expressing both mutant amyloid precursor protein and mutant presenilin 1 transgenes. *Neurobiol. Dis.* **6**, 231–244

13. Wyss-Coray, T., Masliah, E., Mallory, M., McConlogue, L., Johnson-Wood, K., Lin, C. and Mucke, L. (1997) Amyloidogenic role of cytokine TGF-beta1 in transgenic mice and in Alzheimer's disease. *Nature (London)* **389**, 603–606

14. Oyama, F., Sawamura, N., Kobayashi, K., Morishima-Kawashima, M., Kuramochi, T., Ito, M., Tomita, T., Maruyama, K., Saido, T.C., Iwatsubo, T., et al. (1998) Mutant presenilin 2 transgenic mouse: effect on an age-dependent increase of amyloid beta-protein 42 in the brain. *J. Neurochem.* **71**, 313–322

15. Wolfe, M.S., Xia, W., Ostaszewski, B.L., Diehl, T.S., Kimberly, W.T. and Selkoe, D.J. (1999) Two transmembrane aspartates in presenilin-1 required for presenilin endoproteolysis and gamma-secretase activity. *Nature (London)* **398**, 513–517

16. Wong, P.C., Zheng, H., Chen, H., Becher, M.W., Sirinathsinghji, D.J., Trumbauer, M.E., Chen, H.Y., Price, D.L., Van der Ploeg, L.H. and Sisodia, S.S. (1997) Presenilin 1 is required for Notch1 and DII1 expression in the paraxial mesoderm. *Nature (London)* **387**, 288–292

17. Shen, J., Bronson, R.T., Chen, D.F., Xia, W., Selkoe, D.J. and Tonegawa, S. (1997) Skeletal and CNS defects in Presenilin-1-deficient mice. *Cell* **89**, 629–639

18. Conlon, R.A., Reaume, A.G. and Rossant, J. (1995) Notch1 is required for the coordinate segmentation of somites. *Development* **121**, 1533–1545

19. Hardy, J. and Israel, A. (1999) In search of gamma secretase. *Nature (London)* **398**, 466–467

20. Zhou, J., Liyanage, U., Medina, M., Ho, C., Simmons, A.D., Lovett, M. and Kosik, K.S. (1997) Presenilin 1 interaction in the brain with a novel member of the Armadillo family. *NeuroReport* **8**, 2085–2090

21. Zhang, Z., Hartmann, H., Do, V.M., Abramowski, D., Sturchler-Pierrat, C., Staufenbiel, M., Sommer, B., van de Wetering, M., Clevers, H., Saftig, P., et al. (1998) Destabilization of beta-catenin by mutations in presenilin-1 potentiates neuronal apoptosis. *Nature (London)* **395**, 698–702

22. Murayama, M., Tanaka, S., Palacino, J., Murayama, O., Honda, T., Sun, X., Yasutake, K., Nihonmatsu, N., Wolozin, B. and Takashima, A. (1998) Direct association of presenilin-1 with beta-catenin. *FEBS Lett.* **433**, 73–77

23. Kang, D.E., Soriano, S., Frosch, M.P., Collins, T., Naruse, S., Sisodia, S.S., Leibowitz, G., Levine, F. and Koo, E.H. (1999) Presenilin 1 facilitates the constitutive turnover of beta-catenin: differential activity of Alzheimer's disease-linked PS1 mutants in the beta-catenin-signaling pathway. *J. Neurosci.* **19**, 4229–4237

24. Nishimura, M., Yu, G., Levesque, G., Zhang, D.M., Ruel, L., Chen, F., Milman, P., Holmes, E., Liang, Y., Kawarai, T., et al. (1999) Presenilin mutations associated with Alzheimer disease cause defective intracellular trafficking of beta-catenin, a component of the presenilin protein complex. *Nat. Med. (N.Y.)* **5**, 164–169

25. Whitehouse, P.J., Price, D.L., Struble, R.G., Clark, A.W., Coyle, J.T. and DeLong, M.R. (1982) Alzheimer's disease and senile dementia: loss of neurons in the basal forebrain, *Science* **215**, 1237–1239

26. Lorenzo, A. and Yankner, B.A. (1994) β-amyloid neurotoxicity requires fibril formation and is inhibited by congo red. *Proc. Natl. Acad. Sci. U.S.A.* **91**, 12243–12247

27. Irizarry, M.C., Soriano, F., McNamara, M., Page, K.J., Schenk, D., Games, D. and Hyman, B.T. (1997) Aβ deposition is associated with neuropil changes, but not with overt neuronal loss in the human amyloid precursor protein V717F (PDAPP) transgenic mouse. *J. Neurosci.* **17**, 7053–7059

28. Irizarry, M.C., McNamara, M., Fedorchak, K., Hsiao, K. and Hyman, B.T. (1997) APPSw transgenic mice develop age-related Aβ deposits and neuropil abnormalities, but no neuronal loss in CA1. *J. Neuropathol. Exp. Neurol.* **56**, 965–973

29. Calhoun, M.E., Wiederhold, K.H., Abramowski, D., Phinney, A.L., Probst, A., Sturchler-Pierrat, C., Staufenbiel, M., Sommer, B. and Jucker, M. (1998) Neuron loss in APP transgenic mice. *Nature (London)* **395**, 755–756

29a. Takeuchi, E., Irizarry, M., Duff, K., Saido, T., HsiaoAshe, K., Hasegawa, M., Mann, D., Hyman, B. and Iwatsubo, T. (2000) Lack of neuronal loss associated with age-related Aβ deposition in the neocortices of transgenic mice overexpressing both Alzheimer mutant presenilin 1 and amyloid precursor protein. *Am. J. Pathol.* **157**, 331–339

30.   Wong, T.P., Debeir, T., Duff, K. and Cuello, A.C. (1999) Reorganization of cholinergic ter-
       minals in the cerebral cortex and hippocampus in transgenic mice carrying mutated prese-
       nilin-1 and amyloid precursor protein transgenes. *J. Neurosci.* **19**, 2706–2716
31.   Dodart, J., Meziane, H., Mathis, C., Bales, K., Paul, S. and Ungerer, A. (1997) Memory and
       learning impairment precede amyloid deposition in the V717F PDAPP transgenic mouse.
       Abs. 636.5, Society for Neurosciences, New Orleans
32.   Justice, A. and Motter, R. (1997) Behavioral characterisation of PDAPP transgenic
       Alzheimer mice. Abs 636.6, Society for Neurosciences, New Orleans
33.   Chapman, P.F., White, G.L., Jones, M.W., Cooper-Blacketer, D., Marshall, V.J., Irizarry,
       M., Younkin, L., Good, M.A., Bliss, T.V., Hyman, B.T., Younkin, S.G. and Hsiao, K.K.
       (1999). Impaired synaptic plasticity and learning in aged amyloid precursor protein trans-
       genic mice. *Nat. Neurosci.* **2**, 271–276
34.   Chen, K.S., Masliah, E., Grajeda, H., Guido, T., Huang, J., Khan, K., Motter, R., Soriano, F.
       and Games, D. (1998) Neurodegenerative Alzheimer-like pathology in PDAPP 717V--}F
       transgenic mice. *Prog. Brain Res.* **117**, 327–334
35.   Shirazi, S.K. and Wood, J.G. (1993) The protein tyrosine kinase, fyn, in Alzheimer's disease
       pathology. *NeuroReport* **4**, 435–437
36.   Lee, G., Newman, S.T., Gard, D.L., Band, H. and Panchamoorthy, G. (1998) Tau interacts
       with src-family non-receptor tyrosine kinases. *J. Cell Sci.* **111**, 3167–3177
37.   Cobb, B.S., Schaller, M.D., Leu, T.H. and Parsons, J.T. (1994) Stable association of pp60src
       and pp59fyn with the focal adhesion-associated protein tyrosine kinase, pp125FAK. *Mol.
       Cell Biol.* **14**, 147–155
38.   Zhang, C., Qiu, H.E., Krafft, G.A. and Klein, W.L. (1996) A beta peptide enhances focal
       adhesion kinase/Fyn association in a rat CNS nerve cell line. *Neurosci. Lett.* **211**, 187–190
39.   Geula, C., Wu, C.K., Saroff, D., Lorenzo, A., Yuan, M. and Yankner, B.A. (1998) Aging
       renders the brain vulnerable to amyloid β-protein neurotoxicity. *Nat. Med. (N.Y.)* **4**,
       827–828
40.   Duff, K., Knight, H., Refolo, L.M., Sanders, S., Yu, X., Picciano, M., Malester, B., Hutton,
       M., Adamson, J., Goedert, M., et al. (2000) Characterization of pathology in transgenic mice
       over-expressing human genomic and cDNA tau transgenes. *Neurobiol. Dis.* **7**, 87–98
41.   Hutton, M., Lendon, C.L., Rizzu, P., Baher, M., Froelich, S., Houlden, H., Pickering-
       Brown, S., Chakraverty, S., Isaacs, A., Grover, A., et al. (1998) Association of missense and
       5'-splice-site mutations in tau with the inherited dementia FTDP-17. *Nature (London)* **393**,
       702–705
42.   Goedert, M., Spillantini, M.G., Crowther, R.A., Chen, S.G., Parchi, P., Tabaton, M.,
       Lanska, D.J., Markesbery, W.R., Wilhelmsen, K.C., Dickson, D.W., et al. (1999) Tau gene
       mutation in familial progressive subcortical gliosis. *Nat. Med. (N.Y.)* **5**, 454–457
43.   Spillantini, M.G., Murrell, J.R., Goedert, M., Farlow, M.R., Klug, A. and Ghetti, B. (1998)
       Mutation in the tau gene in familial multiple system tauopathy with presenile dementia.
       Proc. Natl. Acad. Sci. U.S.A. **95**, 7737–7741

Biochem. Soc. Symp. **67**, 203–210
(Printed in Great Britain)

19

Modelling Alzheimer's disease in multiple transgenic mice

Ilse Dewachter, Dieder Moechars[1], Jo van Dorpe, Ina Tesseur, Chris Van den Haute, Kurt Spittaels and Fred Van Leuven[2]

Experimental Genetics Group, Center for Human Genetics, Flemish Institute for Biotechnology (VIB), K. U. Leuven Campus, Gasthuisberg, B-3000 Leuven, Belgium

Abstract

We have reported transgenic mice with neuronal overexpression of the clinical mutant β-amyloid precursor protein (APP) known as London, which develop an AD-related phenotype [Moechers, Dewachter, Lorent, Reversé, Baekelandt, Nadiu, Tesseur, Spittaels, Van den Haute, Checler, et al. (1999) *J. Biol. Chem.* **274**, 6483–6492]. Characterized early symptoms (3–9 months) include disturbed behaviour, neophobia, aggression, hypersensitivity to kainic acid, hyposensitivity to N-methyl-D-aspartate, defective cognition and memory, and decreased long-term potentiation. Late in life, at 12–15 months, amyloid plaques develop in the brain and correlate with increased levels of β-amyloid (Aβ)40/42 (the 40- and 42-amino-acid forms of Aβ). The formation of amyloid plaques is dissociated in time from and not involved in the early phenotype. Hyperphosphorylated protein tau is present but no tangle pathology is observed. In double-transgenic mice, i.e. APP/London × Presenilin 1, the increased production of Aβ42 results in amyloid plaques developing by the age of 6 months. Transgenic mice with overexpression of either human apolipoprotein E4 (ApoE4) or human protein tau in central neurons develop severe axonopathy in the brain and spinal cord. Progressive degeneration of nerves and muscles is demonstrated by motor problems, wasting and premature death. Tau is hyperphosphorylated but there is no formation of filaments or neurofibrillary tangles. The tangle aspect of AD pathology is still missing from all current transgenic amyloid models. Its implementation will require insight into the cellular signalling pathways which regulate the microtubule-stabilizing function by phosphorylation of neuronal tau.

[1]Present address: Department of Functional Genomics, Janssen Research Foundation, Beerse, Belgium
[2]To whom correspondence should be addressed.

Introduction

Dementia is rapidly becoming a major social and medical problem following the success of modern medicine and the continuous increase in life expectancy. The unique outcome of the disease (dementia literally means 'dehumanizing') has severe psychological implications for the family and the caretakers, in addition to the patient's complete dependence for all essential needs. Clinical diagnosis of Alzheimer's disease (AD) remains an exclusion diagnosis and there is no direct objective diagnostic test available for AD. Only *post mortem* microscopical examination of the brain offers a definitive diagnosis, based on the presence of intracellular neurofibrillary tangles (NFTs) and extracellular amyloid plaques, visualized by silver impregnation of brain sections essentially as performed by A. Alzheimer in 1907 [1]. Despite considerable progress, problems remain with the precise definition of the molecular and pathological components of the neurodogeneration and the precise mechanisms by which the different pathological lesions are generated [2,3].

Genetic studies have contributed significantly to fundamental studies of AD. Early-onset familial AD is inherited in a Mendelian autosomal-dominant manner and caused by mutations in the APP or presenilin (PS) genes [3]. Although familial AD constitutes the minority of cases of AD (5–10%), these cases have proved extremely important for the identification of molecular links that have provided a molecular basis for all current fundamental research involving APP and PS. In more than 40% of late-onset AD cases (> 65 years) the over-representation of the ε4 allele of the *APOE* gene remains the only genetic, albeit indirect link. Practically, APOE ε4 carriers have an increased risk of developing dementia, without a causal relation. Hence, *APOE* genotyping has no practical diagnostic value but identifies the largest fraction of the elderly at risk of developing AD. In these and in the remaining AD cases, the search for other genetic components has not yet been successful, despite many studies and claims.

Most importantly, despite the variable and divergent genetic causes, all AD patients develop a similar clinical picture and, above all, develop the same pathological lesions in the brain, i.e. amyloid plaques and NFTs, mainly in the hippocampus and cerebral cortex. Thus the different genetic causes must all contain a common pathological parameter; identifying this is actually the major challenge for fundamental research.

This common parameter has been proposed to be the amyloid plaques, the amyloid peptides, or even the NFTs, aggregates of paired helical filaments (PHFs) themselves built of the protein tau. Tau isolated from NFTs from the brain of AD patients is hyperphosphorylated on serine and threonine, in sequences of the type Ser/Thr-Pro. This points to a disordered protein kinase–phosphatase balance. The phosphorylation sites have been established as epitopes for monoclonal antibodies and some have been defined as 'AD-specific', e.g. AT8 and Alz50. In combination with biochemical approaches, proline-dependent tau kinases such as glycogen synthase kinase-3β (GSK-3β) and cyclin-dependent kinase 5 (cdk5/p35) were eventually identified. Since tau is involved in the dynamic stabilization of microtubules as part of the axonal cytoskeleton, stabilizing and allowing axonal transport, it is surprising that mice deficient in tau display only minor physiological problems.

In contrast to APP and the presenilins, no genetic link has been found to the role of tau in AD. On the contrary, mutations in the *tau* gene (chromosome 17) cause types of dementia with a variable clinical picture, commonly known as frontotemporal dementia with Parkinsonism linked to chromosome 17 (FTDP-17). In the brains of these patients, NFTs develop that are similar to those in AD brains, but without amyloid plaques. This is important since it demonstrates that NFTs are more than a correlate and that tau itself can cause neurodegeneration and dementia. This reinforces claims from pathologists that formation of intracellular tangles is an early event in AD and of primary pathological importance. The relation of AD and FTDP-17 further identifies important regional differences in pathology and in the clinical outcome, which itself has to be considered in the strategy used to generate transgenic mouse models.

Fundamental aspects of AD research

Among the molecular defects and brain lesions in AD, we are continually confronted with the problem: what is the cause, correlation and consequence? It remains unclear whether dementia and neurodegeneration are due to a loss of neurons or only of synapses, or to a functional disturbance of synaptic transmission. Apoptosis of neurons or synapses is an important issue in the overall pathogenetic process, whereby excitotoxicity and the glutamate neurotransmitter system continues to emerge in many hypotheses.

Fundamentally, we have to be concerned not only with biochemical, physical and cell-biological systems but also with transgenic mouse models that can implement the causes and reflect the pathology of AD and allow their study in molecular terms. We are using converging systems, aimed at the different factors known from biochemical, genetic and epidemiological research to be involved in AD, i.e. APP, PS1, ApoE and tau and its putative kinases. This strategy reflects the divergent causes as well as the convergent pathological characteristics that develop in the brain of AD patients.

Transgenic mice

All transgenic mice used in our studies were of the FVB/N genetic background and expressed either APP/London or PS1 or both under control of the mouse *thy1* promoter. The APP/London, PS1 and other transgenic mice were derived essentially as described [3a,4]. Briefly, cDNA coding for human APP, mutant PS1 (Ala^{246}→Glu) or ApoE4 were ligated in an adapted mouse *thy1* gene construct [4]. In the final construct, the coding sequences and introns 2 and 3 of the mouse *thy1* gene are replaced, leaving the 5′-neuron-specific control elements intact, which steers expression of the embedded transgene very specifically to central neurons. The linearized mini-gene constructs were micro-injected into prenuclear embryos from superovulated FVB/N female mice. The transgenic founders were identified by Southern blotting of tail-biopt DNA by standard procedures [5]. Transgenic strains that transmitted the transgene in a strictly Mendelian fashion without integration-site effects, were compared and high-expressing strains were selected following Western blotting of brain extracts. Double-transgenic mice overexpressing combinations of human transgenes are obtained by cross-breeding.

APP/PS transgenic mice

Transgenic mice that overexpress wild-type or mutant APP demonstrate part of the AD pathology, as shown by the presence of amyloid plaques, cognitive deficits, behavioural deficits and other traits [3a,4–9]. There is no model yet that displays all aspects of AD pathology or all pathological lesions in the brain, with the formation of NFTs still especially lacking. More complete transgenic models can be expected to result from multiple transgenic lines, i.e. mouse strains that express different combinations of human genes. These are being obtained by cross-breeding available single transgenic mouse strains or mouse strains with null or conditionally modified genes. This strategy has already led to the development of double-transgenic mice which co-express human APP and PS, demonstrating essentially the increased production of β-amyloid (Aβ)42 and earlier development of amyloid plaques, reminiscent of early-onset familial AD [10–13].

Transgenic mice that specifically overexpressed different wild-type and mutant isoforms of APP in their central neurons displayed early phenotypic changes. These included a marked cognitive impairment with decreased long-term potentiation, differential glutamatergic responses, and aggression and neophobia among others ([3a] and references therein). In addition, the transgenic strain that expressed the highest levels of the APP/London clinical mutant also developed a robust amyloidopathy in the brain at the age of 12–15 months [3a].

Aging remains the most important and effective, but least understood, parameter or risk-factor for dementia. We have therefore analysed APP/London transgenic mice at the age of 3 months, at 6–9 months and at 15 months. We determined the effect of age on the level of known intermediates and endproducts of APP processing, i.e. the membrane-bound precursor (APPm), the soluble and plaque-associated amyloid peptides Aβ40 and Aβ42, the secreted ectodomain of APP processed by α-secretase (sAPPα) and the C-terminal transmembrane and cytoplasmic domain resulting from β-secretase cleavage, referred to as 'β-C-stubs' [14].

This comparative analysis revealed that aging did not appreciably affect the levels of either the α-secretase-cleaved ectodomain or the residual β-secretase-cleaved C-terminal stubs of APP [14]. Between the age of 3 and 15 months, the only significant change was the expected increased levels of soluble and insoluble amyloid peptides, Aβ40 and Aβ42, as well as an increase in the Aβ42/40 ratio. Thus aging of the APP/London transgenic mice caused precipitation of the amyloid peptides in the physical form of amyloid plaques, an event accompanying or, more likely, following elevation of the levels of amyloid peptides, especially Aβ42. These phenomena did not occur before the age of 12–15 months in the APP/London transgenic mice. These data confirm and extend findings made by others in two unrelated APP transgenic mouse models, in which increased levels of Aβ peptides with age have been documented [7,8].

We have demonstrated that the level of mRNA of both endogenous APP and the APP transgene driven by the mouse *thy1* gene promoter increased somewhat with age in the brain of transgenic mice [4,15]. The level of membrane-bound APP (APPm) increases with age in the brain of APP/London transgenic mice, in a similar amount and in close parallel with mRNA levels [15]. Relative to those in mice of 3 months, concentrations of APPm in older mice were increased to 122% and 169% at 6–9 months and 15 months respectively. This increase appeared to be specific as it was not observed for the 85 kDa subunit of the low-density lipoprotein receptor-related protein (LRP).

The combined data demonstrate that in the brains of the APP/London transgenic mice, aging itself did not cause a marked shift in the normal processing of APP as mediated by α- and β-secretase. Thus the marked increase in both soluble and plaque-associated amyloid peptides, between 12 and 15 months of age [5], was not a direct consequence of a disturbed balance of the two main proteolytic events that govern APP metabolism [14].

Double-transgenic mice, co-expressing human PS1 with APP/London, already contained high levels of insoluble amyloid peptides at the age of 6–9 months, accompanying the formation of amyloid plaques [14]. This was evidently caused by increased levels of Aβ42, while Aβ40 levels remained fairly constant, increasing the Aβ42/40 ratio of soluble peptides from 0.30 ± 0.04 to 0.96 ± 0.06, in single- and double-transgenic mice of 6–9 months old. Insoluble or plaque-associated amyloid peptides were also dramatically increased, correlating with the earlier development of amyloid plaques in the brains of double-transgenic mice, i.e. at the age of 6–9 months versus 12–15 months in single APP/London transgenic mice.

Thus aging did not shift APP metabolism in APP/London transgenic mice into the more amyloidogenic pathway while still causing increased Aβ40 levels. Since addition of the mutant PS1 increased mainly the Aβ42 levels, an affect most likely exerted via γ-secretase, the combined data argue against an aging phenomenon on γ-secretase. Also, since no evidence was obtained for a decreased α-cleavage or a favoured amyloidogenic β-secretase pathway, other mechanisms need to be considered. We propose that accumulation of amyloid peptides results from their failing clearance, particularly of the Aβ42 peptide. It is tempting to speculate that human genes yet to be discovered might be involved in these unknown routes of clearance, which might functionally connect to ApoE4 and its receptor in the brain, LRP.

Finally, in the absence of indications of a major metabolic shift to the amyloidogenic pathway, aging is proposed to act by decreasing the effective clearance of the amyloid peptides, particularly of Aβ42 relative to the less amyloidogenic Aβ40 peptide. As discussed, this is an attractive hypothesis since effective removal of the amyloid peptides can involve or be mediated by many different intracellular and extracellular proteins, i.e. chaperones, assisting or provoking secretion; recycling and adaptor proteins, for endosomal or other vesicles; cell-surface or secreted carriers; and receptors or extracellular matrix proteins. Clearly, the genetic and epidemiological evidence collected over the last decade, for the involvement or association of different genes encoding functionally diverse proteins in sporadic or late-onset AD, would find a very plausible explanation in this hypothesis.

ApoE4 and tau transgenic mice

Whereas work on APP and PS transgenic mice is most advanced, we have also generated transgenic mice that overexpress human tau as well as human ApoE4 in their central neurons. These are discussed here together because, rather surprisingly, both develop a pathological phenotype that includes severe axonopathy and axonal degeneration.

The tau transgenic mice were psychomotorally impaired and developed prominent axonopathy in the brain and spinal cord [16]. Axonal dilations were evident throughout the brain and spinal cord, with accumulating neurofilaments, mitochondria and vesicles. This suggests that overexpression of tau caused defective axonal transport, which in turn caused distal degeneration of the axon and impaired muscular innervation. Tau became hyperphosphorylated progressively with age as demonstrated by reaction with specified monoclonal antibodies, including AT8 and Alz50. Nevertheless intraneuronal fibrils or tangles were not observed, indicating that merely increasing the concentration of tau is sufficient to cause neuronal injury [16]. Double-transgenic mice expressing APP/London and human tau have been generated and are being observed. Despite their relatively young age (< 3 months) these mice have already developed neurological symptoms that are much more severe than the single APP or tau transgenic parent even at old age, indicating a synergistic effect of the transgenes. Premature death, however, is high, which will necessitate different strategies of analysis for these double-transgenic mice.

The mechanism by which ApoE4 contributes to the development of neurodegeneration remains unknown. To test one specific mode of action of ApoE, we have generated transgenic mice that overexpress human ApoE4 in different cell-types in the brain using four distinct gene promoter constructs. Overexpression of human ApoE4 in neurons of transgenic mice, by way of the *thy1* gene promoter, produced mice with a severe phenotype as opposed to overexpression by the GFAP promoter, which was innocuous even to the age of 20 months [17]. The *thy1*–ApoE4 transgenic mice developed severe motor problems from the age of 3 months, accompanied by muscle wasting, loss of body weight and premature death. Since this resembled in several aspects the pathology in the tau transgenic mice described above, we analysed endogenous mouse tau protein for hyperphosphorylation. In three independent transgenic lines, increased phosphorylation of tau correlated with neuronal ApoE4 expression levels [17]. Hyperphosphorylation of tau increased with age, in parallel with astrogliosis and ubiquitin-positive inclusions in hippocampal neurons. Although unexpected, the finding that neuronal expression of ApoE can increase hyperphosphorylation of tau offers a potential model for the role of ApoE in AD.

In conclusion, crossing the different transgenic mouse strains will make it possible to define and study novel synergistic interactions between the major players that are known to be involved in AD, i.e. APP, PS, tau and ApoE4. Other factors are being introduced genetically by breeding with other transgenic mice, such as those expressing the putative tau kinases, GSK-3β or cdk5. Analysis of hyperphosphorylation of tau by the appearance of isoforms with slower electrophoretic mobility and through immunoreaction with monoclonal antibodies AT8 and AT180, certified to recognize typical phosphorylated tau epitopes in AD. Further analysis of the pathology in the brain and spinal cord is needed, while evidently other biological triggers and drugs can be tested. At this moment the tangle aspect of AD pathology is absent in transgenic mice models, as opposed to the amyloid aspect, so defining its importance in the pathology is not yet possible. In addition, it appears that its implementation might be more difficult than by simple overexpression in neurons, which has been successful for APP and the amyloid models. It can be anticipated that understanding the hyperphosphorylation of tau and its impact in AD will require insight into the cellular signalling pathways that regulate the microtubule-stabilizing function by phosphorylation of neuronal tau.

This investigation was supported by the Fonds voor Wetenschappelijk Onderzoek-Vlaanderen (FWO), NFWO-Lotto, the Interuniversity-network for Fundamental Research (IUAP) of the Belgian Government, the Special Biotechnology Program of the Flemish government (IWT/VLAB/COT-008), the Rooms-fund and Leuven Research and Development.

References

1. Alzheimer, A.(1907) *Allg. Z. Psychiatr. Psych. Gerichtl. Med.* **64**, 146–148
2. Hardy, J. (1997) *Trends Neurosci.* **20**, 154–159
3. Selkoe, D.J. (1998) *Trends Cell Biol.* **8**, 447–453
3a. Moechars, D., Dewachter, I., Lorent, K., Reversé, D., Baekelandt, V., Naidu, A., Tesseur, I., Spittaels, K., Van Den Haute, C., Checler, et al. (1999) *J. Biol. Chem.* **274**, 6483–6492
4. Moechars, D., Lorent, K., De Strooper, B., Dewachter, I. and Van Leuven, F. (1996) *EMBO J.* **15**, 1265–1274
5. Moechars, D., Gilis, M., Kuiperi, C., Laenen, I. and Van Leuven, F. (1998) *NeuroReport* **9**, 3561–3564
6. Games, D., Adams, D., Alessandrini, R., Barbour, R., Berthelette, P., Blackwell, C., Carr, T., Clemens, J., Donaldson, T., Gillespie, F., et al (1995) *Nature (London)* **373**, 523–527
7. Hsiao, K., Chapman, P., Nilsen, S., Eckman, C., Harigaya, Y., Younkin, S., Yang, F. and Cole, G. (1996) *Science* **274**, 99–102
8. Johnson-Wood, K., Lee, M., Motter, R., Hu, K., Gordon, G., Barbour, R., Khan, K., Gordon, M., Tan, H., Games, D., et al. (1997) *Proc. Natl. Acad. Sci. U.S.A.* **94**, 1550–1555
9. Sturchler-Pierrat, C., Abramowski, D., Duke, M., Wiederhold, K.H., Mistl, C., Rothacher, S., Ledermann, B., Burki, K., Frey, P., Paganetti, P.A., et al. (1997) *Proc. Natl. Acad. Sci. U.S.A.* **94**, 13287–13292
10. Borchelt, D.R., Thinakaran, G., Eckman, C.B., Lee, M.K., Davenport, F., Ratovitsky, T., Prada, C.M., Kim, G., Seekins, S., Yager, D., et al. (1996) *Neuron* **17**, 1005–1013

11.   Borchelt, D.R., Ratovitski, T., van Lare, J., Lee, M.K., Gonzalez, V., Jenkins, N.A.,
       Copeland, N.G., Price, D.L. and Sisodia, S.S. (1997) *Neuron* **19**, 939–945
12.   Citron, M., Westaway, D., Xia, W., Carlson, G., Diehl, T., Levesque, H., Johnson-Wood,
       K., Lee, M., Seubert, P., Davis, A., et al. (1997) *Nat. Med. (N.Y.)* **3**, 67–72
13.   Holcomb, L., Gordon, M., McGowan, E., Yu, X., Benkovic, S., Jantzen, P., Wright, K.,
       Saad, I., Mueller, R., Morgan, D., et al. (1998) *Nat. Med. (N.Y.)* **4**, 97–100
14.   Dewachter, I., Van Dorpe, J., Smeijers, L., Gilis, M., Kuipéri, C., Laenen, I., Caluwaerts, N.,
       Moechars, D., Checler, F., Venderstichele, H. and Van Leuven, F. (2000) *J. Neurosci.* **20**,
       6452–6458
15.   Moechars, D., Lorent, K. and Van Leuven, F. (1999) *Neuroscience* **91**, 819–830
16.   Spittaels, K., Van den Haute, C., Van Dorpe, J., Vandezande, K., Laenen, I., Geerts, H.,
       Mercken, M., Sciot, R., Van Lommer, A., Loos, R. and Van Leuven, F. (1999) *Am. J. Pathol.*
       155, 2153–2165
17.   Tesseur, I., Van Dorpe, J., Spittaels, K., Van den Haute, C., Moechars, D. and Van Leuven,
       F. (2000) *Am. J. Pathol.*, **156**, 951–964

Subject index